CRACK THE CORE EXAM

VOLUME 2

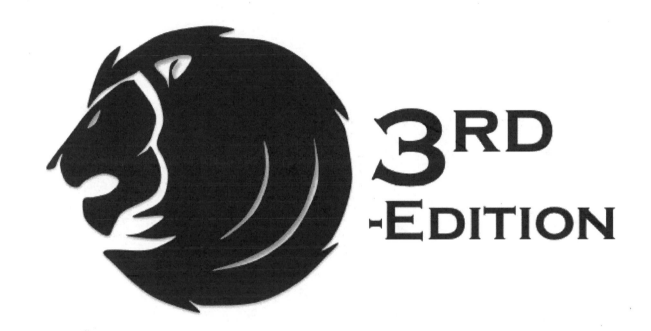

3RD -EDITION

-PROMETHEUS LIONHART, M.D.

Crack the Core Exam - Vol 2 -

Third Ed.

Disclaimer:

Readers are advised - this book is **NOT to be used for clinical decision making**. Human error does occur, and it is your responsibility to double check all facts provided. To the fullest extent of the law, the Author assumes no responsibility for any injury and/or damage to persons or property arising out or related to any use of the material contained in this book.

Published by: Prometheus Lionhart

Title ID: 4815986

ISBN-13: 978-1499618464

CONTENTS

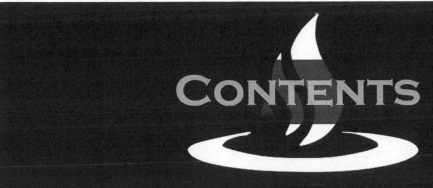

All chapters were written by Prometheus Lionhart, M.D.

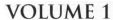 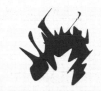

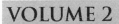 
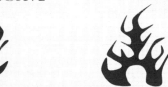
  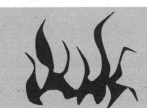
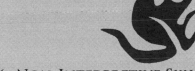 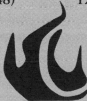 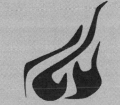

Introduction

As described by the ABR, the "CORE" Exam will cover 18 categories. The categories include: breast, cardiac, gastrointestinal, interventional, musculoskeletal, neuroradiology, nuclear, pediatric, reproductive/endocrinology, thoracic, genitourinary, vascular, computed tomography, magnetic resonance, radiography/fluoroscopy, ultrasound, physics, and safety. This book is outlined to cover the above sections, with the modalities of CT, MRI, Radiography, Fluoroscopy, and Ultrasound integrated into the system based chapters as one would reasonably expect.

On the CORE exam, Physics questions are integrated into each category with no distinct physics examination administered. However, the physics section is still considered a virtual section, and you can fail it. In fact, the physics portion is actually the overall largest section.

Useless trivia from a portion of the RadioIsotope Safety Exam (RISE), one of the requirements for Authorized User Eligibility Status, is also included within the Core Exam.

The official statement is that you can condition up to five categories, which will have to be repeated (for a small additional fee to the ABR). If you fail more than five you have to take the entire test again (for a small additional fee to the ABR). Having said that, historically your results will come in one of three flavors: (1) Pass, (2) Fail, or (3) Conditioned Physics. At this point in time it is incredibly uncommon to fail an individual section (other than physics).

The exam is given twice yearly, in select testing centers.

What makes this book unique?

The Impetus for this book was to not write a reference text or standard review book, but instead, strategy manual for solving multiple choice questions for Radiology. The author wishes to convey that the multiple choice test is different than oral boards in that you can't ask the same kinds of open ended essay type questions. *"What's your differential?"*

Questioning the contents of one's differential was the only real question on oral boards. Now that simple question becomes nearly impossible to format into a multiple choice test. Instead, the focus for training for such a test should be on things that can be asked. For example, anatomy facts - what is it? ... OR... trivia facts - what is the most common location, or age, or association, or syndrome? ... OR... What's the next step in management? Think back to medical school USMLE style, that is what you are dealing with once again. In this book, the author tried to cover all the material that could be asked (reasonably), and then approximate how questions might be asked about the various topics. Throughout the book, the author will intimate, "this could be asked like this" , and "this fact lends itself well to a question." Included in the second volume of the set is a strategy chapter focusing on high yield "buzzwords" that lend well to certain questions.

This is NOT a reference book.
This book is NOT designed for patient care.
This book is designed for studying specifically for multiple choice tests, case conference, and view-box pimping/quizing.

Are there recalls in this book? ABSOLUTELY NOT.

The author has made a considerable effort (it's the outright purpose of the text), to speculate how questions might be asked. A PhD in biochemistry can fail a med school biochemistry test or biochem section on the USMLE, in spite of clearly knowing more biochem than a medical student. This is because they are not used to medicine style questions. The aim of this text is to explore the likely style of board questions and include material likely to be covered, informed by the ABR's study guide.

Throughout the text the author will attempt to fathom the manner of questioning and include the corresponding high yield material. A correct estimation will be wholly coincidental.

Legal Stuff

Readers are advised - **this book is NOT to be used for clinical decision making**. Human error does occur, and it is your responsibility to double check all facts provided. To the fullest extent of the law, the Author assumes no responsibility for any injury and/or damage to persons or property arising out or related to any use of the material contained in this book.

I FIGHT FOR THE USERS

-TRON 1982

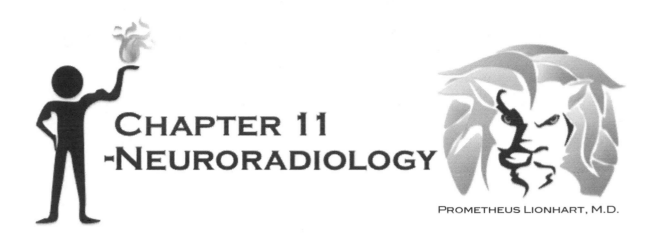

CHAPTER 11 -NEURORADIOLOGY

PROMETHEUS LIONHART, M.D.

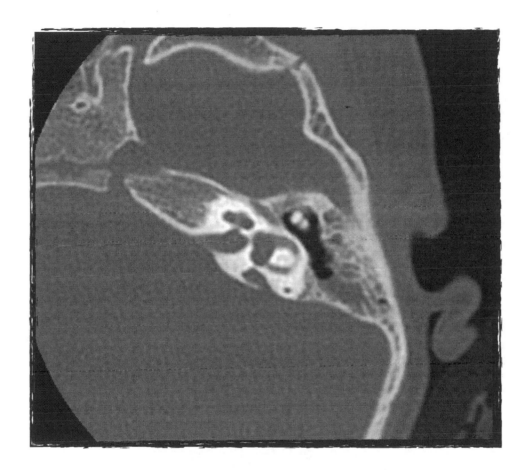

Highest Yield Tip:

Neuroradiology has one of the deepest wells for obscure trivia. A lot of neuro is differential diagnosis, which I've stated over and over again makes for a bad multiple choice question. I think the questions will mainly fall into two categories (1) Anatomy / Aunt Minnie - What is it? and (2) Associated trivia / syndrome.

SECTION 1: BRAIN

Anatomy

There is a ton of anatomy that can be asked on a multiple choice test. My idea is to break it down into three categories: (1) soft tissue – brain parenchyma (*including normal development*), (2) bony anatomy – which is basically foramina, and (3) vascular anatomy.

Soft Tissue Brain Anatomy:

Central Sulcus - This anatomic landmark separates the frontal lobe from the parietal lobe. Old school grey bearded Radiologists (likely the ones who are important enough to write test questions) love to ask how you find this important structure. There are about 10 ways to do this, which brings me to the main reason this is a great pimping question. Even if you can name 9 ways to do it, they can still correct you by naming the 10th way. I noticed during my time as a "trainee" that Attendings tend to be excellent at knowing the answers to the questions they are asking.

Practically speaking this is the strategy I use for findings the central sulcus:

Pretty high up on the brain, maybe the 3rd or 4th cut, I <u>find the cingulate sulcus</u>. This is called the **"pars bracket sign"** - because the bi-hemispheric symmetric pars marginalis form an anteriorly open bracket. The bracket is immediately behind the central sulcus. This is *present about 95% of the time* - it's actually pretty reliable.

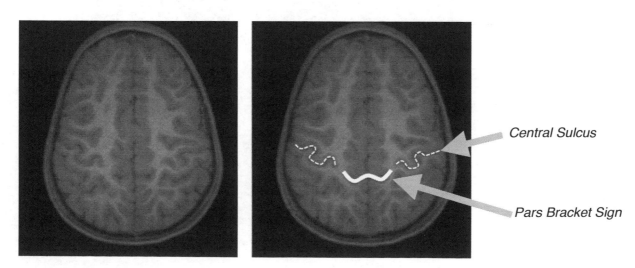

Central Sulcus

Pars Bracket Sign

Central Sulcus Trivia - Here are the other less practical ways to do it.

- Superior frontal sulcus / Pre-central sulcus sign: The posterior end of the superior frontal sulcus, joins the pre-central sulcus
- Inverted omega (sigmoid hook) corresponds to the motor hand
- Bifid posterior central sulcus: Posterior CS has a bifid appearance about 85%
- *Thin post-central gyrus sign* – The precentral gyrus is thicker than the post central gyrus (ratio 1 : 1.5).
- *Intersection* – The intraparietal sulcus intersects the post central sulcus (works almost always)
- *Midline sulcus sign* – The most prominent sulcus that reaches the midline is the central sulcus (works about 70%).

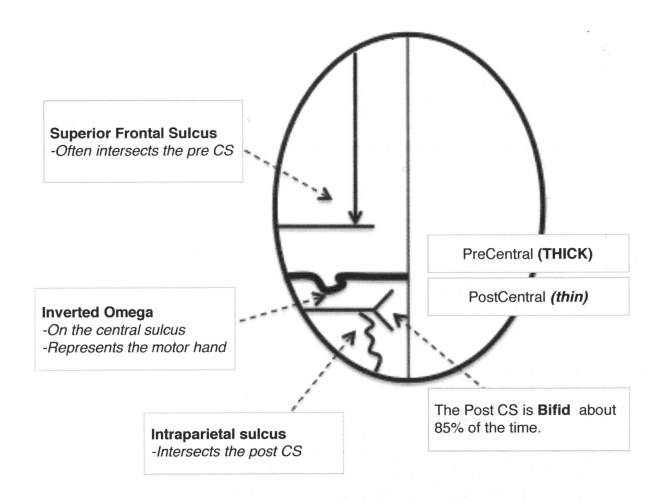

Superior Frontal Sulcus
-Often intersects the pre CS

PreCentral **(THICK)**

PostCentral *(thin)*

Inverted Omega
-On the central sulcus
-Represents the motor hand

Intraparietal sulcus
-Intersects the post CS

The Post CS is **Bifid** about 85% of the time.

Homoculous Trivia:

- The inverted omega (posteriorly directed knob) on the central sulcus / gyrus designates the motor cortex controlling hand function.

- ACA territory gets legs, MCA territory hits the rest.

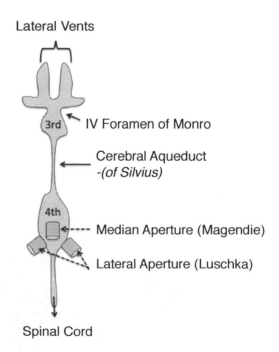

Normal Cerebral Cortex: As a point of trivia, the cortex is normally 6 layers thick, and the hippocampus is normally 3 layers thick. I only mention this because the hippocampus can look slightly brighter on FLAIR compared to other cortical areas, and this is the reason why (supposedly).

Dilated Perivascular Spaces (Virchow-Robins): These are fluid filled spaces that accompany perforating vessels. They are a normal variant and very common. They can be enlarged and associated with multiple pathologies; mucopolysaccharidoses (Hurlers and Hunters), "gelatinous pseudocysts" in cryptococcal meningitis, and atrophy with advancing age. They don't contain CSF, but instead have interstitial fluid. The common locations for these are: around the lenticulostriate arteries in the lower third of the basal ganglia, in the centrum semiovale, and in the midbrain.

Ventricular Anatomy: Just a quick refresher on this. You have two lateral ventricles that communicate with the third ventricle via the interventricular foramen (of Monroe), which in turn communicates with the fourth ventricle via the cerebral aqueduct. The fluid in the fourth ventricle escapes via the median aperture (foramen of Magendie), and the lateral apertures (foramen of Luschka). A small amount of fluid will pass downward into the spinal subarachnoid spaces, but most will rise through the tentorial notch and over the surface of the brain where it is reabsorbed by the arachnoid vili and granulations into the venous sinus system. Blockage at any site will cause a noncommunicating hydrocephalus. Blockage of reabsorption at the vili / granulation will also cause a noncommunicating hydrocephalus.

Arachnoid Granulations: These are regions where the arachnoid projects into the venous system allowing for CSF to be reabsorbed. There are hypodense on CT (similar to CSF), and usually round or oval. This round shape helps distinguish them from clot in a venous sinus (which is going to be linear). On MR they are typically T2 bright (iso to CSF), but can be bright on FLAIR (although this varies a lot an therefore probably won't be tested). These things can scallop the inner table (probably from CSF pulsation)

Cavum Variants:

- *Cavum Septum Pellucidum* - Seen in 100% of preterm infants, 80% of term infants, and 15% of adults. Rarely, can dilate and cause obstructive hydrocephalus
- *Cavum Vergae* – A posterior continuation of the cavum septum pellucidum (*never exists without a cavum septum pellucidum*)
- *Cavum Velum Interpositum* - Extension of the quadrigeminal plate cistern to foramen of Monro. Seen on sagittal as above the 3rd ventricle and below the fornices.

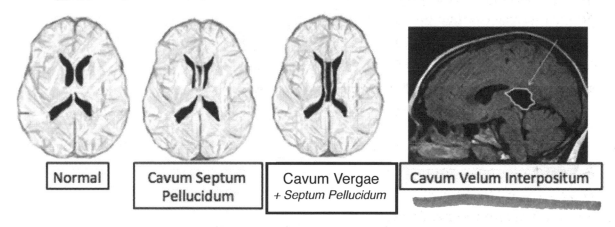

| Normal | Cavum Septum Pellucidum | Cavum Vergae + Septum Pellucidum | Cavum Velum Interpositum |

Basal cisterns: The basal cisterns are good for two things (1) looking for mass effect and (2) anatomy questions. Some people say the suprasellar cisterns look like a pentagon. The five corners of the star lend themselves easily to multiple choice questions: the top of the star is the interhemispheric fissure, the anterior points are the sylvian cisterns, and the posterior points are the ambient cisterns. The quadrigeminal plate looks like a smile.

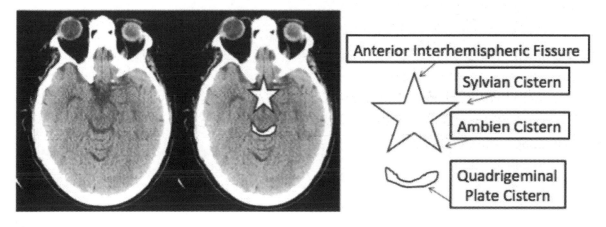

Anterior Interhemispheric Fissure
Sylvian Cistern
Ambien Cistern
Quadrigeminal Plate Cistern

Brain Development:

Brain Myelination: The baby brain has essentially the opposite signal characteristics as the adult brain. **The T1 pattern of a baby, is similar to the T2 pattern of an adult.** The T2 pattern of a baby, is similar to the T1 pattern of an adult. This appearance is the result of myelination changes. The process of myelination occurs in a predetermined order, and therefore lends itself easily to multiple choice testing. The basic concept to understand first is that immature myelin has a higher water content relative to mature myelin and therefore is brighter on T2 and darker on T1. During the maturation process water will decrease, and fat (brain cholesterol and glycolipids) will increase. Therefore mature white matter will be brighter on T1 and darker on T2.

Immature Myelin	*Mature Myelin*
High Water, Low Fat	Low Water, High Fat
Relatively T1 dark, T2 bright	Relatively T1 bright, T2 dark

As a point of highly testable trivia: the T1 changes precede the T2 changes (adult T1 pattern seen around age 1, adult T2 pattern seen around age 2). Should be easy to remember *(1 for T1, 2 for T2)*.

Take Home Point: T1 is most useful for assessing myelination in the first year (especially 0-6 months), T2 is most useful for assessing myelination in the second year (especially 6 months to 18 months).

Order of progression: Just remember, inferior to superior, posterior to anterior, central to peripheral, and sensory fibers prior to motor fibers. The testable trivia, is that **the subcortical white matter is the last part of the brain to myelinate**, with the occipital white matter around 12 months, and the frontal regions finishing around 18 months. The "terminal zones" of myelination occur in the subcortical frontotemporoparietal regions – finishing around 40 months. Another high yield piece of testable trivia is that the **brainstem, and posterior limb of the internal capsule are normally myelinated at birth.**

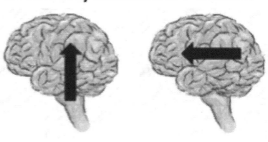

Brain Myelination Pattern

Inferior to Superior, Posterior to Anterior

16

Corpus Callosum: I'll touch on this again in the developmental/congenital section but it's high yield enough to repeat. **The corpus callosum forms front to back (then rostrum last).** Therefore hypoplasia of the corpus callosum is usually absence of the splenium (with the genu intact).

High Yield Points Regarding Brain Development
Myelination Occurs Inferior to Superior, and Posterior to Anterior
The Corpus Callosum Forms Front to Back (with the rostrum last)
Both the Anterior and Posterior Pituitary are Bright at Birth (posterior only bright around 2 months – 2 years)
Calverial Bone Marrow will be active (T1 hypointense) in young kids and fatty (T1 hyperintense) in older kids
The sinuses form in the following order: Maxillary, Ethmoid, Sphenoid, and Frontal Last
Brain Iron increases with age (globus pallidus darkens up).

Bony Anatomy:

Skull Base: The most likely multiple choice questions regarding the skull base are anatomy questions. Specifically, the *"what goes where?"* question is very easy to write.

Foramen	Contents
Foramen Ovale	CN V3, and Accessory Meningeal Artery
Foramen Rotundum	CN V2 ("**R2V2**"),
Superior Orbital Fissure	CN 3, CN 4, CN V1, CN6
Inferior Orbital Fissure	CN V2
Foramen Spinosum	Middle Meningeal Artery
Jugular Foramen	*Pars Nervosa:* Jugular Vein, CN 9, *Pars Vascularis:* CN 10, CN 11
Hypoglossal Canal	CN12
Optic Canal	CN 2, and Opthalmic Artery

The Jugular Foramen

The jugular foramen has two parts which are separated by a bony "jugular spine"

Pars Nervosa - The nervous guy in the front. This contains the Glossopharyngeal nerve (CN9), along with it's tympanic brach - the "Jacobson's Nerve"

Pars Vascularis - This is the "vascular part" which actually contains the jugular bulb, along with the Vagus nerve (CN 10), along with it's auricular branch "Arnold's Nerve," and the Spinal Accessory Nerve (CN 11)

Remember, that they don't have to show you the hole in the axial plane. They can be sneaky and show it in the coronal or sagittal planes. In fact, showing foramen rotundum in the coronal and sagittal planes is a very common sneaky trick.

With regard to the relationship between **spinosum and ovale**, I like to think of this as the foot print a woman's high heeled shoe might make in the snow, with the oval part being ovale, and the pointy heel as spinosum.

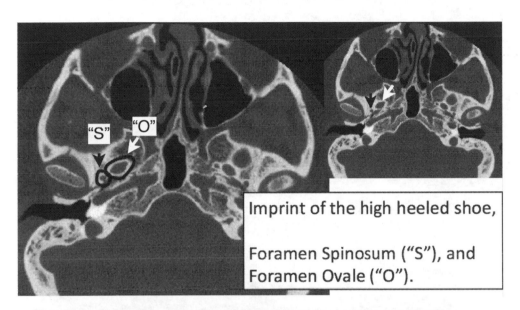

Imprint of the high heeled shoe,

Foramen Spinosum ("S"), and
Foramen Ovale ("O").

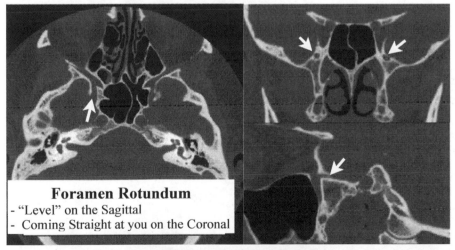

Foramen Rotundum
- "Level" on the Sagittal
- Coming Straight at you on the Coronal

With regard to **Rotundum**, think about it as being totally level or horizontal on the sagittal view.

On the coronal view, it looks like you are staring into a gun

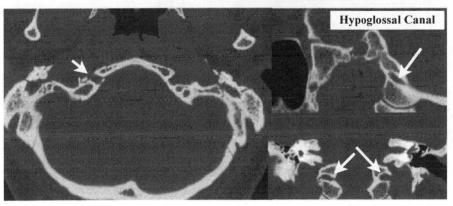

Hypoglossal Canal

The **hypoglossal canal** is very posterior and inferior.

This makes it unique as a skull base foramen.

The relationship between the superior orbital fissure (SOF), the inferior orbital fissure (IOF), foramen rotundum (FR), and the pterygopalatine fossa (PPF) is an important one, that can really lead to some sneaky multiple choice questions (mainly what goes through what). I've attempted to outline this relationship on both sagittal and coronal views.

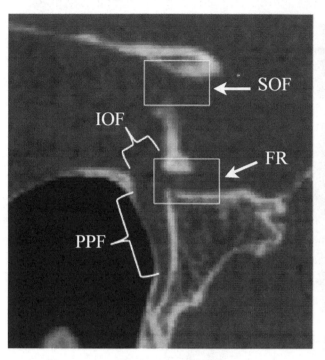

Sagittal

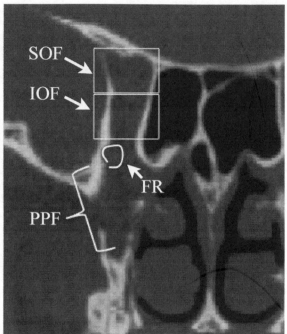

Coronal

Cavernous Sinus: - The question is going to be, what's in it (probably asked as what is NOT in it). CN3, 4, CN V1, CNV2, CN6, and the carotid. **CN2 and CN V3 do NOT run through it**.

The only other anatomy trivia I can think of is that CN6 runs next to the carotid, the rest of the nerves are along the wall. This is why you can get lateral rectus palsy earlier with cavernous sinus pathologies.

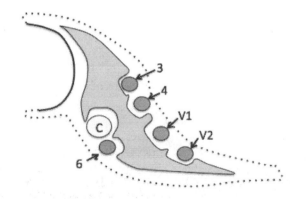

Skull fusion (Craniosynostosis): The craniosynostoses are discussed in more detail in the congenital section. I'll briefly touch on what is normal. The sutures exist to allow for rapid brain growth over the first few years of life. The brain will double in size within the first 6 months, and double again by the second year of life. The majority of skull growth occurs by age 3, at which time most of the sutures will fuse. Some, like the petro-occipital, will remain open into adulthood. When they fuse too early that causes a problem. The long Latin / French sounding word that goes along with that fusion problem makes for a good multiple choice test question (more on this later).

IAC - Nerve Orientation

The thing to remember is "7UP, and COKE Down" - with the 7th cranial nerve superior to the 8th cranial nerve (the cochlear nerve component). As you might guess, the superior vestibular branch is superior to the inferior one.

If it is shown, it is always shown in this orientation. The ideal sequence to find it is a heavily T2 weighted sequence with super thin cuts through the IAC.

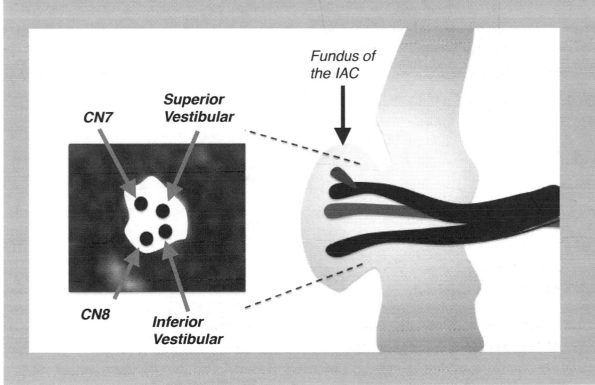

Vascular Anatomy:

Vascular anatomy can be thought of in four sections. (1) The branches of the external carotid (most commonly tested as the order in which the arise from the common carotid). (2) Segments of the internal carotid, with pathology at each level and variants. (3) Vertebral artery, with pathology. (4) Circle of Willis, with pathology and variants.

What are the branches of the external carotid ?

- *Some Administrative assistants Like Fucking Over Poor Medical Students*
  - o Superior Thyroid
  - o Ascending Pharyngeal
  - o Lingual
  - o Facial
  - o Occipital
  - o Posterior Auricular
  - o Maxillary
  - o Superficial Temporal

Anterior Circulation (Carotids):

Some Trivia about the ICA (Internal Carotid):

- The Bifurcation of the IAC and ECA usually occurs at C3-C4

- Cervical ICA has no branches in the neck - if you see branches either (a) they are anomalous or more likely (b) you are a dumb ass and actually looking at the external carotid. Remember the presence of branches is a way you can tell ICA from ECA on ultrasound.

- Flow reversal in the carotid bulb is common

Segment by Segment Trivia:

C1 (Cervical): 4 main pathologies of interest at this level:

- Atherosclerosis: The origin is a very common location
- Dissection: Can be spontaneous (women), and in Marfans or Ehlers-Danlos, and result in a partial Horner's (ptosis and miosis), followed by MCA territory stroke.
- Can have a retropharyngeal course and get "drained" by ENT accidentally.
- Pharyngeal infection may cause pseudoaneurysm at this level.

C2 (Petrous): - Not much goes on at this level. Sometimes aneurysms (which can be surprisingly big).

C3 (Lacerum): Not much here as far as vascular pathology. The anatomic location is important to neurosurgeons for exposing Meckel's cave via a transfacial approach.

C4 (Cavernous): Aneurysms here are strongly associated with hypertension. This segment is affected by multiple pathologies including the development of cavernous – carotid fistula.

C5 (Clinoid): An aneurysm here could compress the optic nerve and cause blindness.

C6: (Ophthalmic - Supraclinoid): Common site for aneurysm formation. **Origin at the "dural ring" is a buzzword** for this artery.

C7 (Communicating - terminal): An aneurysm here may compress CN III and present with a palsy.

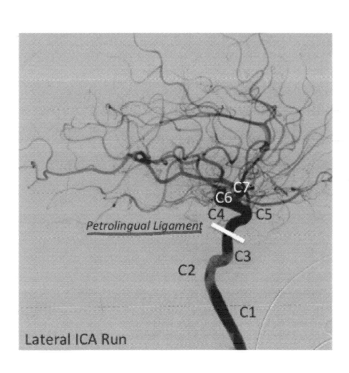

Lateral ICA Run

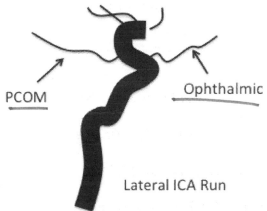

Lateral ICA Run

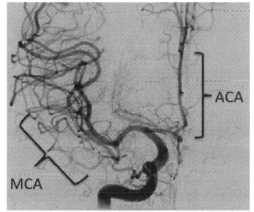

AP ICA Run

Posterior Circulation:

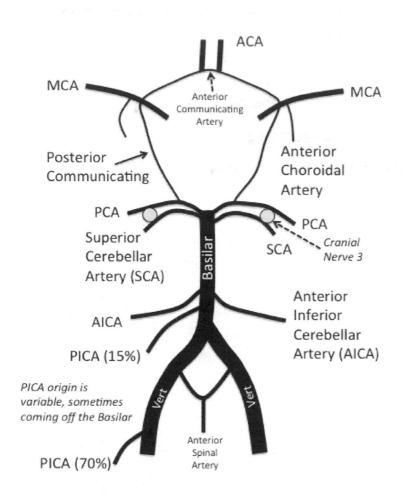

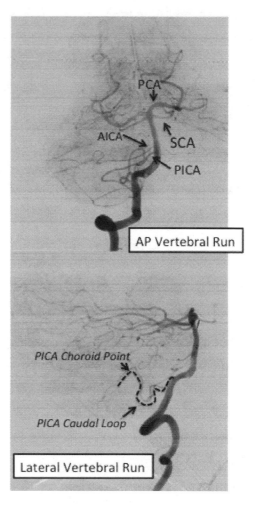

AP Vertebral Run

PICA Choroid Point

PICA Caudal Loop

Lateral Vertebral Run

Vascular Variants:

Fetal Origin of PCA: Most common vascular variant (probably) - seen in up to 30% of general population. The term "fetal PCOM" is typically used to refer to a situation where the PCOM is larger (or the same size) as P1. Another piece of trivia is that *anatomy with a fetal PCA has the PCOM superior / lateral to CN3 (instead of superior / medial - in normal anatomy).*

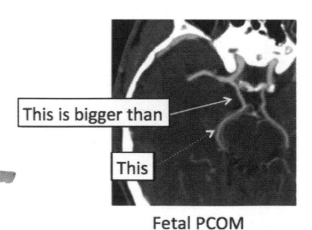

Fetal PCOM

Persistent Trigeminal Artery: Persistent fetal connection between the cavernous ICA to the basilar artery. A characteristic *"tau sign"* on Sagittal MRI has been described. It **increases the risk of aneurysm** (anytime you have branch points).

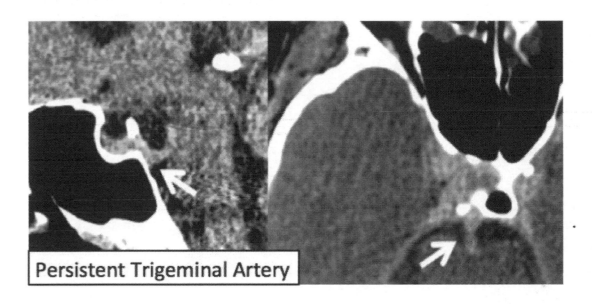

Persistent Trigeminal Artery

Aberrant Carotid Artery: Typically represents an enlarged inferior tympanic artery anastomosis with an enlarged caroticotympanic artery (with underdevelopment of the cervical ICA). This vessel courses though the tympanic cavity and joins the horizontal carotid canal. It can cause pulsatile tinnitus. The oldest trick in the book is to try and fool you into calling it a paraganglioma.

Don't biopsy it !

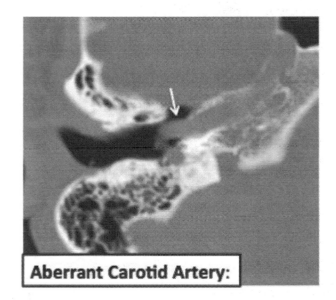

Aberrant Carotid Artery:

Venous Anatomy:

You can ask questions about the venous anatomy in roughly three ways (1) what is it – on a picture, (2) what is a deep vein vs what is a superficial vein, (3) trivia.

What is it?

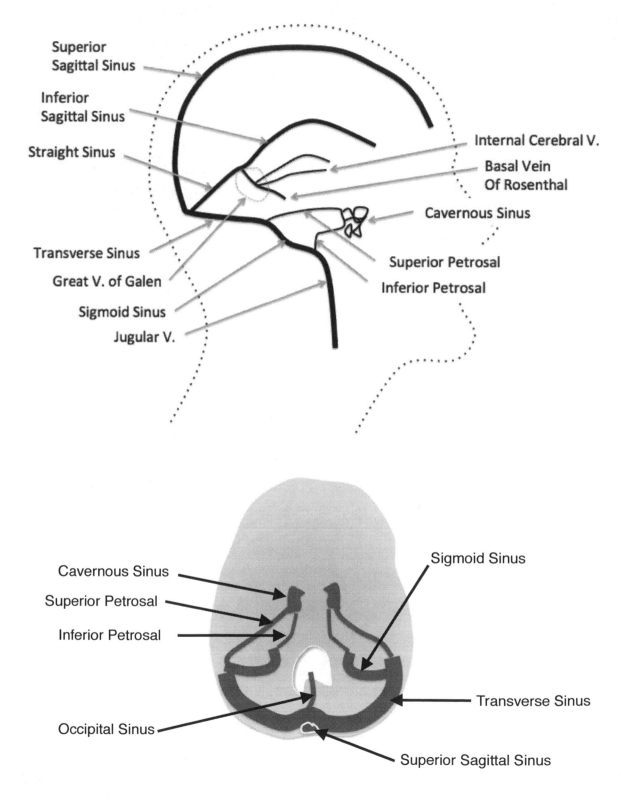

Anastomotic Superficial Veins:

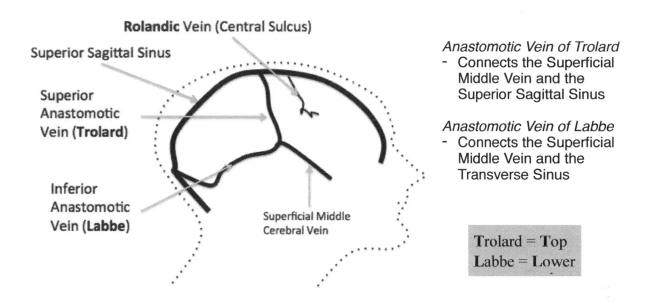

Rolandic Vein (Central Sulcus)

Superior Sagittal Sinus

Superior Anastomotic Vein (**Trolard**)

Inferior Anastomotic Vein (**Labbe**)

Superficial Middle Cerebral Vein

Anastomotic Vein of Trolard
- Connects the Superficial Middle Vein and the Superior Sagittal Sinus

Anastomotic Vein of Labbe
- Connects the Superficial Middle Vein and the Transverse Sinus

Trolard = Top
Labbe = Lower

Here is a way to schematically think about the venous drainage -

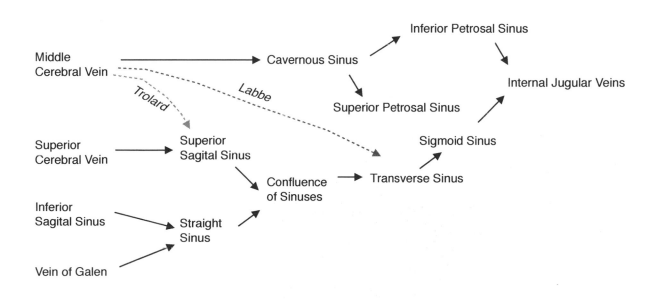

Superficial vs Deep

There is a superficial venous system and a deep venous system. The easiest way to test material like this is your *"which of the following is not?"* or *"which of the following is ?"* type question.

The big ones to remember are in the chart.

Superficial	Deep
Superior Cerebral Veins	Basal Vein of Rosenthal
Superior Anastomotic Vein of Trolard	Vein of Galen
Inferior Anastomotic Vein of Labbe	Inferior Petrosal Sinus
Superficial Middle Cerebral Veins	

Venous Trivia:

Collateral Pathways: The dural sinuses have accessory drainage pathways (other than the jugular veins) that allow for connection to extracranial veins. These are good because they can help regulate temperature, and equalize pressure. These are bad because they allow for passage of sinus infection / inflammation, which can result in venous sinus thrombosis.

Inverse Relationship: There is a relationship between the Vein of Labbe, and the Anastomotic Vein of Trolard. Since these dudes share drainage of the same territory, as one gets large the others get small.

Sounds Latin or French: As a general rule, anything that sounds Latin or French has an increased chance of being on the test.

- *Vein of Labbe:* Large draining vein, connecting the superficial middle vein and the transverse sinus

- *Vein of Trolard:* Smaller (usually) vein, connecting the superficial middle vein and sagittal sinus

- *Basal vein of Rosenthal:* Deep vein that passes lateral to the midbrain through the ambient cistern and drains into the vein of Galen. Its course is similar to the PCA.

- *Vein of Galen:* Big vein ("great") formed by the union of two internal cerebral veins.

Sinus Trivial Anatomy Bonus - The Concha Bullosa

This is a common variant where the middle concha is pneumatized. It's pretty much of no consequence clinically unless it's fucking huge - then it can cause obstructive symptoms.

When I was in private practice there was this ENT who told me he wanted it mentioned in all his CT sinus reports.

That way he could justify doing FESS…

He drove a nice car.

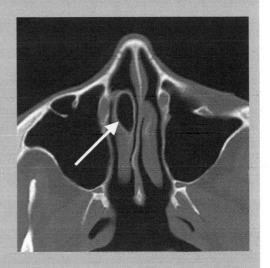

Gamesmanship for Neuro Anatomy

- **First Order Trivia:**
  - *"What is it?"* Style questions are most likely; with possibilities including CTA, MRA, or Angiograms. Considering when the people writing the questions trained, angiograms are probably the most likely.
  - *"What goes through there?"* Neuro foramina
  - *"What doesn't?"* Style questions - CN 2 and CN V3 don't go through the cavernous sinus.

- **Second Order Trivia:**
  - CN 3 Palsy - Think Posterior Communicating Artery Aneurysm
  - CN 6 Palsy - Think increased ICP

Misc Brain Conditions:

Monro-Kellie Doctrine:

The Monro-Kellie doctrine is the idea that the head is a closed shell, and that the three major components: (1) brain, (2) blood – both arterial and venous, and (3) CSF, are in a state of dynamic equilibrium. As the volume of one goes up, the volume of another must go down.

Intracranial Hypotension: If you are leaking CSF, this will decrease the overall fixed volume, the volume of venous blood will increase to maintain the equilibrium. The result is meningeal engorgement (enhancement), distention of the dural venous sinuses, prominence of the intracranial vessels and engorgement of the pituitary. The development of subdural hematoma and hygromas is also a classic look (again, compensating for lost volume).

Idiopathic Intracrainal Hypertension (Pseudotumor Cerebri): Classic scenario of a fat middle aged women with a headache. Etiology is not well understood (making too much CSF, or not absorbing it correctly). It has a lot of associations (hypothyroid, cushings, vitamin A toxicity). The findings follow the equilibrium idea. With increased CSF the ventricles become slit like, the pituitary shrinks (partially empty sella), and the venous sinuses appear compressed. You can also have the appearance of vertical tortuosity of the optic nerves and flattening of the posterior sclera.

Edema:

Cytotoxic: This type of edema can be thought about as intracellular swelling, secondary to malfunction of the Na/K pump. It tends to favor the gray matter, and **looks like loss of the gray-white differentiation.** This is classically **seen with stroke** (or trauma), and is why early signs of stroke involve loss of the GM-WM interface.

Vasogenic: This type of edema is extracellular, secondary to disruption of the blood brain barrier. It looks like **edema tracking through the white matter** (which is less tightly packed than the gray matter). This is classically **seen with tumor and infection**. A response to steroids is characteristic of vasogenic edema.

Communicating: This is an obstruction at the level of villi / granulation, blocking reabsorption. All the ventricles will be dilated (25% of the time the fourth ventricle is normal). There are 4 main causes.

- **Normal Pressure Hydrocephalus:** It's not well understood – and idopathic. The buzz-phrase is "ventricular size out of proportion to atrophy." The frontal and temporal horns of the lateral ventricles are the most affected. "Upward bowing of the corpus callosum" is another catch phrase. On MRI you may see transependymal flow and/or a flow void in the aqueduct and 3rd ventricle. The step 1 trivia is "wet, wacky, and wobbly" – describing the clinical triad of urinary incontinence, confusion, and ataxia. This is treated with surgical shunting.

- **Blood, Pus, and Cancer** – Anything that plugs up the villi – the three most common causes being SAH, Meningitis, and Carcinomatous Meningitis.

Non- Obstructive:

This is sort of a trick question, with the only answer being something that produces CSF. The only answer you need to know is Choroid Plexus Papilloma (discussed in detail in the tumor section).

Quiz: Is transependymal flow seem more with acute hydrocephalus or chronic hydrocephalus?

Answer: Acute.

Brain Herniation:

Subfalcine Herniation: This is just a fancy way of saying midline shift (deviation of ipsilateral ventricle and bowing of the falx). The trivia to know is that the ACA may be compressed, and can result in infarct.

Descending Transtentorial Herniation: The uncus and hippocampus herniated through the tentorial incisura. Effacement of the ipsilateral suprasellar cistern occurs first:

Things to know:

- Perforating basilar artery branches get compressed resulting in *"Duret Hemorrhages"* - classically located in the midline at the pontomesencephalic junction (in reality they can also effect cerebellar peduncles).

- CN3 gets compressed between the PCA and Superior Cerebellar Artery causing ipsilateral pupil dilation and ptosis

- "Kernohan's Notch / Phenomenon" – The midbrain on the tentorium forming an indentation (notch) and the physical exam finding of ipsilateral hemiparesis – which Neurologist's call a *"false localizing sign."* Of course, localization on physical exam is stupid in the age of MRI, but it gives Neurologists a reason to carry a reflex hammer and how can one fault them for that.

Ascending Transtentorial Herniation: Think about this in the setting of a posterior fossa mass. The vermis will herniate upward through the tentorial incisura often resulting in severe obstructive hydrocephalus.

Things to know
- The "Smile" of the quadrigeminal cistern will be flattened or reversed
- *"Spinning Top"* is a buzzword, for the appearance of the midbrain from bilateral compression along its posterior aspect
- Severe hydrocephalus (at the level of the aqueduct).

Cerebellar Tonsil Herniation: Can be from severe herniation after downward transtentorial herniation). Alternatively, if in isolation you are thinking more along the lines of Chiari (Chiari I = 1 tonsil 5mm, or both tonsils 3mm).

Neuro-Degenerative / Toxic Metabolic

Multiple Sclerosis:

By far the most common acquired demyelinating disease. Usually affects women 20-40. As a point of trivia in children there is no gender difference. There are multiple types with the relapsing-remitting form being by far the most common (85%). Clinical history of "separated by time and space" is critical. Findings are the classic T2/FLAIR oval and periventricular perpendicularly oriented lesions. Involvement of the calloso-septal interface is 98% specific for MS (and helps differentiate it from vascular lesions and ADEM). In children the posterior fossa is more commonly involved. Acute demyelinating plaques should enhance and restrict diffusion (on multiple choice tests and occasionally in the real world). Brain atrophy is accelerated in MS.

You can sometimes get a big MS plaque that looks like a tumor. **It will ring enhance but classically incomplete (*like a horseshoe*)**, with a leading demyelinating edge. Solitary spinal cord involvement can be seen but it usually is seen in addition to brain lesions. The cervical spine is the most common location in the spine (65%). Spinal cord lesions tend to be peripherally located.

Multiple Sclerosis Variants:

ADEM (Acute Disseminated Encephalomyelitis): Typically presents in childhood or adolescents, after a viral illness or vaccination. Classically has multiple LARGE T2 bright lesions, which enhance in a nodular or ring pattern (open ring). Lesions do NOT involve the calloso-septal interface.

Acute Hemorrhagic Leukoencephalitis (Hurst Disease): This a fulminant form of ADEM with massive brain swelling and death. The hemorrhagic part is only seen on autopsy (not imaging).

Devics (neuromyelitis optica): Transverse Myelitis + Optic Neuritis.
Lesions in the Cord and the Optic Nerve

Marburg Variant: Childhood variant that is fulminant and terrible leading to rapid death. It usually has a febrile prodrome. "MARBURG!!!" = DEATH

Toxic / Metabolic

PRES (Posterior Reversible Encephalopathy Syndrome): Seen with hypertension or chemotherapy. Features include asymmetric cortical and subcortical white matter edema (usually in parietal occipital regions). PRES does NOT restrict on diffusion (helps tell you it's not a stroke).

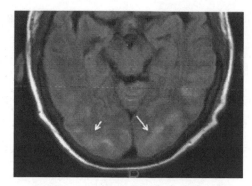

PRES – *T2/FLAIR High Signal*

Radiation-Induced Demyelination: Seen as T2 bright areas and atrophy corresponding to the radiation portal. Can be seen with hemosiderin deposition, and mineralizing microangiopathy (calcifications involving the basal ganglia and subcortical white matter).

Osmotic Demylination Syndrome (CPM): Seen with rapid correction of sodium (usually in a drunk). Usually T2 bright in the central pons (spares the periphery). Can also have an extra-pontine presentation involving the basal ganglia, external capsule, amygdala, and cerebellum.

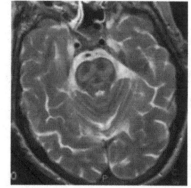

CPM – *T2 Bright Central Pons*

Wernicke Encephalopathy: Caused by thiamine deficiency. Just think contrast **enhancement of the mammillary bodies** (seen more in alcoholics).

Additionally, think increased T2/FLAIR signal in the bilateral medial thalamus and periaqueductal gray.

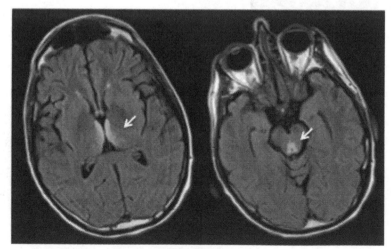

Wernicke
High Signal in Medial Thalamus and Periaqueductal Gray

CNS Findings Secondary to Drugs or Toxins:

- **Carbon Monoxide:** CT Hypodensity / T2 Bright Globus Pallidus (*carbon monoxide causes "globus" warming*).

- **Alcohol:** Brain atrophy , especially the cerebellar vermis.

- **Marchiafava-Bignami**: Seen in drunks. Swelling and T2 bright signal affecting the **corpus callosum** (typically beginning in the body, then genu, and lastly splenium). Will involve the central fibers and spare the dorsal and ventrals fibers (called a **"sandwich sign" on sagittal imaging**).

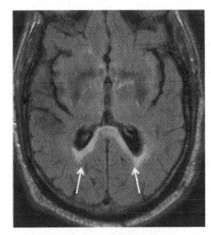

Marchiafava-Bignami
-High T2/FLAIR in the Corpus Callosum

- **Methanol**: Optic nerve atrophy, hemorrhagic **putaminal** and subcortical white matter necrosis.

Post-Radiation: There is a latent period, so imaging findings don't typically show up for about two months post therapy.

- *Whole Brain Radiation* changes are typically T2 bright in the periventricular white matter, sparing the subcortical regions early on. Peripheral extension to the subcortical regions occurs later.

- *Localized Radiation:* Usually we are talking about severe focal edema with mass effect and enhancement. Differentiation from residual tumor can be a sneaky sneaky thing, and MR perfusion may be useful in differentiating.

Post Chemotherapy: You will have T2 effects acutely in the white matter, that can progress to atrophy. Enhancement or mass effect is rare unless it is very severe. Children receiving both radiation and chemotherapy can sometimes develop calcifications - "mineralizing microangiopathy."

Disseminated necrotizing leukoencephalopathy: Severe white matter changes, which demonstrate ring enhancement , classically seen with leukemia patients undergoing radiation and chemotherapy. This is bad news and can be fatal.

Neurodegenerative Disorders:

You can do dementia imaging with a variety of imaging modalities, including CT and MRI for structure, and FDG PET and SPECT for function. **Pearl: On FDG PET the motor strip is always preserved in dementia.**

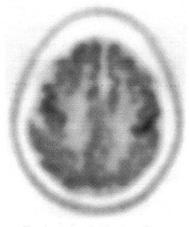

Preserved Motor Strip
—*Seen in degenerative dementias*

> *Mimics*:
>
> Depression can mimic Fontotemporal Dementia.
>
> Lymes, HIV, and Vasculitis can mimic Vascular Dementia

- **Alzheimer Disease:** Most common cause of dementia. Most likely question is **hippocampal atrophy** (which is first), and out of proportion to the rest of the brain atrophy. They could ask temporal horn atrophy > 3mm , which is seen in more than 65% of cases.

- **Multi-infarct Dementia:** This is the second most common cause of dementia. Cortical infarcts and lacunar infarcts are seen on MRI. Most likely to be shown as a PET-FDG case, demonstrating multiple scattered areas of decreased activity

Crossed Cerebellar Diaschisis (CCD): Depressed blood flow and metabolism affecting the cerebellar hemisphere after a contralateral supratentorial insult (infarct, tumor resection, radiation). Creates anAunt Minnie Appearance:

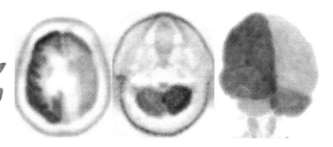

Crossed Cerebellar Diaschisis

- **Dementia with Lewy Bodies:** This is the third most common cause of dementia (second most common neurodegenerative), with a very similar clinical picture to the dementia seen with Parkinsons, with the major difference being that in DLB, the dementia comes first. The hippocampi remain normal in size and you have some decreased FDG uptake in the lateral occipital cortex, with sparing of the mid posterior cingulate gyrus (**Cingulate Island Sign**).

Binswanger Disease: This is a subcortical leukoencephalopathy that affects older people (55 and up), strongly associated with HTN. It's basically a form of *small vessel vascular dementia*. It classically spares the subcortical U fibers *(see page #39 for an explanation on WTF " U Fibers" are)*.

FDG PET - Brain		
Alzheimer	Low posterior temporoparietal cortical activity	Identical to Parkinson Dementia
Multi Infarct	Scattered areas of decreased activity	*Lyme, HIV, and Vasculitis are mimics*
Dementia with Lewy Bodies	Low in lateral occipital cortex	Preservation of the mid posterior cingulate gyrus (**Cingulate Island Sign**)
Picks / Frontotemporal / Depression	Low frontal lobe	*Depression is a mimic*
Huntingtons	Low activity in caudate nucleus and putamen	

Infections

My idea for discussing intracranial infections is to think of a few "testable" scenarios. The neonatal infections, the infections related to HIV, the "characteristic" infections, and lastly meningitis and cerebral abscess.

Neonatal Infections:

We are talking about TORCH infections. The first critical thing is that they only really matter in the first two trimesters (doesn't cause as much harm in third trimester). Calcifications and microcephaly are basically present in all of them.

Here are some high yield points regarding the TORCH infections:

CMV: This is the most common TORCH (by far!, it's 3x more common than Toxo – which is the second most common). It likes to affect the germinal matrix and causes periventricular tissue necrosis. The result is the most likely test question = **Periventricular calcifications.** Another high yield piece of trivia is that of all the TORCHs **CMV has the highest association with polymircogyria .**

Toxoplasmosis: This is the second most common TORCH. It's seen in women who clean up cat shit. The calcification pattern is more random, and affects the basal ganglia (like most other TORCH infections). The frequency is increased in the 3rd trimester (but only causes a problem in the first two). The most likely test question = **hydrocephalus.**

Rubella: Less common because of vaccines. Calcifications are less common than in other TORCHS. On MR, focal high T2 signal might be seen in white matter (related to vasculopathy and ischemic injury).

HSV: As a point of trivia, it's usually HSV-2 in 90% of cases. Unlike adults, the virus does not primarily affect the limbic system but instead affects the endothelial cells resulting in **thrombus and hemorrhagic infarction** with resulting encephalomalcia and atrophy.

HIV: This is not a TORCH but does occur during pregnancy, at delivery, or through breast feeding. **Brain atrophy predominantly in the frontal lobes is** the main testable piece of trivia. You may also have faint basal ganglia enhancement seen on CT and MRI preceding the appearance of basal ganglia calcification.

CNS TORCH - What you need to remember

- **CMV** = *Most Common, Periventricular Calcifications, Polymicrogyria*
- **Toxo** = *Hydrocephalus, Basal Ganglia Calcifications*
- **Rubella** = *Vasculopathy / Ischemia. High T2 signal - Less Calcifications*
- **HSV** = *Hemorrhagic Infarct, and lead to bad encephalomalcia (hydranencephaly)*
- **HIV** = *Brain Atrophy in frontal lobes*

Infections Immunosuppressed Patients Get (people with AIDS)

The most common opportunistic infection in patients with AIDS is toxo. The most common fungal infection (in people with AIDS) is Cryptococcus. Two other infections worth talking about are JC Virus, and CMV.

HIV Encephalitis: I'll lead with the encephalitis people with AIDS get. This is actually pretty common and affects about 50% of AIDS patients. Usually we are talking about a situation with a CD4 < 200. What you are going to see is symmetric increased T2 / FLAIR signal in the deep white matter. T1 will be normal. The lesions will not enhance. There may be associated brain atrophy. These tend to spare the subcortical U-fibers *(PML will involve them)*.

Progressive Multifocal Leukoencephalopathy (PML): This is caused by the JC virus. We are talking about a situation with a CD4 less than 50. The imaging manifestations are a single or multiple scattered hypodensities, with corresponding T1 hypointensity (remember HIV was T1 normal), and T2/FLAIR hyperintensities out of proportion to mass effect - buzzword. The lesions have a predilections for the subcortical U-fibers. The asymmetry of these lesions helps differentiate them from HIV.

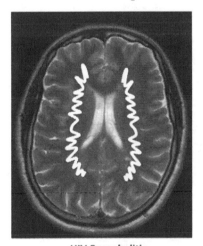
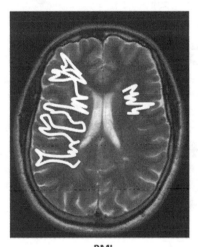
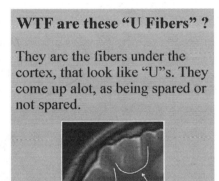

WTF are these "U Fibers" ?

They are the fibers under the cortex, that look like "U"s. They come up alot, as being spared or not spared.

HIV Encephalitis
Symmetric, and Spare Cortical U Fibers

PML
-Asymmetric, and Involves Cortical U Fibers

CMV: Think about brain **atrophy**, periventricular hypodensities (that are T2/FLAIR bright), and **ependymal enhancement**.

Cryptococcus: The most common fungal infection in AIDS. The most common presentation is meningitis that involves the base of the brain (leptomenigneal enhancement). The most likely way this will be shown on a multiple choice exam is **dilated perivascular spaces filled with mucoid gelatinous crap (these will not enhance).** The second most likely way this will be shown is lesions in the basal ganglia "cryptococcomas" – these are T1 dark, T2 bright, and may ring enhance.

Toxo: Most common opportunistic infection in AIDS. Classically we are talking about T1 dark, T2 bright, ring enhancing (when larger than 1cm) lesions. These guys will **NOT** show restricted diffusion. Just think **"ring enhancing lesion, with LOTS of edema."** Most likely test question is that Toxo is Thallium Cold, and Lymphoma is thallium hot.

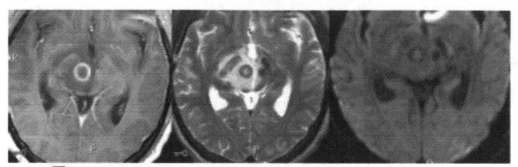

Toxo: *Ring Enhancing, Lots of Edema, Not Restricted*

Wait - I thought abscess restricted diffusion?
Typical abscess does. However, atypical infections like Toxo or fungal don't always do this, and showing that it does NOT restrict might be a sneaky way to test this.

Toxo	Lymphoma
Ring Enhancing	Ring Enhancing
Hemorrhage more common after treatment	Hemorrhage less common after treatment
Thallium Cold	**Thallium HOT**
PET Cold	Pet Hot
MR Perfusion: Decreased CBV	MR Perfusion: Increased (or Decreased) CBV

Summary:

AIDS Encephalitis	PML	CMV	Toxo	Cryptococcus
Symmetric T2 Bright	Asymmetric T2 Bright	Periventricular T2 Bright	Ring Enhancement	Dilated Perivascular Spaces
	T1 dark	Ependymal Enhancement	Thallium Cold	Basilar Meningitis

In general, to solve MR puzzles you will need to be able to work through some MR sequences. The trick is to have a list of things that are T1 bright, T2 bright, Restrict diffusion, and Enhance. Plus you should know the basic enhancement patterns (homogenous, heterogenous, ring, and incomplete ring).

STROKE vs TUMOR vs ABSCESS vs MS Plaque

T2: For the most part, T2 is not helpful for lesion characterization - as tumors, stroke, MS, infections all have edema.

DWI: This is helpful only if they follow the classic rules. Out of those 4 (Tumor, Abscess, MS, and Stroke) the classical diffusion restrictors are: Abscess, and Stroke. Certain hypercellular tumors (classically lymphoma) can restrict, and demyelinating lesions with acute features can restrict.

Enhancement: In this situation this is probably the most helpful. Out of those 4 (Tumor, Abscess, MS, and Stroke) each should have a different pattern.

• *Tumor* could be heterogeneous or homogenous if high grade (or none if low grade).

• *Abscess* will classically have RING pattern.

• *MS* will classically have an Incomplete RING pattern.

• *Stroke* will have cortical ribbon (gyriform) type enhancement in the sub-acute time period (around 1 week).

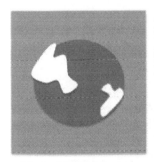 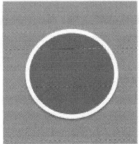 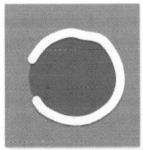 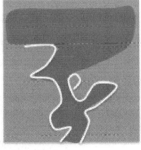

Heterogeneous
-Most likely Tumor (higher grade)

Ring
-Can be lots of stuff: <u>Abscess</u> and Tumor are both prime suspects

Incomplete Ring
-Classic for <u>demyelinating lesion</u>

Gyriform
-Classic for <u>subacute stroke</u> *(can also be seen with PRES or encephalopathy / encephalitis)*

The Characteristic Infections:

TB Meningitis: TB meningitis looks just like regular meningitis, except that it has a predilection for the basal cisterns and may have dystrophic calcifications. There may be **enhancement of the basilar meninges with minimal nodularity.** Complications include vasculitis which may result in infarct (more common in children). Obstructive hydrocephalus is common. *Most likely way to show this is enhancement of the basilar meninges (sarcoid can do that too - so it won't be a distractor unless he/she also has hydrocephalus - in which case pick TB).*

HSV: It's HSV 1 in adults and HSV 2 in neonates. I mention that because (1) it seems like testable trivia and (2) they actually have different imaging appearances (as mentioned above type 2 doesn't love the limbic like type 1). For the purpose of multiple choice test you are going to have a swollen (unilateral or bilateral) **medial temporal lobe**, which will be T2 bright. *Earliest sign is actually restricted diffusion* – related to vasogenic edema. This could be tested by asking "what sequence is more sensitive?", with the answer being the **diffusion is more sensitive than T2.** Blooming on gradient means it's bleeding (common in adults, rare in neonate form). Other trivia is that it **spares the basal ganglia** (distinguishes it from MCA stroke).

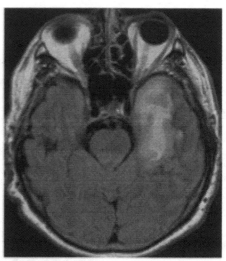

Herpes –
Edema in the temporal lobe

Limbic Encephalitis: Not an infection, but a commonly tested mimic. It is a **paraneoplastic syndrome (usually small cell lung cancer**), that looks very **similar to HSV.** This could be asked by showing a classic HSV image, but then saying HSV titer negative. The second order question would be to ask for lung cancer screening.

West Nile: Several viruses characteristically involve the basal ganglia (Japanese Encephalitis, Murray Valley Fever, West Nile…) , the only one realistically testable is West Nile. We are talking about **T2 bright basal ganglia and thalamus, with corresponding restricted diffusion**. Hemorrhage is sometimes seen.

CJD: There are 3 types: sporadic (80-90%), variant (rare), and familial (10%). Random factoid is that it has a characteristic appearance on EEG, and this "14-3-3" protein assay is a CSF test neurologists order. The imaging features are variable and can be unilateral, bilateral, symmetric, or asymmetric. I want to concentrate on the most likely testable appearances of which I think there are 3.

(1) DWI Showing Cortical Gyriform restricted signal – supposedly diffusion is the most sensitive sign, and the cortex is the most common early site of manifestation.

(2) "Hockey Stick Sign / Pulvinar Sign" – Restricted diffusion in the dorsal medial thalamus (which looks like a hockey stick), or in the pulvinar

(3) A series of MRs or CTs showing rapidly progressive atrophy

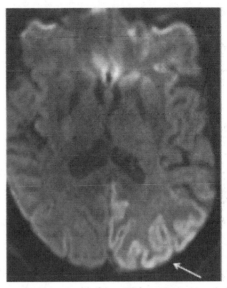

CJD: Gyriform Restricted Diffusion

Neurocysticercosis: Caused by eating pig shit (or undercooked pork). The bug is tinea solium. The most common locations of involvement are the subarachnoid space over the cerebral hemispheres, basal cisterns, brain parenchyma, and ventricles (in that descending order). As a point of trivia, involvement of the basal cisterns carries the worst outcome.

It has 4 stages which could be written in the form of a multiple choice questions (that would be really dirty, and therefore likely):

- Vesicular – thin walled cyst (iso-iso T1/T2 + no edema)
- Colloidal – hyperdense cyst (bright-bright T1/T2 + edema)
- Granular – cyst shrinks, wall thickens (less edema)
- Nodular - small calcified lesion (no edema)

Meningitis and Cerebral Abscess

You can think of meningitis in 4 main categories: bacterial (acute pyogenic), viral (lymphocytic), chronic (TB or Fungal), and non-infectious (sarcoid).

Essentially, we are talking about thick leptomeningeal enhancement, in the appropriate clinical setting. The complications are numerous and include venous thrombosis, vasospasm (leading to the stroke), empyema, ventriculitis, hydrocephalus, abscess etc… and so on and so forth.

Abscess Facts (trivia)
- *DWI - Restricts*
- *MRS – Lactate High*
- *PET FDG – Increased Metabolic*

A very testable piece of trivia is that infants will often get sterile reactive subdurals (much less common than in adults).

Empyema: Can be subdural or epidural (just like blood). Follows the same rules as far as crossing dural attachments (epidurals don't) and crossing the falx (subdurals don't). Subdurals are more common and have more complications relative to epidurals. The vast majority of subdurals are the sequela of frontal sinusitis. The same is true of epidurals with some sources claiming 2/3 of epidurals are secondary to sinusitis. They are often T1 bright and can **restrict on diffusion**.

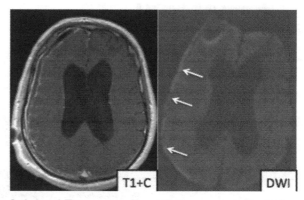

Subdural Empyema: *Dural Enhancement, Restricts*

Intraaxial Infections; We are talking Cerebritis, Abscess, and Ventriculitis:

Again lots of causes via direct spread, or hematogenous spread. The causes worth thinking about include right to left shunts, and pulmonary AVMs. Cerebritis is the early form of intra-axial infection, which can lead to abscess if not treated.

Ventriculits: Usually the result of a shunt placement, or intrathecal chemo. The ventricle will enhance and you can sometimes see ventricular fluid-fluid levels. If septa start to develop you can end up with obstructive patterns of hydrocephalus. The intraventricular extension of abscess is a very serious / ominous "pre-terminal event".

Brain Tumors - The Promethean Method:

I want to introduce my idea for brain tumor diagnosis. The strategy is as follows; (1) decide if it's single or multiple, (2) look at the age of the patient - *adults and kids have different differentials*, (3) look at the location - *different tumors occur in different spots,* (4) now use the characteristics to separate them. The strategy centers around narrowing the differential based off age and location till you are only dealing with 3-4 common things, then using the imaging characteristics to separate them. It's so much easier to do it that way.

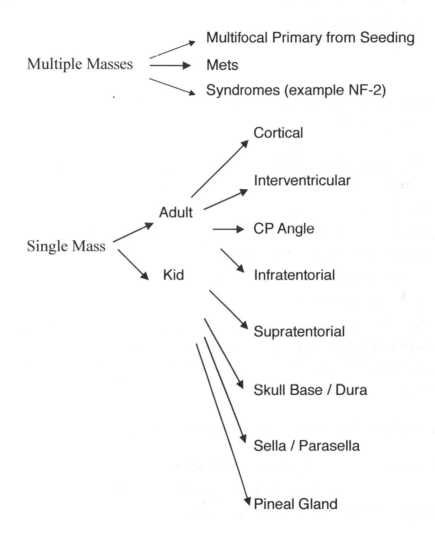

Before we get rolling, the first thing to do is to ask yourself is this a tumor, or is it a mimic? Mimics would be abscess, infarct, or a big MS plaque. This can be tricky. If you see an incomplete ring - you should think giant MS plaque. If they show you diffusion it is either lymphoma or a stroke (or an abscess) - you'll need to use enhancement to straighten that out (remember lymphoma enhances homogeneously).

Two more high yield topics before we start crushing the differentials:

"Intra-axial" vs *"Extra-axial"*

The Brant and Helms discussion on brain tumors will have you asking "intra-axial" vs "extra-axial" first. This is not always that simple, but it does lend itself very well to multiple choice test questions (therefore it's high yield).

Basically you need to memorize the "signs of extra-axial location"

- CSF Cleft
- Displaced Subarachnoid Vessels
- Cortical Gray matter between the mass and white matter
- Displaced and expanded Subarachnoid spaces
- Broad Dural Base / Tail
- Bony Reaction

Why Do Things Enhance?

Understanding the WHY is very helpful for problem solving. Let me first answer the question "why DON'T things enhance?" They DON'T enhance because of the blood brain barrier. So, when things DO enhance it's because either (a) they are outside the blood brain barrier (they are extra-axial), or (b) because they have melted the blood brain barrier.

In other words, extra axial things (classic example is the meningioma) will enhance. High grade tumors (and infections) enhance. Low grade tumors just aren't nasty enough to take the blood brain barrier down.

Are their exceptions? HA! There always are. And Yes... they are ALWAYS testable.

Gangliogliomas and Pilocytic Astrocytomas are the exceptions - they are low-grade tumors, but they enhance.

Multiple Masses

In adults or kids if you see multiple masses you are dealing with mets (or infection). Differentiating between mets and infection is gonna be done with diffusion (infection will restrict). If they want you to decide between those two they must show you the diffusion otherwise only one or the other will be listed as a choice.

Trivia on Mets

- Most common CNS met in a kid = neuroblastoma (BONES, DURA, ORBIT - not brain)

- Most common location for mets = Supratentorial at the Grey-White Junction (this area has a lot of blood flow + an abrupt vessel caliber change... so you also see hematogenous infection / septic emboli go there first too).

- Most common morphology is "round" or "spherical"

- Remember that mets do NOT have to be multiple. In fact 50% of mets are solitary. In an adult a solitary mass is much more likely to be a met than a primary CNS neoplasm.

- **MRCT** in the mnemonic for bleeding mets (**M**elanoma, **R**enal, **C**arcinoid / Choriocarcinoma, **T**hyroid).

- Usually Mets have more surrounding edema than primary neoplasms of similar size.

- *"Next Step Gamesmanship"* - Because the most common intra-axial mass in an adult is a met, if they show you a solitary mass (or multiple masses) and want a next step it's gonna be go hunting for the primary (think lung, breast, colon... the common stuff).

What about a multifocal primary brain tumor, can that happen? Oh yeah there are a few that like to do that (you should still think Met first).

- *Tumors that like to be multifocal:* Lymphoma, Multicentric GBM, Gliomatosis Cerebri
- *Tumors that are multifocal from seeding:* Medulloblastoma, Ependymoma, GBM, Oligodendroglioma
- *Syndromes:* - Tumors with syndromes are more likely to be multifocal.

NF 1	NF 2 "MSME"	Tuberous Sclerosis	VHL
Optic Gliomas	Multiple Schwannomas	Subependymal Tubers	Hemangioblastomas
Astrocytomas	Meningiomas	IV Giant Cell Astrocytomas	
	Ependymomas		

Cortically Based *(P-DOG):*

Most intra-axial tumors are located in the white matter. So when a tumor spreads to or is primarily located in the gray matter you get a shorter DDx. High yield piece of trivia regarding the cortical tumor / cortical met is that they often have *very little edema* and so a *small cortical met can be occult without IV contrast.*

P-DOG:

- **P**leomorphic Xanthoastrocytoma (PXA)
- **D**ysembryoplastic Neuroepithelial Tumor (DNET)
- **O**ligodendroglioma,
- **G**anglioglioma

Oligodendroglioma*:* Remember this is the guy that **calcifies 90% of the time**. It's most common in the frontal lobe and the buzzword is "**expands the cortex**". This takes after its most specific feature of cortical infiltration and marked thickening. It's likely you could get asked about this **1p/19q deletion** which apparently has a better outcome.

Ganglioglioma: This guy can occur at any age, anywhere, and look like anything. However, for the purpose of multiple choice testing the classic scenario would be a 13 year old with seizures, and a temporal lobe mass that is cystic and solid with focal calcifications. There may be overlying bony remodeling.

DNET (Dysembryoplastic Neuroepithelial Tumor): Kid with **drug resistant seizures.** The mass will always be in the **temporal lobe** (on the test – real life 60% temporal). Focal cortical dysplasia is seen in 80% of the cases. It is hypodense on CT, and on MRI there will be little if any surrounding edema. High T2 signal **"bubbly lesion."**

PXA (Pleomorphic Xanthroastrocytoma): Superficial tumor that is ALWAYS supratentorial and usually involves the **temporal lobe.** They are often in the **cyst with a nodule** category (50%). There is usually no peritumeral T2 signal. The tumor frequently invades the leptomeninges. Looks just like a Desmoplastic Infantile Ganglioglioma - but is not in an infant.

Oligodendroglioma	Ganglioglioma	DNET	PXA
ADULT - (40s-50s)	Any Age	PEDS (< 20)	PEDS (10-20)
Can Enhance	Can Enhance	Does **NOT** Enhance	Will Enhance
Calcification Common	NOT Bubbly	High Signal "Bubbly"	Dural Tail***
"Expands the Cortex"	Can look like Anything		Cyst with Nodule

Interventricular

Tumors can arise from the ventricular wall, septum pellucidum, or choroid plexus.

Ventricular Wall & Septum Pellucidum	Choroid Plexus	Misc
Ependymoma **(PEDS)**	Choroid Plexus Papilloma **(PEDS in Trigone)** **(ADULT in 4th Vent)**	Mets
Medulloblastoma **(PEDS)**	Choroid Plexus Carcinoma **(PEDS)**	Meningioma
SEGA (Subependymal Giant Cell Astrocytoma) = **PEDS**	Xanthogranuloma ("Found "in **ADULTS**)	Colloid Cyst
Subependymoma **(ADULT)**		
Central Neurocytoma **(YOUNG ADULT)**		

—

Ventricular Wall / Septum Pellucidum Origin:

Ependymoma: Bimodal distribution on this one (large peak around 6 years of age, tiny peak around 30 years old). I would basically think of this as a **PEDS tumor.**

They come in two flavors:

(a) 4th Ventricle - which is about 70% of the time. with frequent extension into the foramen of Luschka and Magendie. They are the so called "plastic tumor" or *"tooth paste" tumor* because they squeeze out of the 4th ventricle.

(b) Parenchymal Supratentorial - which is about 30% of the time. These are usually big (> 4cm at presentation).

Medulloblastoma: Lets just assume we are talking about the "Classic Medulloblastoma" which is a type of PNET. If you want to understand the genetic spectrum of these things read Osborn's Brain - but that's probably overkill.

age 6 - 11

This is a **pediatric tumor** - with most occurring before age 10 (technically there is a second peak at 20-40 but for the purpose of multiple choice tests I'm going to ignore it).

These guys are cerebellar (arise from vermis – project into 4th ventricle) tumors that love to met via CSF pathways. The mass is heterogeneous on T1 and T2, and enhances homogeneously. They are much more common than their chief differential consideration the Ependymoma. They are hypercellular and may restrict. They calcify 20% of the time (less than Ependymoma). As mentioned above, they like to "drop met." The buzzword is *"zuckerguss"* which apparently is German for sugar icing, as seen on post contrast imaging of the brain and spinal cord. As a point of absolute trivia, they are *associated with Basal Cell Nevus Syndrome, and Turcots Syndrome.*

CT hyperdense
T2 isointense to gray

Gorlin Syndrome - If you see a **medulloblastoma** next look for **dural calcs**. If you see thick dural calcs you might be dealing with this syndrome. They get **basal cell** skin cancer after radiation, and have odontogenic cysts.

NEXT STEP Trivia: Preoperative imaging of the entire spinal axis should be done in any child with a posterior fossa neoplasm, especially if medulloblastoma or ependymoma is suspected. Evidence of tumor spread is a statically significant predictor of outcome.

Medulloblastoma	Ependymoma
More common	Less Common
Originate from Vermis / FLOOR of the 4th Ventricle	Originate from the ROOF of the 4th ventricle.
Can project into 4th ventricle, do NOT usually extend into basal cisterns	Can extend into basal cisterns like tooth paste pushing though foramina of Luschka and Magendie
Enhance Homogeneously *(more so than Ependymoma anyway)*	Enhance Heterogeneously
Calcify Less (20%)	Calcify More (50%)
Linear "icing-like" enhancement of the brain surface is referred to as "Zuckerguss"	

Subependymal Giant Cell Astrocytoma (SEGA): This is going to be shown in the setting of TS. They will more than likely show you renal AMLs or tell you the kid has seizures / developmental delay.

Because it's syndromic you see it in kids (average age 11).

It will arise from the wall of the lateral wall of the ventricle (near the foramen of Monro), often causing hydrocephalus. It enhances homogeneously.

This vs That: SEGA vs Subependymal Nodule (SEN)- The SEN will stay stable in size, the SEGA will grow. The SEGA is found in the lateral ventricle near the foramen of Monroe, the SEN can occur anywhere along the ventricle. SENs are way more common. Both SEN and SEGA can calcify.

Pearl - Enhancing, partially calcified lesion at the foramen of Monro bigger than 5mm is a SEGA not a SEN.

— (the next 2 IV tumors are in ADULTS) —

Subependymoma: Found in ADULTS. Well circumscribed IV masses **most commonly at the foramen of Monro and the 4th ventricle**. They can cause hydrocephalus. They typically don't enhance. They are T2 bright (like most tumors).

Central Neurocytoma: This is the *most common IV mass in an ADULT aged 20-40.* The buzzword is "swiss cheese," because of the numerous cystic spaces on T2. They **calcify a lot** (almost like oligodendrogliomas).

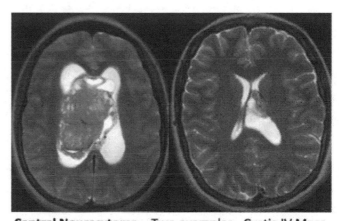

Central Neurocytoma – Two examples , Cystic IV Mass

Choroid Plexus Origin:

Choroid Plexus Papilloma / Carcinoma: Can occur in peds (85% under the age of 5) or adults. They make up about 15% of brain tumors in kids under one. Basically you are dealing with an intraventricular mass, which is often making CSF, so it causes hydrocephalus. *Here is the trick, brain tumors are usually supratentorial in adults and posterior fossa in kids. This tumor is an exception.* Remember exceptions to rules are highly testable.

Trivia -

- **In Adults it's in the 4ᵗʰ Ventricle, in Kids it's in the lateral ventricle (usually trigone).**

- Carcinoma type is ONLY SEE IN KIDS - and are therefore basically ONLY SEEN IN LATERAL VENTRICLE / TRIGONE

- Carcinoma Association with Li-Fraumeni syndrome (bad p53)

- Angiography may show enlarged chorodial arteries which shunt blood to the tumor,

- Carcinoma type of this tumor looks very similar (unless it's invading the parenchyma) and is almost exclusively seen in kids.

- The tumor is typically solitary but rarely you can have CSF dissemination

Xanthogranuloma – This is a benign choroid plexus mass. You see it all the time (7%) and don't even notice it. **The trick is that they restrict on diffusion,** so they are trying to trick you into working them up. They are benign… leave them alone.

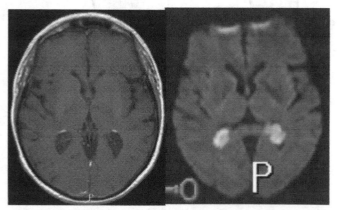

Xanthogranuloma – *Note the Restricted Diffusion*

Misc:

Mets - The most common location of intraventricular metastasis is the trigone of lateral ventricles (because of vascular supply of choroid plexus). The most common primary is controversial - and either lung or renal. If forced to pick I'd go Lung because it's more common overall. I think all things equal renal goes more - but there are less renal cancers. It all depends on how the question is worded.

Colloid Cyst – These are found almost exclusively in the anterior part of the 3rd ventricle behind the foramen of Monro. They **can cause sudden death via acute onset hydrocephalus**. Their appearance is somewhat variable and depends on what they are made of. If they have cholesterol they will be T1 bright, T2 dark. If they don't, they can be T2 bright. The trick is a round well circumscribed mass in the anterior 3rd ventricle. If shown on CT, it will be pretty dense.

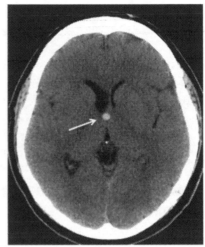

Colloid Cyst –
- *Anterior 3rd Ventricle*
– *Hyperdense on CT*

Meningioma – Can occur in an intraventricular location, most commonly (80%) at the trigone of the lateral ventricles (slightly more on the left). Details on meningiomas are discussed below.

Cerebellar Pontine Angle (CPA)

Age is actually less of an issue here because the DDx isn't that big. Most of these are adult tumors, but in the setting of NF-2 you could have earlier onset.

Epidemiology: Vestibular Schwannoma is #1 - making up 75% of the CPA masses, #2 is the meningioma making up 10%, and the Epidermoid is #3 making up about 5%. The rest are uncommon.

Vestibular Schwannoma – These guys account for 75% of CPA masses. When they are bilateral you should immediately think **NF-2** (*one for each side*). Enhances strongly but more heterogeneous than meningomas. May widen the porus acousticus resulting in a "trumpet shaped" IAC.

Meningioma – Second more common CPA mass. One of the few brain tumors that is more common in women. They can calcify, and if you are lucky they will have a dural tail (which is pretty close to pathognomonic – with a few rare exceptions). Because they are extradural they will enhance strongly. Radiation of the head is known to cause meningiomas.

Meningioma	Schwannoma
Enhance Homogeneously	Enhance Less Homogeneously
Don't Usually Invade IAC	Invade IAC
Calcify more often	IAC can have "trumpeted" appearance

Trivia:

- Most common location of a meningioma is over the cerebral convexity.

- They take up octreotide and Tc-MDP on Nuclear Medicine tests (sneaky).

Epidermoid – Can be congenital or **acquired** (after trauma – classically after LP in the spine). Unlike dermoids they are usually off midline. They will follow CSF density and intensity on CT and MRI (*the exception is this zebra called a "white epidermoid" which is T1 bright – just forget I ever mentioned it*). The key points are (1) unlike an arachnoid cyst they are bright on FLAIR (sometimes warm - *they don't completely null)*, and (2) they **will restrict with diffusion**.

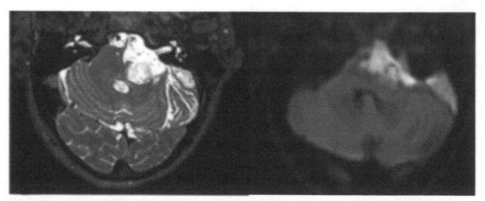

Epidermoid : *Follows CSF Signal – Restricts Diffusion*

Dermoid Cyst – This is about 4x less common than an epidermoid. It's more common in kids / young adults. Usually midline, and usually are found in 3rd decade. They contain lipoid material and are usually hypodense on CT and very bright on T1. They are associated with NF2.

Trivia -

- These are usually midline

- Most common location for a dermoid cyst is the suprasellar cistern (posterior fossa is #2)

This vs That: Dermoid vs Epidermoid — The easy way to think of this is that the Epidermoid behaves like CSF, and the Dermoid behaves like fat.

IAC Lipoma - It can occur, and is basically the only reason you get a T1 when you are working up CPA masses. It will fat sat out - because its a lipoma. There is an association with sensorineural hearing loss, as the vestibulocochlear nerve often courses through it.

Arachnoid Cyst – Common benign lesions that is located within the subarachnoid space and contains CSF. They are increased in frequency in mucopolysaccharidoses (as are perivascular spaces). They are **dark on FLAIR** (like CSF), and **will NOT restrict with diffusion.**

> *How can you tell an epidermoid from an arachnoid cyst?*
>
> The epidermoid restricts, the arachnoid cyst does NOT.

Infratentorial - Most are PEDS (Hemangioblastoma is the exception).

Atypical Teratoma / Rhabdoid – These are highly malignant tumors (WHO IV), and rarely occur in patient's older than 6 years. The average age is actually 2 years, but they certainly occur in the first year of life. They can occur in supra and infratentorial locations (most common in the cerebellum). These are usually **large, pissed off looking tumors with necrosis** and heterogeneous enhancement.

Juvenile Pilocytic Astrocytoma (JPA): Just think cyst with a nodule in a kid. They are WHO grade 1, but the nodule will still enhance. This will be located in the posterior fossa (or optic chiasm).

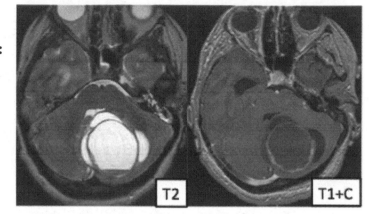

Pilocytic Astrocytoma : *Cyst + Nodule in Kid*

Diffuse Brain Stem Glioma (DPG): Seen in kids age 3-10. Most common location is the pons, which is usually a high grade fibrillary glioma. It's going to be T2 bright with subtle or no enhancement. The 4th ventricle will be flattened. The imaging features are so classic that no biopsy is needed.

Ganglioglioma: This guy can occur at any age, anywhere, and look like anything… and was discussed under the cortical lesions (page 48)

Medulloblastoma: *Discussed with the IV lesions (page 50)*

Ependymoma: *Discussed with the IV lesions (page 49)*

Hemangioblastoma: First things first – immediately think about this when you see **cyst with a nodule** in an ADULT. Then think **Von Hippel Lindau**, especially if they are multiple. These things are slow growing, indolent vascular tumors, that can cause hydrocephalus from mass effect. About 90% of the time they are found in the cerebellum.

I Say Posterior Fossa Cyst with a Nodule - PEDS, you say JPA

I say Posterior Fossa Cyst with a Nodule - ADULT, you say Hemangioblastoma

Supratentorial - Most are Adults (DIG, DNET, PXA are exceptions).

Mets - The most common supratentorial mass - discussed on page 47

Astrocytoma: Most common primary brain tumor in adults. Tumors fitting in the category include Pilocytic Astrocytoma (WHO1), Diffuse Astrocytoma (WHO 2), Anaplastic Astrocytoma (WHO 3) , and GBM (WHO 4). Remember that low grade tumors don't typically enhance (WHO2) and higher grades do (GBM and some Anaplastics). The exception to this rule is the pilocytic astrocytoma which often has an enhancing nodule. GBM is the beast that cannot be stopped. It grows rapidly, it necrosis, it crosses the midline, and it can restrict on diffusion. Remember Turcot Syndrome (*that GI polyp thing*) is associated with GBMs.

Gliomatosis Cerebri: A diffuse glioma with extensive infiltration. It involves at least 3 lobes and is often bilateral. The finding is usually mild blurring of the gray-white differentiation of CT, with extensive T2 hyperintensity and little mass effect on MR. It's low grade, so it **doesn't typically enhance**.

Oligodendroglioma: Discussed under the cortical tumors - page 48.

Primary CNS Lymphoma: Seen in end stage AIDS patients, and those post-transplant. EB virus plays a role. Most common type in non-hodgkin B cell. *Classic picture would be an intensely enhancing homogeneous solid mass in the periventricular region, with **restricted diffusion**.* However, it can literally look like and do anything. Classic Multiple choice test question is that it is Thallium Positive on Spect (toxo is not).

I say restricting brain tumor, you say Lymphoma.

— These next 3 are most common in Peds PEDS —

PXA (Pleomorphic Xanthroastrocytoma): *Discussed under the cortical tumors - page 48.*

DNET :*Discussed under the cortical tumors - page 48.*

Desmoplastic Infantile Ganglioglioma / Astrocytoma "DIG": These guys are large cystic tumors that like to involve the superficial cerebral cortex and leptomeninges. Unlike the Atypical Teratoma / Rhabdoid, these have an ok prognosis. They **ALWAYS arise in the supratentorial location** usually involving more than one lobe (frontal and parietal most commonly), and usually present before the first birthday.

-Buzzword is "rapidly increasing head circumference."

Skull Base:

Chordoma – This is a locally aggressive tumor that originates from the notochord.

WTF is the "notochord" ? It's an embryology thing thats related to spine development.

The thing you need to know is that the notochord is a midline structure. Therefore all Chordomas are midline - either in the clivus, vertebral bodies (especially C2), or Sacrum. You can NOT get them in the hips, ribs, legs, arms, or any other structure that is not totally midline along the axis of the axial skeleton.

Things to know:
- It is most common in the sacrum (#2 is the clivus)
- When it involves the spine it's most common at C2 - but typically extends across a disc space to involve the adjacent vertebral body.
- It's T2 Bright
- It's ALWAYS Midline.

Chondrosarcoma – This is the main differential of the chordoma in the clivus. The thing to know is that it is **nearly always lateral to midline** *(chordoma is midline)*. These are also T2 bright, but will have the classic "arcs and rings" matrix on a chondrosarcoma. Obviously you'll need a CT to describe that matrix.

—

Dura:

Meningioma – As described above it is common and enhances homogeneously. The most common location is over the cerebral convexity and it has been <u>known to cause hyperostosis</u>.

Hemangiopericytoma – This is a soft tissue sarcoma that can **mimic an aggressive meningioma**, because they both enhance homogeneously. They also can mimic a dural tail, with a narrow base of dural attachment. They **won't calcify or cause hyperostosis , but will invade the skull.**

Mets – The most common met to the dura is from breast cancer. 80% will be at the gray-white junction. They will have more edema than a primary tumor of similar size.

Sella / Parasella - Adults

Pituitary Adenoma – The most common tumor of the sella. They are seen 97% of the time in adults. If they are greater than 1cm they are "macroadenomas." When functional, most are prolactin secreting (especially in women). Symptoms are easy to pick up in women (menstrual irregularity, galactorrhea). Men tend to present later because their symptoms are more vague (decreased libido). On MR, 80% are T1 dark and T2 bright. They take up contrast more slowly than normal brain parenchyma.

Pituitary Anatomy Refresher
FLAT - PEG
FLAT is in the front -FSH, LSH, ADH, TSH
PEG is back -Prolactin, Endorphins, GSH

Things to know (about Pituitary adenomas):

- *Microadenoma under 10mm,*
- *Macroadenoma over 10mm.*
- *Microadenomas typically form in the adenohypophysis (front 2/3).*
- *Prolactinoma is the most common functional type.*
- *Typically they enhance less than normal pituitary.*

Pituitary Apoplexy – Hemorrhage or Infarction of the pituitary, usually into an enlarged gland (either from pregnancy or a macroadenoma). Here are the multiple choice trivia association: taking bromocriptine (or other prolactin drugs), "Sheehan Syndrome" in pregnant woman, Cerebral Angiography. They will be **T1 bright** (remember adenoma is usually T1 dark). Supposedly this is an emergent finding because the lack of hormones can cause hypotension.

Rathke Cleft Cyst – Usually an incidental finding, that is rarely symptomatic. They are variable on T1 and T2, but are usually very bright on T2. They do NOT enhance.

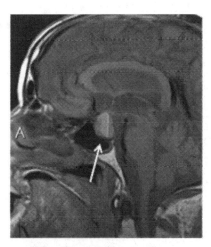

Pituitary Apoplexy
-Shown on T1
-T1 Bright Pituitary

Epidermoid - Discussed on page 54. Remember these guys restrict on diffusion.

Craniopharyngioma – They come in two flavors: (a) Papillary and (b) Adamantinomatous. The Papillary type is the adult type (Papi for Pappi). They are solid and do not have calcifications. They recur less frequently than the Adamantinomatous form (because they are encapsulated). They strongly enhance. The relationship to the optic chiasm is key for surgery. Pediatric type is discussed below (under on the next page with the peds tumors).

Sella / Parasella - Peds

Craniopharyngioma – As stated above, they come in two flavors: (a) Papillary and (b) Adamantinomatous. The kid type is the Adamantinomatous form. These guys are **calcified** (papillary is not). These guys recur more (Papillary does less – because it has a capsule). *Buzzword is "machinery oil."*

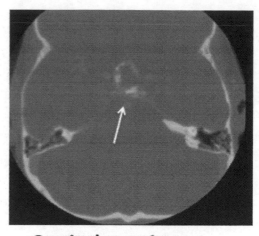

Craniopharyngioma
-*Shown on bone window*
-*Calcifications in the Sella*

Hypothalamic Hamartoma – A classic Aunt Minnie. This is a hamartoma of the tuber cinereum (part of the hypothalamus located between the mammillary bodies and the optic chiasm). They are T1 and T2 iso and they do NOT enhance.

The classic history is **gelastic seizures** (although precocious puberty is actually more common).

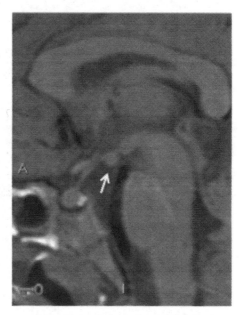

Hamartoma of the Tuber Cinereum

Pineal Region -

There are 3 main characters here, all of which can present with "vertical gaze palsy" (dorsal Parinaud syndrome).

Germinoma: The **more common of the 3**, and seen almost exclusively in boys (Germinomas in the suprasellar region are usually in girls). Precocious puberty may occur from secretion of hCG. Characteristic findings are a **mass containing fat and calcification** with variable contrast enhancement. It is heterogeneous on T1 and T2 (because of its mixed components).

Pineoblastoma: Does occur in childhood. Unlike the pineocytoma these guys are **highly invasive.** Some people like to think of these as PNETs in the pineal gland. They are **associated with retinoblastoma.** They are heterogeneous and enhance vividly.

Pineocytoma: Rare in childhood. Well-circumscribed, and **non-invasive.** Tend to be more solid, and the solid components do typically enhance.

Calcification Patterns in Pineal Tumors

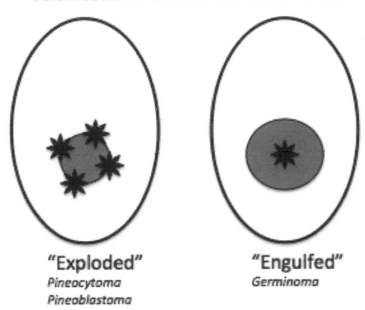

"Exploded"
Pineocytoma
Pineoblastoma

"Engulfed"
Germinoma

Pineal Cyst - An incidental findings that is meaningless... although frequently obsessed over.

Special Topics - A Few Extra Tips on Characterization:

"Restriction"

If they show a supratentorial case with restriction it's likely to be one of two things (1) **Abscess** or (2) **Lymphoma**. Technically any hypercellular tumor can restrict (**GBM, & Medulloblastoma**), but lymphoma is the one they classically show restricting.

If it's a CP angle case, then it's an **epidermoid**.

Lastly, a dirty move could be to show **Herpes** encephalitis restricting in the temporal horns.

"Midline Crossing"

If they show it crossing the midline its most likely going to be a **GBM or Lymphoma**. Alternatively sneaky things they could show doing this would be **radiation necrosis**, a big **MS** plaque in the corpus callosum, or Meningioma of the falx simulating a midline cross.

"Calcification"

If they show it in the brain it is probably an **Oligodendroglioma**. The trick is that Oligodendrogliomas calcify 90% of the time by CT (and 100% by histopathology), whereas astrocytoma only calcify 20% of the time. But astrocytoma is very common and oligodendroglioma is not. So in other words in real life it's probably still an astrocytoma.

"T1 Bright"

Most tumors are T1 dark (or intermediate). Exceptions might include a tumor that has bled (Pituitary apoplexy, or hemorrhagic mets). Hemorrhagic mets are classically seen on **MR** and **CT** (**M**elanoma, **R**enal, **C**arcinoid / **C**horiocarcinoma , **T**hyroid). Tumors with fat will also be T1 bright (Lipoma, Dermoid). Melanin is T1 bright (Melanoma). Lastly think about cholesterol in a colloid cyst.

> **T1 Bright:**
>
> *Fat:* Dermoid, Lipoma
> *Melanin:* Melanoma
> *Blood:* Bleeding Met or Tumor
> *Cholesterol:* Colloid Cyst

Special Topic Syndromes:

NF-1	Optic Nerve Gliomas
NF-2	MSME: Multiple Schwannomas, Meningiomas, Ependymomas
VHL	Hemangioblastoma (brain and retina)
TS	Subependymal Giant Cell Astrocytoma, Cortical Tubers
Nevoid Basal Cell Syndrome (Gorlin)	Medulloblastoma
Turcot	GBM, Medulloblastoma
Cowdens	Lhermitte-Dulcos (Dysplastic cerebellar gangliocytoma)

MSME

If you see tumors EVERYWHERE then you are dealing with <u>NF-2</u>. Ironically there are no neurofibromas in neurofibromatosis type 2 (obviously that would make a great distractor).

Just remember **MSME**
> **M**ultiple **S**chwannomas,
> **M**eningiomas,
> **E**pendymomas

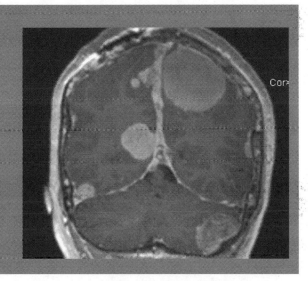

Lhermitte-Dulcos *(Dysplastic cerebellar gangliocytoma)*
- This thing is very uncommon, but when you see it you need to have the following thoughts:

> Hey! Thats Lhermitte Dulcos....
>
> I guess she has Cowdens syndrome....
>
> I guess she has breast CA

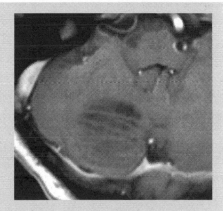

Next Step? - Mammogram

The appearance is classic, with a "tiger stripe" mass, typically contained on one cerebellar hemisphere (occasionally crosses the vermis). It's not a "cancer", but actually a hamartoma - which makes sense since Cowdens is a hamartoma syndrome.

Trauma

Parenchymal Contusion: The rough part of the skull base can scrape the brain as it slides around in a high speed MVA. Typical locations include the anterior temporal lobes and inferior frontal lobes. The concept of coup (site of direct injury) and contre-coup (opposite side of brain along vector of force). Contusion can look like blood with associated edema in the expected regions.

Diffuse Axonal Injury/Shear Injury: There are multiple theories on why this happens (different density of white and gray matter etc...) they don't matter for practical purposes or for multiple choice.

Things to know:

- *Initial Head CT is often normal*
- *Favorite sites of DAI are the posterior corpus callosum, and GM-WM junction in the frontal and temporal lobes*
- *Multiple small T2 bright foci on MRI*

Subarachnoid Hemorrhage: Trauma is the most common cause. FLAIR is the most sensitive sequence. This is discussed in more detail below.

Subdural vs Epidural	
Epidural	**Subdural**
Trauma Patient – with a skull fracture	Old man or alcoholic with an atrophic brain who likes to fall a lot, and stretch / tear those bridging veins.
"Bi-convex" or Lenticular	"Bi-concave"
Can cross the midline	Does not cross the midline, may extend into interhemispheric fissure
Can NOT cross a suture	Can cross a suture
Usually arterial	Usually venous
Can rapidly expand and kill you	

The LeFort Fracture Pattern System: In the dark ages, Rene LeFort beat the skull of cadavers with clubs and threw them off buildings. He then described three facial fracture patterns that interns in ENT and people who write multiple test questions think are important. It can be overly complicated but the most common way a test question is written about these is either by asking the buzzword, or the essential component.

Buzzwords:

- LeFort 1: "The Palate Separated from the Maxilla" or "Floating Palate"
- LeFort 2: "The Maxilla Separated from the Face" or "Pyramidal"
- LeFort 3: "The Face Separated from the Cranium"

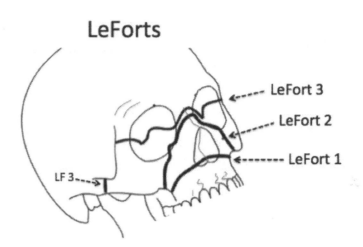

Essential Elements: All three fracture types share the pterygoid process fracture. If the pterygoid process is not involved, you don't have a LeFort. Each has a unique feature (which lends itself easily to multiple choice.

- * LeFort 1: Lateral Nasal Aperture
- * LeFort 2: Inferior Orbital Rim and Orbital Floor
- * LeFort 3: Zygomatic Arch and Lateral Orbital Rim/Wall

Things to Know About Facial Fractures:

- Nasal Bone is the most common fracture
- Zygomaticomaxillary Complex Fracture (Tripod) is the most common fracture pattern, and involves the zygoma, inferior orbit, and lateral orbit.
- Le-Fort Fractures are both a stupid and a high yield topic in facial trauma – for multiple choice. Floating Palate = 1, Pyramidal = 2, Separated Face = 3
- Transverse vs Longitudinal Temporal Bone Fractures – this classification system is stupid and outdated since most are mixed and otic capsule violation is a way better predictive factor… but this is still extremely high yield – see chart on the next page (66).

Mucocele: If you have a fracture that disrupts the frontal sinus outflow tract (usually nasal-orbital-ethmoid types) you can develop adhesions, and obstruction of the sinus resulting in mucocele development. The **buzzword is "airless expanded sinus."** They are usually T1 bright, with a thin rim of enhancement (tumors more often have solid enhancement). The frontal sinus is the most common location – occurring secondary to trauma (as described above).

Temporal Bone Fractures: The traditional way to classify these is longitudinal and transverse and this is almost certainly how the questions will be written. In the real world that system is old and worthless, as most fractures are complex with components of both. The real predictive finding of value is violation of the otic capsule - as described in more modern papers.

Longitudinal	Transverse
Long Axis of T-Bone	Short Axis of T-Bone
More Common	Less Common
More Ossicular Dislocation	More Vascular Injury (Carotid / Jugular)
Less Facial Nerve Damage (around 20%)	More Facial Nerve Damage (>30%)
More Conductive Hearing Loss	More Sensorineural Hearing Loss

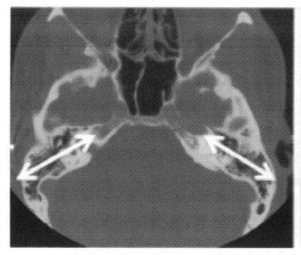

Longitudinal

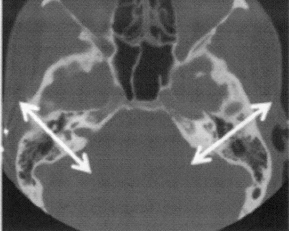

Transverse

How old is that blood?

This is an extremely high yield topic. Maybe the most high yield topic in all of neuro, with regard to multiple choice. The question can be asked with CT or MRI (MRI more likely). If they do ask the question with CT it's most likely to be the subacute subdural that is isointense to brain, with loss sulci along the margins. They could also show the "swirl sign" – see below.

Blood on CT	
Hyperacute Acute (< 1 hour)	Hypodense
Acute (1 hour – 3 days)	Hyperdense
Subacute (4 days – 3 weeks)	Progressively less dense, eventually becoming isodense to brain. **Peripheral rim enhancement may occur with contrast.**
Chronic (> 3 weeks)	Hypodense

Swirl Sign – This is an ominous sign of active bleeding. The central low attenuation blood represents acute non-clotted blood, with surrounding more acute blood.

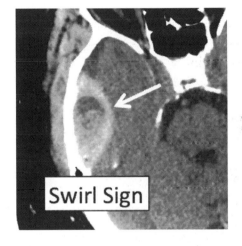

MRI is more difficult to remember. Some people use the mnemonic "IB, ID, BD, BB, DD" or "**I**t **B**e **I**ddy **B**iddy, **BaB**y, **D**oo-**D**oo" which I find very irritating. I prefer mnemonics that employ known words (just my opinion). Another one with actual words is "**G**eorge **W**ashington **B**ridge" For T1 (Gray, White, Black), and Oreo Cookie for T2 (Black, White, Black).

Instead of memorizing baby babbling noises, I use this graph showing a clockwise movement. This thing may seem tricky and too much to bear, at first, but it does actually work and once you draw it twice, you'll have it memorized. You'll also notice a few things: (1) you won't feel like a dipshit for making baby noises, (2) you'll have a renewed sense of self-esteem, and (3) you are likely to notice marked improvement in your golf-swing.

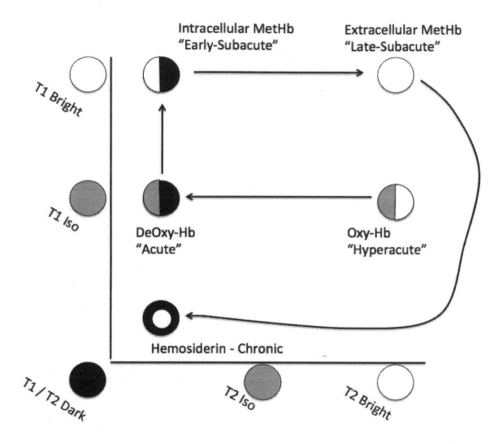

Another strategy is to actually try and understand the MRI changes (I strongly discourage this).

Hyperacute	< 24 hours	Oxyhemoglobin, Intracellular	T1- Iso, T2 Bright
Acute	1-3 days	Deoxyhemoglobin, Intracellular	T1 – Iso, T2 Dark
Early Subacute	> 3 days	Methemoglobin, Intracellular	T1 Bright, T2 Dark
Late Subacute	>7 days	Methemoglobin, Extracellular	T1 Bright, T2 Bright
Chronic	> 14 days	Ferritin and Hemosiderin, Extracellular	T1/ T2 Dark Peripherally, Center may be T2 bright

Hemorrhage (Non-Traumatic)

Subarachnoid Hemorrhage:

Yes, the most common cause is trauma. A common point of trivia is that the **most sensitive sequence on MRI for acute SAH is FLAIR** (because it won't suppress out - making it hyperintense). Be aware that **supplemental oxygen** (usually 50-100%) **can give you a fake out that looks like SAH on FLAIR**. When the blood is real, in the absence of trauma, there are a few other things to think about.

> **Sequella of SAH**
>
> (1) Hydrocephalus - Early
> (2) Vasospasm - 7-10 days
> (3) Superficial Siderosis - Late

- *Aneurysm – Discussed below.*

- **Benign Non-Aneurysm Perimesencephalic hemorrhage**: This is a well described entity (although not well understood). This is NOT associated with aneurysm (usually – 95%), and may be associated with a venous bleed. The location of the blood – around the midbrain and pons without extension into the lateral Sylvian cisterns or interhemispheric fissures is classic. **Just think anterior to the brainstem**. Re-bleeding and ischemia are rare- and they do extremely well.

- **Superficial Siderosis**: This is a side effect of repeated episodes of SAH. I like to think about this as *"staining the surface of the brain with hemosiderin."* The classic look is curvilinear **low signal on gradient coating the surface of the brain**. The classic history is sensorineural hearing loss and ataxia.

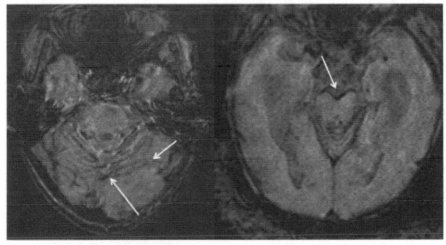

Superficial Siderosis – *Hemosiderin Staining*

Intraparenchymal Hemorrhage:

- **Hypertensive Hemorrhage:** Common locations are the basal ganglia, pons, and cerebellum. For the purpose of multiple choice tests the **basal ganglia is the most common location (specifically the putamen).** You typically have intraventricular extension of blood.

- **Amyloid Angiopathy:** History of an old dialysis patient (or some other history to think Amyloid). *The classic look is multiple lobes at different ages with scattered microbleeds on gradient.*

- **Septic Emboli:** These are seen in certain clinical scenarios (**IV drug user**, organ transplant, cyanotic heart disease, AIDS patients, people with lung AVMs). **The classic look is numerous small foci of restricted diffusion.** Septic emboli to the brain result in abscess, mycotic aneurysms (most commonly in the distal MCAs), The location favors the gray-white interface and the basal ganglia. There will be surrounding edema around the tiny abscesses. The classic scenario should be parenchymal bleed in a patient with infection.

- **Other random causes:** This would include AVMs, vasculitis, brain tumors (primary and mets) - these are discussed in greater detail in various section of the text.

Intraventricular Hemorrhage:

- Not as exciting. Just think about trauma, tumor, hypertension, AVMs, and aneurysms – all the usual players.

Epidural / Subdural Hemorrhage:

- Obviously these are usually post-traumatic.

- **Dural AVFs and High Flow AVMs** can bleed causing subdurals / subarachnoid spaces. These are discussed further, later in the chapter.

Vascular

Stroke –

Stroke is a high yield topic. You can broadly categorize stroke into ischemic (80%) and hemorrhagic (20%). It's critical to remember that stroke is a clinical diagnosis and that imaging findings compliment the diagnosis.

WaterShed Zones: Below is a diagram showing the various vascular territories. The junction between these zones is sometimes referred to as a "Watershed". These areas are prone to ischemic injury, especially in the setting of hypotension or low oxygen states (near drowning or Roger Gracie's cross choke from the mount).

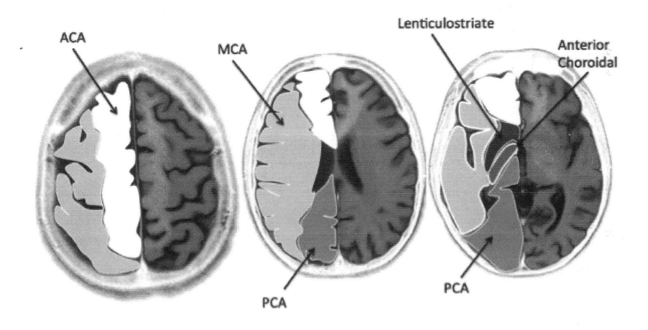

Gamesmanship: **Watershed Infarcts in a Kid = Moyamoya**

Imaging Signs on CT:

Dense MCA Sign	Intraluminal thrombus is dense, usually in the M1 and/or M2 segments
Insular Ribbon Sign	Loss of normal high density insular cortex from cytotoxic edema
Loss of GM-WM differentiation	Basal Ganglia / Internal Capsular Region and Subcortical regions
Mass Effect	Peaks to 3-5 days
Enhancement	Rule of 3s: Starts in 3 days, peaks in 3 weeks, gone by 3 months.

"Fogging" - This is a phase in the evolution of stroke when the infarcted brain looks like normal tissue. This is seen around 2-3 weeks post infarct. "Fogging" is classically described with non-contrast CT, but T2 MRI sequences have a similar effect (typically occurring around day 10). In the real world, you could give IV contrast to demarcate the area of infarct or just understand that fogging occurs.

Imaging Signs on MRI:

Restricted Diffusion: Acute infarcts usually are bright from about 30 mins after the stroke to about 2 weeks. **Restricted diffusion without bright signal on FLAIR should make you think hyperacute (< 6 hours).**

Not Everything That Restricts is a Stroke —
Bacterial Abscess, CJD (cortical), Herpes, Epidermoids, Hypercellular Brain Tumors (Classic is lymphoma), Acute MS lesions, Oxyhemoglobin, and Post Ictal States. Also artifacts (susceptibility and T2 shine through).

Enhancement: The rule of 3's is still useful. Enhancement starts around day 3, it peaks around 3 weeks, and is gone by 3 months.

	0-6 hours	6-24 hours	24 hours -1 week
Diffusion	Bright	Bright	Bright
FLAIR	**NOT BRIGHT**	Bright	Bright
T1	Iso	Dark	Dark, with Bright Cortical Necrosis
T2	Iso	Bright	Bright

Hemorrhagic Transformation – This occurs in about 50% of infarcts, with the typical time period between 6 hours and 4 days. If you got TPA it's usually within 24 hours of treatment. People break these into (1) tiny specs in the gray matter called "petechial" which is the majority (90%) and (2) full on hematoma – about 10%.

Who gets it? People on anticoagulation, people who get TPA, people with embolic strokes (especially large ones), venous infarcts.

Predictors of Hemorrhagic Transformation in Patients Getting TPA
Multiple Strokes, Proximal MCA occlusion, **Greater than 1/3 of the MCA territory**, Greater than 6 hours since onset "delayed recanalization", Absent collateral flow

Venous Infarct: Not all infarcts are arterial, you can also stroke secondary to venous occlusion (usually the sequelae of dural venous sinus thrombosis or deep cerebral vein thrombosis). In general, venous infarcts are at higher risk for hemorrhagic transformation. In little babies think dehydration, in older children think about mastoiditis, in adults think about coagulopathies (protein C & S def) and oral contraceptives. The most common site of thrombosis is the sagittal sinus, with associated infarct occurring 75% of the time.

Venous thrombosis can present as a dense sinus or "empty delta" on contrast. Venous infarcts tend to have *heterogeneous restricted diffusion*. Venous thrombosis can result in vasogenic edema that eventually progresses to stroke and cytotoxic edema.

- Arterial stroke = Cytotoxic Edema

- Venous Stroke = Vasogenic Edema + Cytotoxic Edema

Stigmata of chronic venous thrombosis include the development of a a dural AVF, or increased CSF pressure from impaired drainage.

Aneurysm

Who gets them? People who smoke, polycystic kidney disease, connection tissue disorders (Marfans, Ehlers-Danlos), people with aortic coarctation, NF, FMD, and AVMs.

Where do they occur? They occur at branch points (why do persistent trigeminals get more aneurysms ? – because they have more branch points). They favor the anterior circulation (90%) – with the **anterior communicating artery being the most common site**. As a piece of random trivia the basilar is the most common posterior circulation location (PICA origin is the second most common).

When do they rupture? Rupture risk is increased with size, a posterior location, history of prior SAH, smoking history, and female gender.

Which one did it? A common dilemma is SAH in the setting of multiple aneurysms. The things that can help you are location of the SAH/Clot, location of the vasospasm, size, and which one is the most irregular (*Focal out-pouching - "Murphy's tit"*)

Aneurysm Types:

Saccular (Berry): The most common type. They are commonly seen at bifurcations. The underlying pathology may be a congenital deficiency of the internal elastic lamina and tunica media (at branch points). Remember that most are idiopathic (with the associations listed above). They are multiple 15-20% of the time.

Fusiform Aneurysm – Associated with PAN, Connective Tissue Disorders, or Syphilis. These more commonly affect the posterior circulation. May mimic a CPA mass.

Pseudo Aneurysm – Think about this with an irregular (often sacular) arterial out-pouching at a strange / atypical location. You may see focal hematoma next to the vessel on non-contrast.

- *Traumatic* – Often distal secondary to penetrating trauma or adjacent fracture.

- *Mycotic* – Often distal (most commonly in the MCA), with the associated history of endocarditis, meningitis, or thrombophlebitis.

Pedicle Aneurysm – Aneurysm associated with an AVM. The trivia to know is that it's **found on the artery feeding the AVM** (75% of the time). *These may be higher risk to bleed than the AVM itself (because they are high flow).*

Blister Aneurysm – This is a sneaky little dude (the angio is often negative). It's broad-based at a non-branch point (supraclinoid ICA is the most common site).

Infundibular Widening – Not a true aneurysm, but instead a funnel-shaped enlargement at the origin of the Posterior Communicating Artery at the junction with the ICA. *Thing to know is "not greater than 3mm."*

Saccular (Berry)	Branch Points – in the Anterior Circulation
Fusiform	Posterior Circulation
Pedicle Aneurysm	Artery feeding the AVM
Mycotic	Distal MCAs
Blister Aneurysm	Broad Based Non-Branch Point (Supraclinoid ICA)

Maximum Bleeding – Aneurysm Location	
ACOM	Interhemispheric Fissure
PCOM	Ipsilateral Basal Cistern
MCA Trifurcation	Sylvian Fissure
Basilar Tip	Interpeduncular Cistern, or Intraventricular
PICA	Posterior Fossa or Intraventricular

Vascular Malformation:

There are 6 different kinds, and I will actually touch on all 6 – some in more detail than others.

(1) High Flow AVMs: This is the most common type of high flow lesion. They favor a supratentorial location and are the result of a congenital malformation in the development of the capillary bed. As the name "high flow" implies there is an arterial component (arterial component -> nidus -> draining veins). Hemorrhage is the most common complication, and has a bleeding incidence of about 3% per year. Seizure would be the second most common complication, and the adjacent brain may be atrophic and gliotic.

- *Increased Bleeding Risk: Small size of AVM (actually higher pressure), single draining vein, intranidal/perinidal aneurysm, basal ganglia/thalamic/ periventricular locations.*

(2) Dural AVF: These can be high flow or low flow. They are less common than the high flow AVMs. Unlike the AVM these are thought to be acquired secondary to dural sinus thrombosis. Unlike AVMs there is no nidus. This presents in the 50s-60s (AVMs present in 20s-30s). **Classic symptom is pulsatile tinnitus, when it involves the sigmoid sinus**. May have vision problems if the cavernous sinus is involved.

- *Increased Bleeding Risk: Direct cortical venous drainage.*
- *Can be occult on MRI/MRA - need catheter angio if suspicion high*

- *SPINAL AVFs are actually the most common type of AVFs - a helpful hint is the classic clinical history of "gradual onset LE weakness"*

(3) DVA: This is not actually a vascular malformation, just a variation in normal venous drainage. If you tried to resect one, you would end up with a nice venous infarct. Some buzzwords are "caput medusa" or "large tree with multiple small branches" – to describe its appearance. The big thing to remember is the **association with cavernous malformations.**

(4) Cavernous Malformation: These things are also called "cavernomas" and "cavernous angiomas." These are low flow lesions with a dilated capillary bed **without intervening normal brain tissue.** They can be single or multiple (more common in Hispanics). Buzzword is "popcorn-like" with "peripheral rim of hemosiderin." Look for them on gradient (because of the hemosiderin). They can ooze some blood, but typically don't have full-on catastrophic bleeds. As mentioned above, they may have a nearby DVA.

(5) Capillary Telangiectasia: This is another slow flow lesion, that unlike the cavernoma does have intervening normal brain tissue. They don't bleed and are usually totally incidental. The most common look for this is a single lesion in the pons. Again these are best seen on gradient (slow flow and deoxyhemoglobin). The buzzword is "brush-like" or "stippled pattern" of enhancement. Key high yield fact is that **these can develop as a complication of radiation therapy**.

(6) Mixed – This is a wastebasket term, most often used for DVA with AV shunting or DVAs with telangiectasias.

Vasospasm

Vessels do not like to be bathed in blood (SAH), it makes them freak out (spasm). The **classic timing for this is 4-14 days after SAH (NOT immediately)**. It usually looks like smooth, long segments of stenosis. It typically involves multiple vascular territories. It can lead to stroke.

Who gets it? It's usually for SAH and the more volume of SAH the greater the risk. In 1980 some neurosurgeon came up with this thing called the Fisher Score, which grades vasospasm risk. The gist of it is greater than 1mm in thickness or intraventricular / parenchymal extension is at higher risk.

Are there Non-SAH causes of vasospasm? Yep. Meningitis, PRES, and Migraine Headache.

Critical Take Home Point - Vasospasm is a delayed side effect of SAH. It does NOT occur immediately after a bleed. You see it 4-14 days after SAH.

Vascular Dissection

Vascular dissection can occur from a variety of etiologies (usually penetrating trauma, or a trip to the chiropractor). Penetrating trauma tends to favor the carotids, and blunt trauma tends to favor the vertebrals. This would be way too easy to show on CT as a flap, so if it's shown it's much more likely to be the T1 bright "crescent sign", or intramural hematoma.

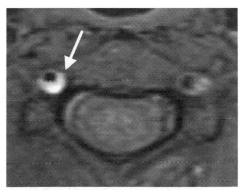

"Crescent Sign" of Dissection
- it's the T1 bright intramural blood.

Vasculitis

You can have a variety of causes of CNS vasculitis. One way to think about it is by clumping it into (a) Primary CNS vasculitis, (b) Secondary CNS vasculitis from infection, or sarcoid, (c) systemic vasculitis with CNS involvement, and (d) CNS vasculitis from a systemic disease.

Primary CNS vasculitis	Primary Angiitis of the CNS (PACNS)
Secondary CNS vasculitis from infection, or sarcoid	**Meningitis** (bacterial, TB, Fungal). Septic Embolus, Sarcoid,
Systemic vasculitis with CNS involvement	**PAN**, Temporal Arteritis, Wegeners, Takayasu's,
CNS vasculitis from a Systemic Disease	**Cocaine Use**, RA, SLE, Lyme's

They all pretty much look the same with multiple segmental areas of vessel narrowing, with alternating dilation ("beaded appearance"). You can have focal areas of vascular occlusion.

Trivia:

- *PAN is the Most Common systemic vasculitis to involve the CNS (although it is a late finding).*

- *SLE is the Most Common Collagen Vascular Disease*

Misc Vascular Conditions

Moyamoya – This non-atherosclerotic poorly understood entity (originally described in Japan – hence the name), is characterized by progressive stenosis of the supraclinoid ICA eventually leading to occlusion. The progressive stenosis results in an enlargement of the basal perforating arteries.

Things to know:

- *Buzzword = "Puff of Smoke" – for angiographic appearance*
- *Watershed Distribution*
- *In a child think sickle cell*
- *Other notable associations include: NF, prior radiation, Downs syndrome*
- *Bi-Modal Age Distribution (early childhood, and middle age)*
- *Children Stroke, Adults Bleed*

CADASIL – *(Cerebral Autosomal Dominant Arteriopathy with Subcortical Infarcts and Leukoencephalopathy)*. Think about a 40 year old **presenting with migraine headaches**, then eventually dementia. The MRI will show severe white matter disease involving multiple vascular territories, in the frontal and **temporal lobe**. The occipital lobes are often spared.

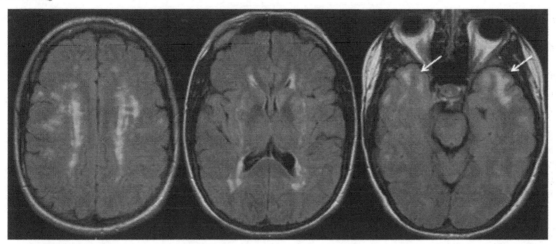

CADASIL – *Diffuse White Matter Disease, Hitting the Temporals, Sparing Occipitals*

NASCET Criteria: The North American Symptomatic Carotid Endarterectomy Trial (NASCET) criteria, is used for carotid stenosis.

The rule is: measure the degree of stenosis using the maximum internal carotid artery stenosis ("A") compared to a parallel (non-curved) segment of the distal, cervical internal carotid artery ("B").

You then use the formula [1- A/B] X 100%.

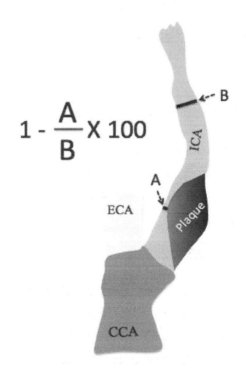

$$1 - \frac{A}{B} \times 100$$

Developmental / Congenital

Congenital malformations is a very confusing and complicated topic, full of lots of long Latin and French sounding words. If we want to keep it simple and somewhat high yield you can look at it in 6 basic categories: (1) Failure to form, (2) Failure to cleave, (3) Failure to migrate, (4) Normal forming but massive insult makes you look like you didn't form (5) Herniation syndromes, and (6) Craniosynostosis.

Failure to Form:

A classic point of trivia is that the corpus callosum forms front to back (then rostrum last). Therefore hypoplasia of the corpus callosum is usually absence of the splenium (with the genu intact).

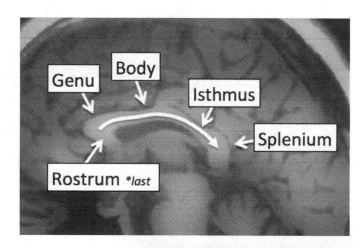

With agenesis of the corpus callosum, a common trick is to show colpocephaly (asymmetric dilation of the occipital horns).

When you see this picture you should say two things:

(1) Corpus Callosum Agenesis
(2) Pericallosal Lipoma

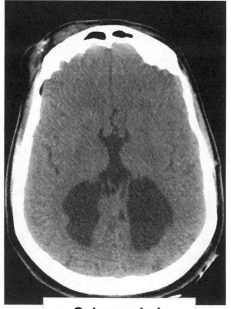

Colpocephaly
(asymmetric dilation of the occipital horns).

Callosal Dysgenesis / Agenesis: This is associated with lots of other syndromes/ malformations (Lipoma, heterotopias, schizencephaly, lissencephaly etc…). **"Most common anomaly seen with other CNS malformations."** If they ask this, it will either be the colpocephaly picture, the **steer horn** appearance of coronal, or the **vertical ventricles** widely spaced (racing car) on axial.

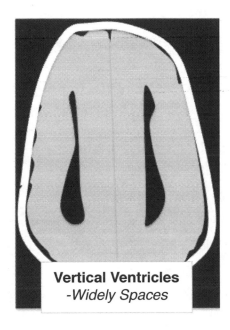

Vertical Ventricles
-Widely Spaces

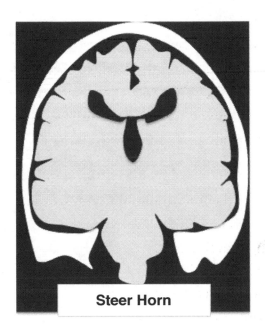

Steer Horn

Why are the lateral ventricles widely spaced when you have no Corpus Callosum ? There are these things called **"Probst bundles"** which are densely packed WM tracts - destined to cross the CC - but can't (because it isn't there). So instead they run parallel to the interhemispheric fissure -making the vents look widely spaced.

Intracranial Lipoma: Associated with callosal dysgenesis. 50% are found in the interhemispheric fissure and if they show it that's where is will be.

Trivia: CNS Lipomas are congenital malformations, not true neoplasms. The tubulonodular type frequently calcify.

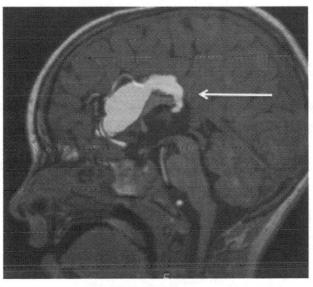

Intracranial Lipoma

Anencephaly: Neural tube fails to close on the cranial end leading to reduced or absent cerebrum and cerebellum. The hindbrain will be present. Obviously this is not compatible with life. Trivia: **AFP will be elevated, polyhydraminos** will be present (hard to swallow without a brain). If they show it, it will have to be antenatal ultrasound and will likely be polyhydramnios plus the incredibly creepy **"frog eye" appearance** on the coronal plane (due to absent cranial bone / brain with bulging orbits).

Iniencephaly: Rare neural defect with the main features including deficit of the occipital bones. This results in an enlarged foramen magnum. These guys also have really jacked up spines. **"Star Gazing Fetus"** is the buzzword because they are contorted in a way that makes their face turn upward (hyper-extended cervical spine, short neck, and upturned face).

Arhinencephaly: No olfactory bulbs and tracts. Seen with **Kallmann Syndrome** (hypogondaism, mental retardation).

Rhombencephalosynapsis: Congenital anomaly of the cerebellum, where the vermis doesn't develop and instead you just fuse your cerebellum. Classically a transversely oriented singe lobed cerebellum is shown (this is an Aunt Minnie).

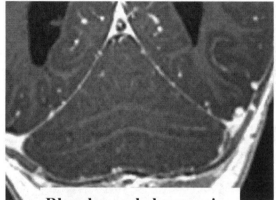

Rhombencephalosynapsis
-Note the Vertical Line Across the Cerebellum

Joubert Syndrome: OK so this is another Aunt Minnie, because of the **"Molar Tooth" appearance** of the superior cerebellar peduncles (they are elongated like the roots of a tooth). There is going to be a small or aplastic cerebellar vermis, and there will be absence of pyramindal decussation. It has a **strong association (50%) with retinal dysplasia.** There is also an association with multicystic dysplastic kidneys (30%). When you see it in combination with liver fibrosis it's a total zebra (near unicorn) called COACH syndrome.

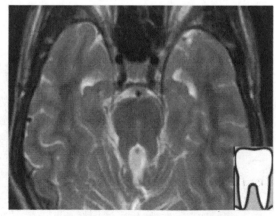

Joubert – Molar Tooth

Dandy Walker:

Radiologists love to nitpick and obsess over details. Usually, the more meaningless the detail the more ferocious the debate. Along those lines...

This is a "spectrum" that leads to much confusion and argument. For the purpose of the multiple choice tests I would just say that Dandy Walker = Absent Vermis. **The buzzword is "torcular-lambdoid inversion."** *The torcular is above the level of the lambdoid due to abnormally high tentorium.*

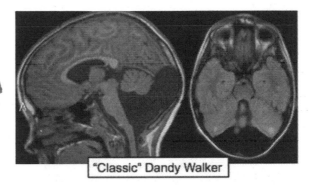

"Classic" Dandy Walker

The following chart is just for the sake of addressing the ridiculousness of this posterior fossa situation. It ought to be very low yield for the exam (which probably means it is high-yield). It may also be useful if you want to join in the debate.

Morphology (Most Severe -> Least Severe)	**Features**			
"Ventriculocele" DWM Variant	Cystic Dilation of 4th	Complete or partial Agenesis of the Vermis	Enlarged Posterior Fossa PLUS erosion into the occipital bone -> encephalocele	
"Classic" DWM	Cystic Dilation of 4th	Complete or partial Agenesis of the Vermis	Enlarged Posterior Fossa	Superiorly rotated vermian remnant
"Variant" DWM	Partially obstructed 4th Ventricle	Variable Hypoplasia of the Vermis (*less severe*)	Posterior Fossa **NOT enlarged**	
Persistent Blake Pouch	Cyst below and posterior to the vermis	Normal Vermis	Posterior Fossa **NOT enlarged**	The tentorium is elevated
Mega Cisterna Magna	Retro-Cerebellar CSF Space > 10mm	Cerebellum Normal	Enlarged posterior fossa caused by enlarged cisterna magna	

Failure To Cleave

Holoprosencephaly (HPE): This is a midline cleaving problem with the brain failing to cleave into two separate hemispheres. The cleavage apparently occurs back to front (opposite of the formation of the corpus callosum), so in milder forms the posterior cortex is normal and the anterior cortex is fused.

It is classified as a spectrum:

Lobar ⟶ Semilobar ⟶ Alobar (most severe)

Lobar (mild)	Semi-Lobar	Alobar (severe)
Right and Left Hemispheres are separate (anterior/inferior frontal still sometimes fused)	Basic structure present but **fused at the thalami**. Posterior brain is normal.	There is a **single large ventricle**, with fusion of the thalami and basal ganglia.
May be limited to absent septum pellucidum	Olfactory tracts and bulbs are gone	No Falx. No corpus callosum.
Pituitary Problems are common		

The old saying "face predicts brain, but brain doesn't predict face" is actually mostly true. In other words, monster Cyclops babies usually have some midline defect (holoprosencephaly). There are several other associations that are frequently shown and often testable:

HPE Associations:

- Single Midline Monster Eye
- Solitary Median Maxillary Incisor (MEGA-Incisor)
- Nasal Process Overgrowth leading to Pyriform Aperture Stenosis

 : **Meckel-Gruber Syndrome:**
- Classic triad:
    - o   Holoprosencephaly,
    - o   Multiple Renal Cysts and
    - o   Polydactyly

Anencephaly: This actually means "no –brain". This is basically the extreme end of the Holoprosencephaly spectrum. You are going to have no brain (only a brainstem), no skull, and no scalp. *See the reproductive chapter in Volume 1 for more on this.*

Failure to Migrate / Proliferate:

Hemimegalencephaly: Rare but unique (Aunt Minnie) malformation characterized by **enlargement of all or part/s of one cerebral hemisphere**. The cause of this condition is speculated to be problem of neuronal differentiation and cell migration in a single hemisphere. The affected hemisphere may have focal or diffuse neuronal migration defects, including areas of polymicrogyria, pachygyria, and heterotopia.

Here is the trick: Look at which side (the big side or the little side) has the ventriculomegaly.

- *Small Side + Big Ventricle = Atrophy (as might be seen with Rasmussen's Encephalitis)*
- *Big Side + Big Ventricle = Hemimegalencephaly*

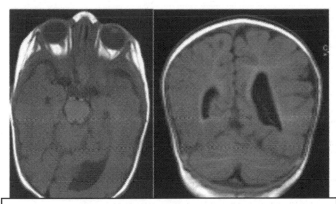

Hemimegalencephaly - *Big Side Big Ventricle*

Lissencephaly-Pachygyria Spectrum: The spectrum of diseases that cause relative smoothness of the brain surface. Vocabulary includes agyria (no gyri), pachygyria (broad gyri) and lissencephaly (smooth brain surface).

You can think about it as either:

- Type 1/Classic form = Smooth Brain. This results from arrest of migration. Buzzwords include "figure 8", "hours glass appearance", "vertically oriented shallow Sylvian fissures". This one is associated with band heterotopias.

- Type II as a cobblestone brain. This results from over migration. There is not band heterotopia and the cortex is thinner than type I.

Grey Matter Heterotopias:
"Normal Neurons in Abnormal Locations" These guys can be grouped and then grouped and then subgrouped into groups.

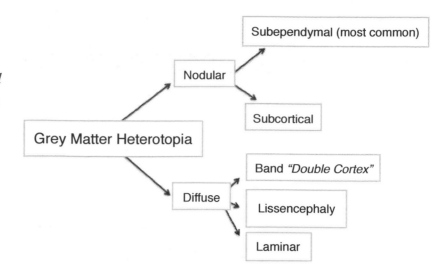

They are associated with other congenital neurologic conditions. A random point of trivia: if you are trying to compare subependymal heterotopias with the subependymal tubers of TS, the tubers are usually higher on T2 signal than gray matter and are often calcified (except in early childhood).

Schizencephaly: Migrational disorder that results in a grey matter lined cleft that will extend through the entire hemisphere. It comes in two main flavors: (1) Closed Lip (20%) and (2) Open Lip (80%).

Highly Testable Associations:
- *Optic Nerve Hypoplasia (30%)*
- *Absent Septum Pellucidum (70%)*
- *Epilepsy (demonic possession) 50-80%*

Classic THIS vs THAT: Porencephalic Cyst vs Open Lip Schizencephaly.

They look very similar, but the schizencephalic cleft should be lined with gray matter, and is a true malformation. The porencephalic cyst is a just a hole from a prior encephaloclastic event (ischemia). *Normal forming but massive insult makes you look like you didn't form.*

Hydranencephaly: Devastating condition characterized by destruction of the cerebral hemispheres. Basically this turns the skull into a bag of CSF. It is thought to be secondary to a vascular insult in utero (**think double MCA infarct**). This could be seen in the setting of a TORCH causing a necrotizing vasculitis (HSV does this). The key point is that you did have a normal brain, so you have a falx, but the cortical mantle is gone.

"Lots of CSF" - Brain Strategy

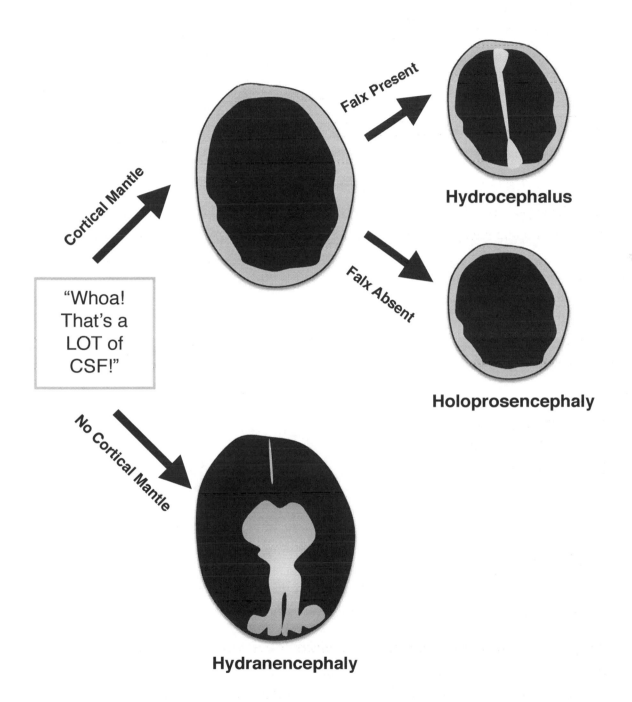

Herniation Syndrome Vocab

Cephaloceles – Herniation of the cranial contents through a defect in the skull.

- Meningoencephalocele – brain + Meninges
- Meningocele – just meninges (no brain)

Chiari Malformations:

Chiari malformation essentially occurs because of a mismatch between size and content of the posterior fossa.

Type 1: These guys have headaches. Criteria is one cerebellar tonsil **more than 5mm below the foramen magnum**. This is often accompanied by crowding of the posterior fossa and you should look for syringohydromyelia (seen in about 50% of cases). As you age, the tonsils ascend, so 3mm below the foramen in a 90 year old would be abnormal. There are several associations but the one that is most often asked is with Klippel-Feil syndrome (congenital C-spine fusion).

Type 2: This type is more complicated and there are like 20 findings. Hydrocephalus is found in more than 90% of cases. I'm going to try and pick the five I think they are most likely to ask or show.

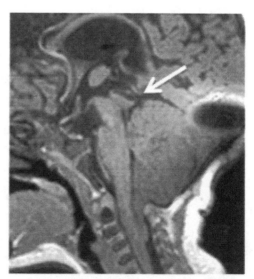

Tectal Beaking – Chiari 2

- Myelomenigocele – Lumbar Spine
- Towering Cerebellum
- Tectal Plate Beaking
- Long Skinny 4th Ventricle (*elongated craniocaudally, short in other dimensions*) --- a normal 4th ventricle may suggest shunt malfunction
- Interdigitated Cerebral Gyri (most likely shown on axial CT, single image)

Type 3: Just think Chiari II + Encephalocele (either high cervical or low occipital)

Craniosynostosis

Premature fusion of one or more of the cranial sutures can result in a weird shaped head. I have just a few high yield points regarding the subject. Scaphocephaly (Sagittal Suture) is the most common subtype and is often referred to a dolichocephaly. Brachycephaly (Coronal and/or Lambdoid) is often associated with syndromes.

Of course they are all zebras but a few are worth knowing:

- **Aperts:** *Brachycephaly + Fused Fingers*
- **Crouzons:** *Usually Brachycepahly (but not always) + First Arch (Maxilla and Mandible Hypoplasia)*
- **Cleidocranial Dysostosis**: *Brachycephaly + Wormian Bones + Absent Clavicles*

Plagiocephaly can result from unilateral coronal or lambdoid suture fusion (frontal or occipital plagiocephaly). **Ipsilateral coronal fusion can elevate the superior orbital wall and cause a harlequin eye.**

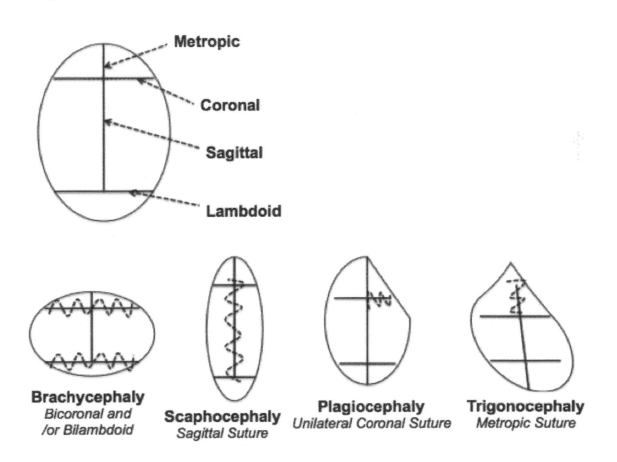

Brachycephaly
Bicoronal and /or Bilambdoid

Scaphocephaly
Sagittal Suture

Plagiocephaly
Unilateral Coronal Suture

Trigonocephaly
Metropic Suture

High Yield Trivia / Buzzwords for Craniosynostosis:

- Most common type = sagittal (dolichocephaly or scaphocephaly)
- Sagittal Suture craniosynostosis almost always (80%) affects boys
- Coronal Suture Craniosynostosis affects more girls.
- "Harlequin Eye" = Unilateral Coronal Suture Craniosynostosis (lifts supra-orbital margin).
- Lambdoid Craniosynostosis favors the right side (70%)
- Turricephaly (the tower) is from both coronal and lambdoid fusion

Misc Peds Brain Conditions:

Enlarged extra-axial fluid spaces: Extra-axial fluid spaces are considered enlarged if greater than 5mm. **BESSI** is the name people throw around for "benign enlargement of the subarachnoid space in infancy." The etiology is supposed to be immature villa (that's why you grow out of it).

BESSI Trivia: (1) It's the most common cause of macrocephaly, (2) it typically resolves after 2 years with no treatment, (3) there is an increased risk of subdural bleed - either spontaneous or with a minor trauma.

> **BESSI vs Subdural Collection**
>
> *BESSI* - Cortical veins are adjacent to the inner table
>
> *Subdural* - Cortical veins are displaced away from the inner table.

Trivia - Pre-mature kids getting tortured on ECMO often get enlarged extra-axial spaces. This isn't really the same thing as BESSI and more related to fluid changes / stress.

Choanal Atresia: This is a malformation of the choanal openings. Buzzwords are *"failure to pass NG tube"* and *"respiratory distress while feeding"* (neonates have to breath through their noses). It's usually unilateral (2/3). There are two different types: bony (90%), and membranous (10%). The appearance is a unilateral or bilateral posterior nasal narrowing, with thickening of the vomer. There are a bunch of syndromic associations: CHARGE, Crouzons, DiGeorge, Treacher Colins, and Fetal Alcohol Syndrome.

Piriform Aperture Stenosis – This can occur in isolation or with choanal atresia. The big thing to know is the high association with hypothalamic-pituitary-adrenal axis dysfunction.

MELAS – This is a mitochondrial disorder with lactic acidosis and stroke like episodes. The SPECT question is always: increased lactate, decreased NAA.

—

Leukodystrophies: These are zebra disorders that affect the white matter in kids. If you see a brain MRI on a kid with jacked up white matter, you should be thinking about one of these guys. The distinction between them is totally academic, since they are all untreatable and fatal.

Here are my tricks:
- *Canavans* is always shown with SPECT – with an elevated NAA.
- *Alexanders* has a big head (like Alexander the Great), and has frontal white matter involvement (frontal because of his personality disorder - metaphorically speaking).
- *Metachromatic* is the most common, and the buzzword is "tigroid." Tigroid refers to dark spots or stripes within the T2 bright demylinated periventricular white matter.

	Head Size	Age	Territory	Trivia
Metachromatic	Normal Head	Infantile form 1-2 yo. Juvenile form 5-7	Diffuse white matter involvement, with **tigroid appearance**.	**Most common Leukodystrophy**. Deficiency of the enzyme arylsulfatase A.
Adreno Leukodystrophy	Normal Head	5-10 yo.	Symmetric occipital and splenium of corpus callosum white matter involvement.	Sex-linked recessive condition (peroxisomal enzyme deficiency) **occurring only in boys.**
Leigh disease	Normal Head	Less than 5 yo.	Focal areas of subcortical white matter. Basal ganglia and periaquaductal gray matter involvement.	Also called subacute necrotizing encephalo-myelopathy. Mitochondrial enzyme defect.
Alexander disease	Big Head	Less than 1 yo.	**Frontal white matter** involvement.	
Canavan disease	Big Head	Less than 1 yo.	Diffuse Bilateral sub cortical U fibers.	Elevated NAA (MRS).

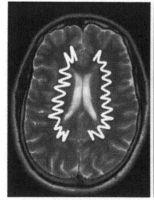
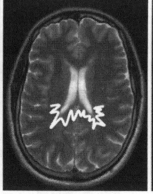
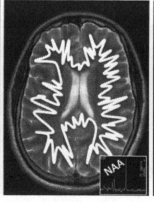
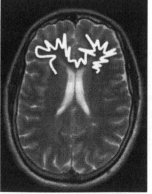

Metachromatic   Adreno   Canavans   Alexander

High Yield MR SPECT Trivia:

- The highest normal peak is NAA.
- The NAA peak will be super high with Canavans.
- Choline is elevated in anything that causes cell turnover (tumor, infarct, or inflammation).
- Lactate and Lipid peaks superimpose - you need to use an intermediate TE (around 140) to causes an "inversion" of the lactate peak (so you can see it).
- Lactate-Lipid peak has a characteristic "double peak" at a long TE (around 280)
- A normal adult head should not have a lactate peak (it's a marker of aerobic metabolism) - so you see it in necrotic tumors (high grade) and infection (cerebral abscess).
- It's normal to see lactate elevated in the first hours of life.**Remember exceptions to rules are always high yield.**
- Myoinositol is elevated with Alzheimer's and low grade gliomas
- Alanine elevation is specific for Meningiomas
- Meningiomas do NOT have elevated NAA.
- Glutamine is elevated in Hepatic Encephalopathy
- High Grade Tumor = Choline Up, NAA down, Lactate and Lipids Up
- Low Grade Tumor = Choline Down, NAA down, Inositol Up
- Radiation Necrosis Pattern: Choline Down, NAA Down, Lactate Up

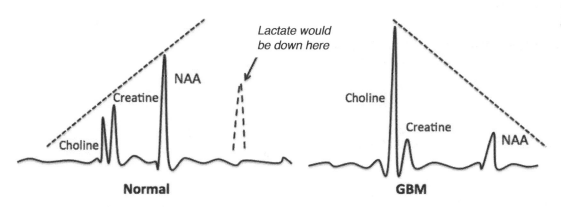

Notice that Choline, Creatine, and NAA fall in alphabetical order. That makes it easy to remember which is which

- *Vocab:* The normal dotted line is called "Hunter's Angle"

SECTION 2: HEAD AND NECK

Temporal Bones:

Petrous Apex:

Anatomic Variation: Variation can occur in the amount of pneumatization, marrow fat, bony continuity, and vascular anatomy.

- *Asymmetric Marrow:* - Typically the petrous apex contains significant fat, closely following the scalp and orbital fat (T1 and T2 bright). When it's asymmetric you can have two problems (1) falsely thinking you've got an infiltrative process, when you don't and (2) overlooking a T1 bright thing (cholesterol granuloma) thinking it's fat. The key is to use STIR or some other fat saturating sequence.

- *Cephaloceles:* - A cephalocoele describes a herniation of CNS content through a defect in the cranium. In the petrous apex they are a slightly different animal. They don't contain any brain tissue, and simply represent cystic expansion and herniation of the posterolateral portion of Meckel's cave into the superomedial aspect of the petrous apex. Describing it as a **herniation of Meckel's Cave would be more accurate**. These are usually unilateral and are classically described as *"smoothly marginated lobulated cystic expansion of the petrous apex."*

- *Variant Anatomy of the Carotid Artery*: - The 2 main variants to be aware of are the persistent stapedial artery, and aberrant internal carotid. For the purpose of the exam the only things to know are **don't biopsy them** *(they aren't glomus tympanicum tumors),* and **they can give pulsatile tinnitus.**

Inflammatory Lesions:

- **Cholesterol Granuloma** – The **most common primary petrous apex lesion**. Mechanism is likely obstruction of the air cell, with repeated cycles of hemorrhage and inflammation leading to expansion and bone remodeling. The most common symptom is hearing loss. On CT the margins will be sharply defined. On MRI it's gonna be **T1 and T2 bright,** with T2 dark hemosiderin rim, and faint peripheral enhancement. The slow growing ones can be watched. The fast growing ones need surgery.

  o *Key Point; Cholesterol Granuloma = **T1** and T2 Bright.*

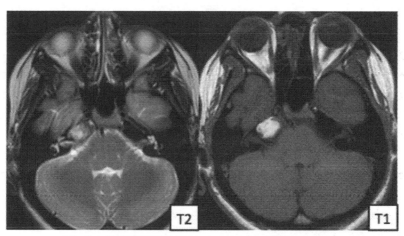

Cholesterol Granuloma = T1 and T2 Bright.

- **Cholesteatoma** - This is basically an epidermoid (ectopic epithelial tissue). They are congenital (not acquired) in the petrous apex. They are typically slow growing, and produce bony changes similar to cholesterol granuloma. The difference is their MRI findings; T1 dark, T2 bright, and restricted diffusion.

  o *Key Point; Cholesteatoma = T1 Dark, T2 Bright, Restricted Diffusion*

Cholesterol Granuloma	*Cholesteatoma*
T1 Bright	T1 Dark
T2 Bright	T2 Bright
Doesn't Restrict	**Does Restrict**
Smooth Expansile Bony Change	Smooth Expansile Bony Change

- **Apical Petrositis** – Infection of the petrous apex is a rare complication of infectious otomastoiditis. It can have some bad complications if it progresses including osteomyelitis of the skull base, vasospasm of the ICA (if it involves the carotid canal), subdural empyema, venous sinus thrombosis, temporal lobe stroke, and full on meningitis. In children, it can present as a primary process. In adults it's usually in the setting of chronic otomastoiditis or recent mastoid surgery.

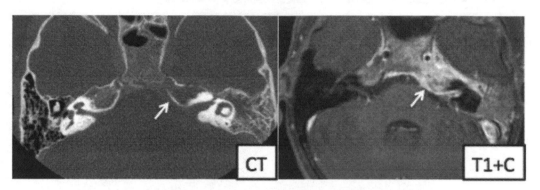

Apical Petrositis

- **Grandenigo Syndrome** – This is a complication of apical petrositis, when Dorello's canal (CN 6) is involved. They will show you (or tell you) that the patient has a lateral rectus palsy. The classic triad = otomastoiditis, face pain (trigeminal neuropathy), and lateral rectus palsy.

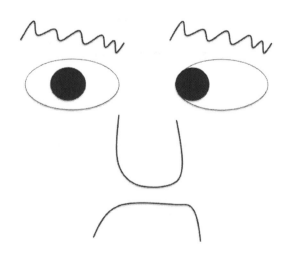

Tumors:

- **Endolymphatic Sac Tumor** – Rare tumor of the endolymphatic sac and duct. Although most are sporadic, when you see this tumor you should immediately think **Von-Hippel-Lindau**. They usually grow into the CPA. They almost always have **internal amorphous calcifications on CT**. There are T2 bright, with **intense enhancement**. They are **very vascular** often with **flow voids**, and **tumor blush** on angiography.

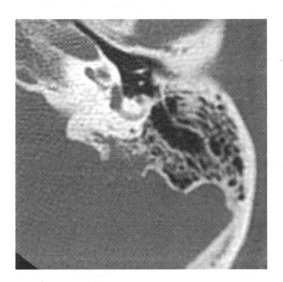

- **Paraganglioma** - On occasion, paraganglioma of the jugular fossa (glomus jugulare or jugulotympanic tumors) can invade the occipital bone and adjacent petrous apex. As much as **40% of the time it's hereditary, and they are multiple**. The **most common presenting symptom in hoarseness** from vagal nerve compression. They are very vascular masses - they enhance avidly with a **"salt and pepper"** appearing on post contrast MRI, with **flow voids**. They are **FDG avid.**

Please see the discussion of the subtypes on page 111.

Inner Ear

Congenital

Large Vestibular Aqueduct Syndrome - The vestibular aqueduct is a bony canal that connects the vestibule (inner ear) with the endolymphatic sac. When this becomes enlarged (> 1.5mm) it is associated with **progressive sensorineural hearing loss**. As a point of trivia, the large vestibular aqueduct syndrome is associated with an **absence of the bony modiolus in more than 90% of patients.** This has an Aunt Minnie appearance. Supposedly this is the result of failure of the endolymphatic sac to resorb endolymph, leading to endolymphatic hydrops and dilation.

Trivia:
- This is the most common cause of congenital sensorineural hearing loss
- The finding is often (usually) bilateral.
- There is an association with cochlear deformity - near 100%

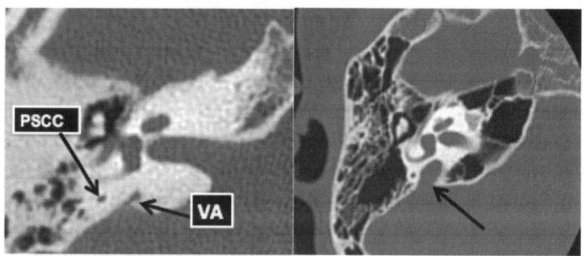

The normal VA is never larger than the adjacent PSCC

Enlarged Vestibular Aqueduct

Infections

Labyrinthitis – This is an inflammation of the membranous labyrinth, most commonly the result of a viral infection. The cochlea and semicircular canals will be shown enhancing on T1 post contrast imaging.

Labyrinthitis Ossificans - This is the sequella of prior infection (typically meningitis). You see it in kids (ages 2-18 months). They will show this on CT – with ossification of the membranous labyrinth. They also get sensorineural hearing loss.

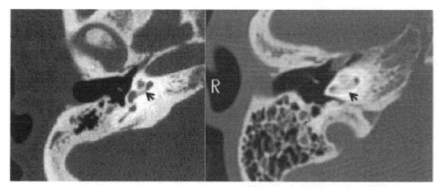

Normal   **Labyrinithitis Ossificans**

Otosclerosis (Fenestral and Retrofenestral): A better term would actually be "oto<u>spong</u>iosus," as the bone becomes more lytic (instead of sclerotic). When I say conductive hearing loss in an adult female, you say this.

- *Fenestral* – This is bony resorption anterior to the oval widow at the fissula ante fenestram. If not addressed, the footplate will fuse to the oval window.

- *Retro-fenestal* – This is a **more severe** form, which has progressed to have **demineralization around the cochlea**. This form usually has a sensorineural component, and is **bilateral and symmetric nearly 100% of the time**.

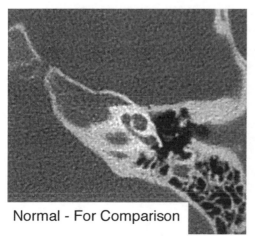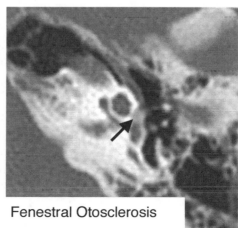

Normal - For Comparison   Fenestral Otosclerosis

Middle Ear

Otitis Media (OM) – This is a common childhood disease with effusion and infection of the middle ear. It's more common in children and patients with Downs Syndrome because of a more horizontal configuration of the Eustacian tube. It's defined as chronic if you have fluid persisting for more than six weeks. The complications are more of an issue (and more amenable to multiple choice questions).

Complications of OM:

- *Coalescent Mastoiditis* –erosion of the mastoid septae with or without intramastoid abscess

- *Facial Nerve Palsy* – Secondary to inflammation of the tympanic segment (more on this below).

- *Dural Sinus Thrombosis* – Adjacent inflammation may cause thrombophlebitis or thrombosis of the sinus. This in itself can lead to complications:

  - *Venous Infarct:* This can occur secondary to dural sinus thrombosis
  - *Otitic Hydrocephalus:* Venous thrombosis can affect resorption of CSF and lead to hypdocephalus.

- *Meningitis, and Labyrinthitis* – can both occur

Cholesteatoma – This is a bunch of exfoliated skin debris growing in the wrong place. It creates a big inflammation ball which wrecks the temporal bone and the ossicles. The idea is basically this, you have two parts to the ear drum, a flimsy whimpy part "Pars Flaccida", and a tougher part "Pars Tensa." The flimsy Flacida is at the top, and the tensa is at the bottom. If you "acquire" a hole with some inflammation / infection involving the pars flaccida you can end up with this ball of epithelial crap growing and causing inflammation in the wrong place.

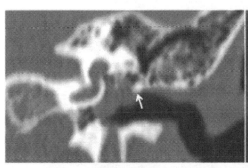 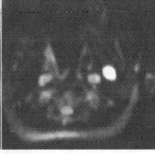

Pars Flaccida – Cholesteatoma
- **Typical location with erosion of scutum (arrow)**
- **They Restrict Diffusion**

Cholesteatoma Order of Destruction predictable (and testable):

(1) The Scutum
(2) The Ossicles (long process of the incus)
(3) The Lateral Segment of the Semi-Circular Canal.

Pars Flaccida Type	*Pars Tensa Type:*
• *Acquired Types are more common – typically involving the pars flaccida. They grow into* **Prussak's Space** • *The* **Scutum is eroded early** *(maybe first)- considered a very specific sign of acquired cholesteatoma* • *The* Malleus head is displaced medially • ***The long process of the incus is the most common segment of the ossicular chain to be eroded.*** • Fistula *to the semi-circular canal most commonly involves the* lateral *segment*	• *The inner ear structures are involved earlier and more often* • *This is less common than the Flaccida Type*

Labyrinthine Fistula: This is a potential complication of cholesteatoma (can also be congenital or iatrogenic), in which there is a bony defect between the inner ear and tympanic cavity. **The lateral semicircular canal is most often involved.**

Anatomy Blitz - Relevant Anatomy for the Cholesteatoma

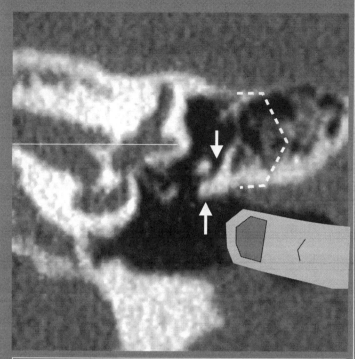

This is a coronal view of the T-Bone. To orient you I drew I cartoon finger in the ear. That finger is running right up to the ear drum (tympanic membrane). The membrane is usually too thin to see, but it's right around there. Remember the flimsy Flacida is at the top and the thicker Tensa is at the bottom.

There are two white arrows here.

The top arrow is pointing to a space between an ossicle (incus) and the lateral temporal bone. This is called "Prussak's space" and is the most common location of a pars flacida Cholesteatoma. Remember the incus was the most common ossicle eroded.

The bottom arrow is pointing to a bony shield shaped bone - "the scutum" which will be the first bone eroded by a pas flaccid

The white dotted bracket is showing where the **"attic"** is. This is also called the "epitympanum" by anatomists.

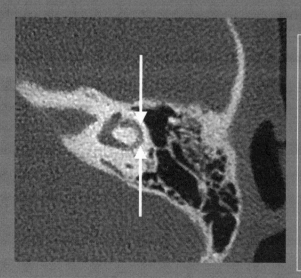

This is an axial through the level of that horizontal line on the coronal image above. The cut is right through the epitympanum.

There are two arrows, both of which are pointing to the horizontal/lateral **portion of the semi-circular canal (SCC)**. This is important because if the cholesteatoma eats the SCC - this is the part it will eat / fistula into.

Superior Semicircular Canal Dehiscence: This is an Aunt Minnie. It's supposedly from long standing ICP although the most likely way this will be asked is either (1) what is it? with a picture or (2) **"Noise Induced Vertigo"** or "Tulio's Phenomenon." You are probably wondering who "Tulio" was.

Pietro Tullio was some mad scientist who drilled holes in the semicircular canals of pigeons then observed that they became off balance when he exposed them to sound. He also created a "pigeon rat" like Hugo Simpson did in the 1996 Simpsons Halloween Special (this is not confirmed).

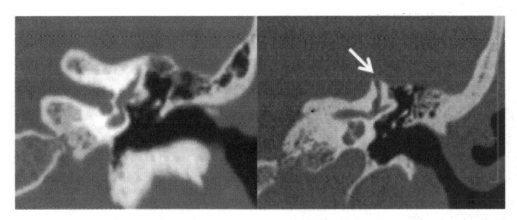

Normal Anatomy   Superior Semicircular Canal Dehiscence

External Ear

Necrotizing External Otitis: This is a raging terrible infection of the external auditory canal. You are going to see swollen EAC soft tissues, probably with a bunch of small abscesses, and adjacent bony destruction . They always (95%) have diabetes and the causative agent is always (98%) Pseudomonas.

The Facial Nerve

There are only 2 or 3 things that are likely to be tested regarding the facial nerve.

(1) *Which parts normally enhance?* - It's easier to remember what does NOT. The cisternal, canalicular, and labyrinthine segments should NOT enhance. The remainder of the nerve - the intratemporal course - can enhance (tympanic, mastoid). Normal enhancement is due to the perineural venous plexus.

(2) *What causes abnormal enhancement?* The big one is Bell's Palsy. Lymes, Ramsay Hunt, and Cancer can do it too.

(3) *When do you damage the facial nerve?* Usually the transverse T-Bone fracture (more than the longitudinal).

Skull Base

Pagets – This is discussed in great depth in the MSK chapter. Having said that, I want to remind you of the Paget skull changes. You can have osteolysis as a well-defined large radiolucent region favoring the frontal and occipital bones. The inner table is affected more than the outer table. The buzzword is **osteolysis circumscripta**.

Paget's Skull related complications:
- Deafness is the most common complication
- Cranial Nerve Paresis
- Basilar Invagination -> Hydrocephalus -> Brainstem Compression
- Secondary (high grade) osteosarcoma.

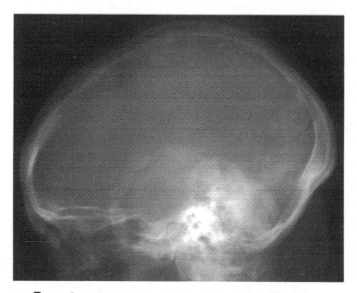

Pagets - Osteolysis Circumscripta (lytic phase)

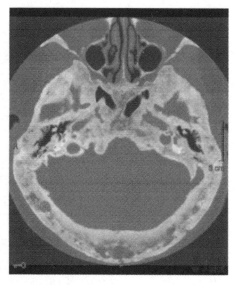

Thickened Expanded Skull (Sclerotic Phase)

Chordoma (midline) and *Chondrosarcoma (off midline) - discussed on page 58.*

Fibrous Dysplasia - The ground glass lesion. If you are getting ready to call it's Pagets stop and look at the age. Paget is typically an older person (8% at 80), where as fibrous dysplasia is usually in someone less than 30.

Trivia:
- Classically fibrous dysplasia of the skull spares the otic capsule
- McCune Albright Syndrome - Multi-focal fibrous dysplasia, cafe-au-lait spots, and precocious puberty.

Sinuses

Juvenile Nasal Angiofibroma (JNA) – Often you can get this one right just from the history. **Male teenager with nose bleeds** (obstruction is actually a more common symptom).

Antrochoanal Polyp – Also seen in young adults (30s-40s), this time with nasal congestion / obstruction symptoms. This one arises within the maxillary sinuses, and passes through and enlarges the sinus ostium (or accessory ostium). Buzzword is "**widening of the maxillary ostium.**" Classically, there is no associated bony destruction but instead smooth enlargement of the sinus. The polyp will extend into the nasopharynx. This thing is basically a monster inflammatory polyp with a thin stalk arising from the maxillary sinus.

JNA Trivia to know:
- Mass is centered on the sphenoplatine foramen
- Expansion of the Pterygopalatine Fossa
- It's very vascular – and they may show an angiogram with a blush (during embolization therapy).
- Its primary vascular supply is from the ascending pharyngeal artery and/or internal maxillary artery

Inverting Papilloma: This uncommon tumor has distinctive imaging features (which therefore make it testable). The **classic location is the lateral wall of the nasal cavity – most frequently related to the middle turbinate.** Impaired maxillary drainage is expected. **A focal hyperostosis tends to occur at the tumor origin. The MRI buzzword is "cerebriform pattern"** – which sorta looks like brain on T1 and T2. **Another high yield pearl is that 10% harbor a squamous cell CA.**

Esthesioneuroblastoma - This is a neuroblastoma of olfactory cells so it's gonna start at the cribiform plate. It classically has a dumbbell appearance with growth up into the skull and growth down into the sinuses, with a waist at the plate. There are often cysts in the mass. There is a bi-modal age distribution.

Things to know:
- *Dumbbell shape with wasting at the cribiform plate is classic*
- *Intracranial posterior cyst is a "diagnostic" look*
- *Octreotide scan will be positive – since it is of neural crest origin*

Squamous Cell / SNUC: Squamous cell is the **most common head and neck cancer.** The maxillary antrum is the most common location. It's highly cellular, and therefore low on T2. Relative to other sinus masses it enhances less. *SNUC (the undifferentiated squamer),* is the monster steroided up version of a regular squamous cell. They are massive and seen more in the ethmoids.

summary chart on sinus tumors in the strategy chapter (page 362)

Epistaxis - This is usually idiopathic, although it can be iatrogenic (picking it too much - or not enough). They could get sneaky and work this into a case of HHT. The most common location is the anterior septal area (Kiesselbach plexus), but because these are anterior they tend to be easy to compress manually. The posterior ones are less common (5%) but tend to be the ones that "bleed like stink" (need angio). Most cases are given a trial of nasal packing. When that fails the N-IR team is activated. *The main supply to the posterior nose is the sphenopalatine artery (terminal internal maxillary artery) and tends to be the first line target.* Watch out for the variant anastomosis between the ECA and ophthalmic artery (you don't want to embolize the eye).

The Mouth

Floor of Mouth Dermoid / Epidermoid - There isn't a lot of trivia about these other than the buzzword and what they classically look like. The **buzzword is "sack of marbles"** - fluid sack with globules of fat. They are typically **midline**.

Ranula - This is a mucous retention cyst. They are typically **lateral**. There are two testable pieces of trivia to know: (1) **they arise from the sublingual gland / space**, and (2) use the word **"plunging" once it's under the mylohyoid muscle.**

Torus Palatinus- This is a normal variant that looks scary. Because it looks scary some multiple choice writer may try and trick you into calling it cancer. **It's just a bony exostosis** that comes off the hard palate in the midline. Classic history "Grandma's dentures won't stay in."

Sialolithiasis - Stones in the salivary ducts. The testable trivia includes: (1) **Most commonly in the submandibular gland duct (wharton's)**, (2) can lead to an infected gland "sialoadenitis", and (3) chronic obstruction can lead to gland fatty atrophy.

Odontogenic Infection – These can be dental or periodontal in origin. If I were writing a question about this topic I would ask three things. The first would be that **infection is more common from an extracted tooth** than an abscess involving an intact tooth.

The second would be that the **attachment of the mylohyoid muscle to the mylohyoid ridge dictates the spread of infection to the sublingual and submandibular spaces**. Above the mylohyoid line (anterior mandibular teeth) goes to the sublingual space, and below the mylohyoid line (second and third molars) goes to the submandibular space.

The third thing I would ask would be that an **odontogenic abscess is the most common masticator space "mass" in an adult.**

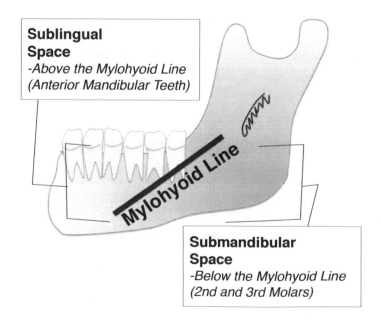

Sublingual Space
-*Above the Mylohyoid Line (Anterior Mandibular Teeth)*

Submandibular Space
-*Below the Mylohyoid Line (2nd and 3rd Molars)*

Ludwig's Angina - This is a super aggressive cellulitis in the floor of the mouth. If they show it, there will be gas everywhere. Trivia: most cases start with an odontogenic infection.

Osteonecrosis of the Mandible- The trivia is most likely gonna be etiology. Just remember it is related to prior radiation, licking a radium paint brush, or **bisphosphonate treatment**

Cancer - Squamous cell is going to be the most common cancer of the mouth (and head and neck). In an older person think drinker and smoker. In a younger person think **HPV**. HPV related SCCs tend to be present with large necrotic level 2a nodes (don't call it a brachial cleft cyst!). *Classic scenario = young adult with new level II neck mass = HPV related SCC.*

Thyroglossal Duct Cyst – This can occur anywhere between the foramen cecum (the base of the tongue) and the thyroid gland. They are usually found in the midline at or above the hyoid. It looks like a thin walled cyst. Further discussion in the endocrine chapter.

Classic Mouth Pictures:

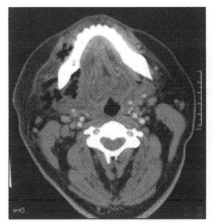
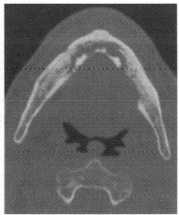
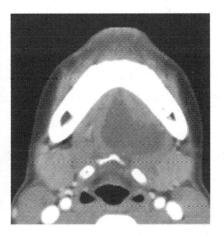

Ludwig's Angina   Osteonecrosis of Jaw   Ranula

Suprahyoid Soft Tissue Neck

The suprahyoid neck is usually taught by using a "spaces" method. This is actually the best way to learn it. What space is it? What is in that space? What pathology can occur as the result of what normal structures are there. Example: lymph nodes are there – thus you can get lymphoma or a met.

Parotid Space:

The parotid space is basically the parotid gland, and portions of the facial nerve. You can't see the facial nerve, but you can see the retromandibular vein (which runs just medial to the facial nerve). Another thing to know is that the parotid is the only salivary gland to have lymph nodes, so pathology involving the gland itself, and anything lymphatic related is fair game.

Parotid Space Contains:
- The Parotid Gland
- Cranial Nerve 7 (Facial)
- Retro-mandibular Vein

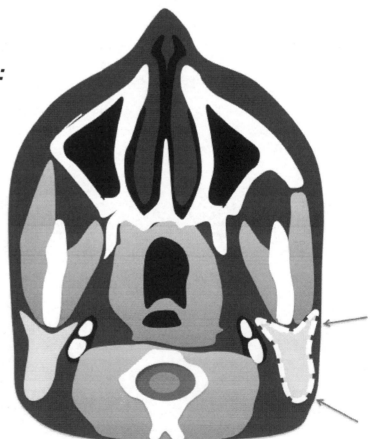

Pathology:

Pleomorphic Adenoma (benign mixed tumor) - This is the most common major *(and minor)* salivary gland tumor. It occurs most commonly in the parotid, but can occur in the submandibular, or sublingual glands. 90% of these tumors occur in the superficial lobe. They are commonly T2 bright, with a rim of low signal. **They have a small malignant potential** and are treated surgically.

- *Superficial vs Deep:* Involvement of the superficial (lateral to the facial nerve) or deep (medial to the facial nerve) lobe is critical to the surgical approach. A line is drawn connecting the lateral surface of the posterior belly of the digastric muscle and the lateral surface of the mandibular ascending ramus to separate superficial from deep.
- Apparently, if you resect these like a clown you can spill them, and they will have a massive ugly recurrence.

Warthins: This is the second most common benign tumor. This one ONLY occurs in the parotid gland. This one is **usually cystic, in a male, bilateral (15%), and in a smoker**. As a point of total trivia, this tumor takes up pertechnetate (it's basically the only tumor in the parotid to do it, *ignoring the ultra rare parotid oncocytoma*).

Mucoepidermoid Carcinoma – This is the most common malignant tumor of minor salivary glands. The general rule is – the smaller the gland the more common the malignant tumors, the bigger the gland the more common the benign tumors. There is a variable appearance based on the histologic grade. There is an association with radiation.

Adenoid Cystic Carcinoma – This is another malignant salivary gland tumor, which favors minor glands but can be seen in the parotid. The number one thing to know is perineural spread. This tumor likes perineural spread. **When I say adenoid cystic you say perineural spread**.

Pearl: I used to think that perineurial tumor spread would widen a neural foramen (foramen ovale for example). It's still might... but it's been my experience that a nerve sheath tumor (schwannoma) is much more likely to do that. Let's just say for the purpose of multiple choice that neural foramina widening is a schwannoma - unless there is overwhelming evidence to the contrary.

Lymphoma – Because the parotid has lymph nodes (it's the only salivary gland that does), you can get lymphoma in the parotid (primary or secondary). If you see it and it's bilateral, you should think Sjogrens. Sjogrens patients have a big risk (like 1000x) of parotid lymphoma. Like lymphoma is elsewhere in the body, the appearance is variable. You might see bilateral homogeneous masses. For the purposes of the exam, **just knowing you can get it in the parotid (primary or secondary) and the relationship with Sjogrens is probably all you need.**

Other Parotid Trivia:

- **Acute Parotitis:** Obstruction of flow of secretions is the most common cause. They will likely show you a stone (or stones) in Stensen's duct, which will be dilated. The stones are calcium phosphate. Post infectious parotitis is usually bacterial. Mumps would be the most common viral cause. As a point of trivia, sialography is contraindicated in the acute setting.

- **Benign Lymphoepithelial Disease:** You have bilateral mixed solid and cystic lesions with diffusely enlarged parotid glands. This is seen in HIV. The condition is painless (unlike parotitis – which can enlarge the glands).

- **Sjogrens** – Autoimmune lymphocyte induced destruction of the gland. "Dry eyes and Dry Mouth." Typically seen in women in their 60s. **Increased risk** (like 1000x) risk of non-Hodgkins MALT type **lymphoma.** There is a **honeycombed appearance of the gland**.

Carotid Space:

Carotid Space Contains:
- Carotid artery,
- Jugular vein,
- Portions of CN 9, CN 10, CN 11,
- Internal jugular chain lymph nodes

There are 3 Classic Carotid Space Tumors:
(1) Paraganglioma
(2) Schwannoma
(3) Neurofibroma

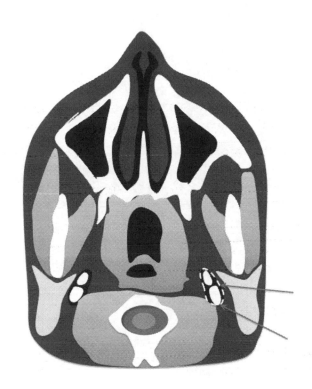

Paragangliomas: There are three different ones worth knowing about – based on location. The imaging features are the same. They are **hypervascular (intense tumor blush)**, with a "**Salt and Pepper" appearance on MRI** from all the heterogeneous stuff and **flow voids**. They can be multiple and bilateral in familial conditions. **[111]In- octreotide accumulates in these tumors** (receptors for somatostatin).

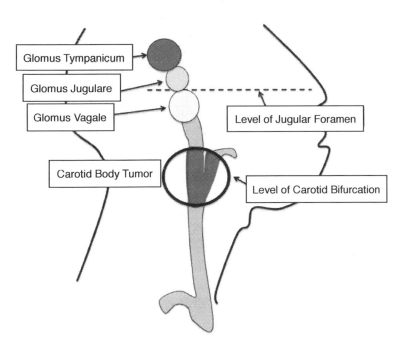

Carotid Body Tumor =Carotid Bifurcation (*Splaying ICA and ECA*)

Glomus Jugulare = Skull Base (*often with destruction of jugular foramen*)

Middle Ear Floor Destroyed = Glomus Jugulare.

Glomus Vagale = Above Carotid Bifurcation, but below the Jugular Foramen

Glomus Tympanicum = Confined to the middle ear. Buzzword is *"overlying the cochlear promontory."*

Middle Ear Floor Intact = Glomus Tympanum

Schwannoma – Can involve the 9, 10, 11, and even 12th CN.

Schwannoma	Paraganglioma
Not all that vascular on Angio	Hypervascular (tumor blush on angio)
No Salt and Pepper	Salt and Pepper Look on MRI
NOT [111]In- octreotide avid	[111]In- octreotide avid
No Flow Voids (target sign)	Flow Voids

Lemierre syndrome – This is a thrombophlebitis of the jugular veins with distant metastatic sepsis (usually septic emboli in the lung). It's found in the setting of oropharyngeal infection (pharyngitis, tonsillitis, peri tonsillar abscess), or recent ENT surgery.

Lymph Nodes = Metastatic lesions from squamous cell cancer frequently involve this area.

—

Masticator Space:

As the name implies this space contains the **muscles of mastication** (masticator, temporalis, medial and lateral pterygoids).

Additionally, you have the angle and **ramus of the mandible**, plus the **inferior aveolar nerve**.

A trick to be aware of is that the space extends superiorly along the side of the skull via the temporalis muscle. So, aggressive neoplasm or infection may ride right up there.

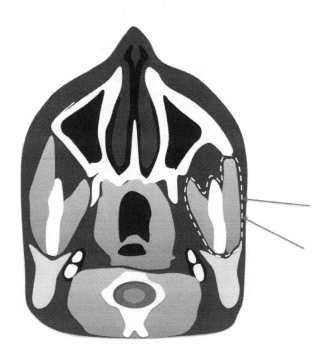

Odontogenic Infection – In an adult this is the most common cause of a masticator space mass. If you see a mass here, the next move should be to look at the mandible on bone windows. Just in general, you should be on the look out for spread via the pterygopalatine fossa to orbital apex and cavernous sinus. The relationship with the mylohyoid makes for good trivia - as discussed above.

Sarcomas – In kids, you can run into nasty angry masses like Rhabdomyosarcomas. You can also get sarcomas from the bone of the mandible (chondrosacroma favors the TMJ).

Cavernous Hemangiomas – These can also occur, and are given away by the presence of pleboliths. Venous or lymphatic malformations may involve multiple compartments / spaces.

Congenital stuff and Aggressive Infection/Cancer tends to be trans-spatial.

Perineural Spread – You can have perineural spread from a head and neck primary along the 5th CN.

When I say "perineural spread" you should think two things:
(1) adenoid cystic minor salivary tumor and
(2) melanoma.

Nerve Sheath Tumors – Since you have a nerve, you can have a schwannoma or neurofibroma of V3. Remember the schwannoma is more likely to cause the foramina expansion vs perineurial tumor spread.

—

Retropharyngeal Space / Danger Space

Behind the middle layer of deep cervical fascia but anterior to the alar fascia, lives this midline space.

Danger Space - The so called "danger space" , is actually just posterior to the "true" retropharyngeal space - behind the alar layer of fascia. It's a potential space - that you can't see unless it's distended. Certain Anatomists like to make the distinction that this space is separate from the "true retropharyngeal space," others lump them together. If forced to choose - simply read the mind of the question writer to decide which camp he/she falls into. I would pick them as separate entities because people who do academics / write questions tend to enjoy making things overly complicated.

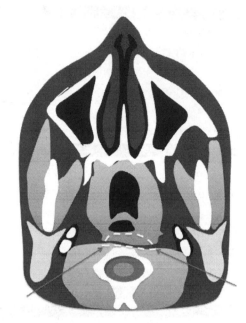

So what's the danger in infection in the danger space?? It tracts down into the mediastinum… so you can dump pus (or cancer) right into the mediastinum (that's bad).

Infection – Involvement of the retropharyngeal space most often occurs from spread from the tonsillar tissue. You are going to have enhancing soft tissue and stranding in the space. You should evaluate for spread of infection into the mediastinum.

Necrotic Nodes - Squamous cell mets or suppurative infection to the lateral retropharyngeal nodes of Rouviere. Papillary thyroid cancer can also met here. Lymphoma can involve these nodes, but won't be necrotic until treated.

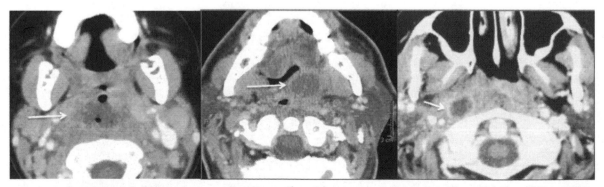

Retropharyngeal Abscess   **Peritonsilar Abscess**   **Suppurative Node of Rouviere**

Parapharyngeal Space

The parapharyngeal space is primarily a ball of fat with a few branches of the trigeminal nerves, and the pterygoid veins. The primary utility of the space is when it is displaced (discussed below). Mets and infections can directly spread into this space (squamous cell cancer from tonsils, tongue, and larynx). Cancer and infection can spread rapidly in a vertical direction through this fat.

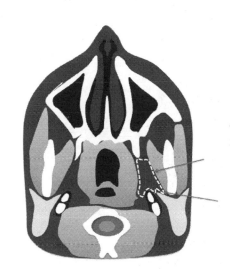

The parapharyngeal space is bordered on four sides by different spaces. If you have a mass dead in the middle, it can be challenging to tell where it's coming from. Using the displacement of fat, you can help problem solve. Much more important than that, this lends itself very well to multiple choice.

Parotid Mass Pushes Medially (PMPM)

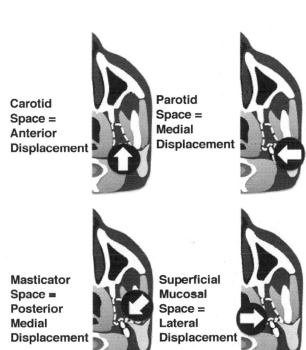

Carotid Space = Anterior Displacement

Parotid Space = Medial Displacement

Masticator Space = Posterior Medial Displacement

Superficial Mucosal Space = Lateral Displacement

Squamous Cell Cancer

When you are talking about head and neck cancer, you are talking about squamous cell cancer. Now, this is a big complex topic and requires a fellowship to truly understand / get good at. Obviously, the purpose of this book is to prepare you for multiple choice test questions not teach you practical radiology. If you want to actually learn about head and neck cancer for a practical sense you can try and find a copy of Harnsberger's legendary handbook (which has been out of print for 20 years). A more modern alternative is probably Raghavan's Manual of Head and Neck Imaging. Now, for the trivia....

Lymph node anatomy:

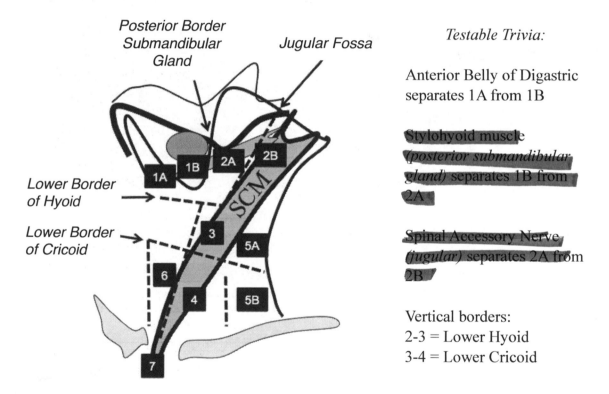

Testable Trivia:

Anterior Belly of Digastric separates 1A from 1B

Stylohyoid muscle (posterior submandibular gland) separates 1B from 2A

Spinal Accessory Nerve (jugular) separates 2A from 2B

Vertical borders:
2-3 = Lower Hyoid
3-4 = Lower Cricoid

Floor of the Mouth SCC: I touched on this once already. Just remember smoker/drinker in an old person. HPV in a young person. Necrotic level 2 nodes can be a presentation (not a brachial cleft cyst).

Nasopharyngeal SCC: This is more common in Asians and has a bi-modal distribution: group 1 (15-30) typically Chinese, and group 2 (> 40). Involvement of the parapharyngeal space results in worse prognosis (compared to nasal cavity or oropharynx invasion). The most common location is the Fossa of Rosenmuller (FOR). If you see (1) a unilateral mastoid effusion, or (2) a pathologic retropharyngeal node look in the FOR. *The "earliest sign" of nasopharyngeal SCC is the effacement of the fat within the FOR.* If you see a supraclavicular node then you should look closely at the bones for mets (especially the clivus).

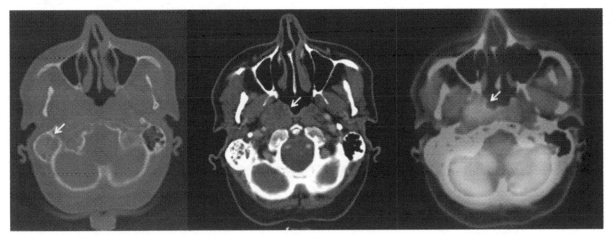

| Unilateral Mastoid Effusion | Fossa of Rosenmuller Mass | PET Avid |

Laryngeal SCC: The role of the Radiologist is not to make the primary cancer diagnosis here, but to assist in staging. Laryngeal cancers are subdivided into (a) supraglottic, (b) glottic, and (c) infraglottic types. "Transglottic" would refer to an aggressive cancer that crosses the laryngeal ventricle.

Things to know about laryngeal SCC:
- Glottic SCC has the best outcome (least lymphatics), and is the most common (60%)
- Subglottic is the least common (5%), and can be clinically silent till you get nodes
- Subglottic tumors are often small compared to nodal burden
- Fixation of the cords indicates at least a T3 tumor
- The only reliable sign of cricoid invasion is tumor on both sides of the cartilage (irregular sclerotic cartilage can be normal).
- Invasion of the cricoid cartilage is a contraindication to all types of laryngeal conservation surgery (cricoid cartilage is necessary for postoperative stability of the vocal cords).
- Paraglottic space involvement makes the tumor T3 and "transglottic." This is best seen in coronals.

Infrahyoid Soft Tissue Neck

Laryngocele: When the laryngeal saccule dilates with fluid or air you call it a laryngocele.

Why does it dilate ? Usually because its obstructed, and the testable point is that 15% of the time that obstruction is a tumor.

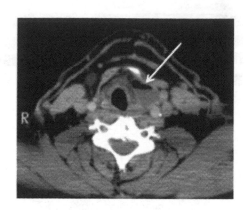

Laryngocele

Vocal Cord Paralysis: The **affected side will have an expanded ventricle** (it's the opposite side with a cancer). If you see it on the left, a good "next step" question would be to look at the chest (for recurrent laryngeal nerve involvement at the AP window).

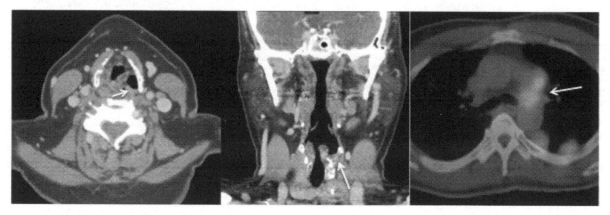

Vocal Cord Paralysis – Ipsilateral Expanded Ventricle   **AP Window PET Avid Node**

Orbit

Congenital

Coloboma: This is a focal discontinuity of the globe (failure of the choroid fissure to close). They are usually posterior. If you see a unilateral one - think sporadic. **If you see bilateral ones - think CHARGE (coloboma, heart, GU, ears).**

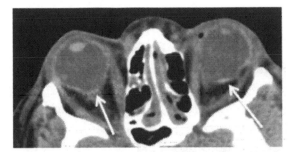

Bilateral Coloboma – CHARGE Syndrome

Persistent Hyperplastic Primary Vitreous (PHPV) - This is a failure of the embryonic ocular blood supply to regress. It can lead to retinal detachment. The classic look is a small eye (microphthalmia) with increased density of the vitreous. No calcification.

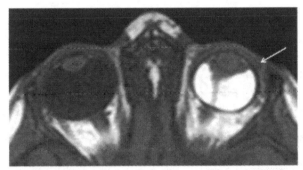

Retinal Detachment in the setting of PHPV

Coat's Disease - The cause of this is a retinal telangiectasis, that results in leaky blood and subretinal exudate. It can lead to retinal detachment. It's seen in young boys and typically unilateral. The key detail is that it is NOT CALCIFIED (retinoblastoma is).

Coats disease has a smaller globe. Retinoblastoma has a normal sized globe.

Retinal Detachment - This can occur secondary to PHPV or Coats. It can also be caused by trauma, sickle cell, or just old age. The imaging finding is a "V" or "Y" shaped appearance due to lifted up retinal leaves and subretinal fluid (as seen in the PHPV case above).

Globe Size - A Source of Possible Trivia

- *Retinoblastoma* - Normal Size
- *Toxocariasis* - Normal Size

- *PHPV* - Small Size *(Normal Birth Age)*
- *Retinopathy of Prematurity* - Bilateral Small
- Coats - Smaller Size

Orbital Tumors:

Optic Nerve Glioma: These almost always (90%) occur under the age of 20. You see expansion / enlargement of the entire nerve. If they are bilateral you think about **NF-1**. They are most often WHO grade 1 *Pilocystic Astrocytomas*. If they are sporadic they can be GBMs and absolutely destroy you.

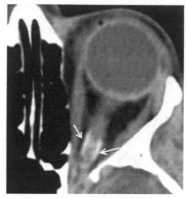

"Tram-Track" = Meningioma

Optic Nerve Sheath Meningioma: The buzzword is *"tram-track" calcifications*. Another buzzword is "doughnut" appearance, with **circumferential enhancement around the optic nerve**.

IgG4 - Orbit

Orbital Pseudotumor: This is one of those IgG4 idiopathic inflammatory conditions that involves the extraoccular muscles. It looks like an expanded muscle. The things to remember are that this thing is painful, unilateral, it **most commonly involves the lateral rectus** and it **does NOT spare the myotendinous insertions**. Remember that Graves does not cause pain, and does spare the myotendinous insertions. It gets better with steroids. It's classically T2 dark.

Tolosa Hunt Syndrome: This is histologically the same thing as orbital pseudotumor but instead involves the cavernous sinus. It is painful (just like pseudotumor), and presents with multiple cranial nerve palsies. It responds to steroids (just like pseudotumor).

Lymphocytic Hypophysitis: This is the same deal as orbital pseudotumor and tolosa hunt, except it's the pituitary gland. Just think enlarged pituitary stalk, in a post partum / 3rd trimester woman. It looks like a pituitary adenoma, but it classically has a T2 dark rim.

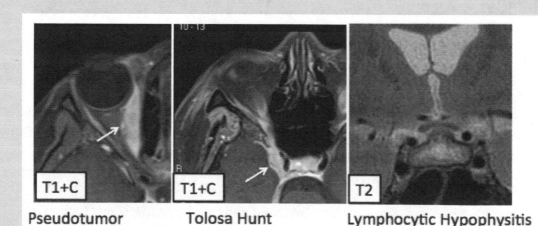

Pseudotumor
-*Involves Cavernous Sinus*

Tolosa Hunt
-*Involves Cavernous Sinus*

Lymphocytic Hypophysitis
-*Dark T2 Signal Around Gland*

Dermoid: This is the most common benign congenital orbital mass. It's usually **superior and lateral,** arising from the frontozygomatic suture, and presenting in the first 10 years of life. It's gonna have fat in it (like any good dermoid). The location is classic.

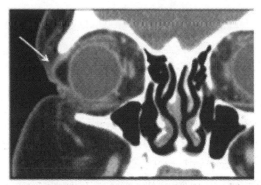

Orbital Dermoid – *Classic Location*

Rhabdomyosarcoma - *Most common extra-occular orbital malignancy in children* (dermoid is most common benign orbital mass in child). When they do occur - 40% of the time it's in the head and neck - and then most commonly it's in the orbit. It's still rare as hell.

Metastatic Neuroblastoma - This has a very classic appearance of **"Raccoon Eyes"** on physical exam. The *classic location is periorbital tumor infiltration with associated proptosis.* Don't forget a basilar skull fracture can also cause Raccoon Eyes... so clinical correlation is advised.

Metastatic Breast Cancer - This is classic gamesmanship here. The important point to know is that unlike primary orbital tumors that are going to cause proptosis, classically the **breast cancer met causes a desmoplastic reaction and enophthalmos.**

Lymphoma - There is an association with **Chlamydia Psittaci** (the bird fever thing) and **MALT lymphoma of the orbit.** It usually involves the **upper outer orbit** - closely associated with the **lacrimal gland.** It will enhance homogeneously and restricts diffusion - just like in the brain.

Globe Tumors:

Melanoma - This is the **most common intra-occular lesion in an adult.** If you see an enhancing soft tissue mass in the **back of an adult's eye** this is the answer. I can only think of three ways you could ask about this: (1) show a picture - what is it?, (2) ask what the most common intra-occular lesion in an adult is, or (3) ask the buzzword *"collar button shaped"* - which is **related to Bruch's membrane.**

Retinoblastoma - This is the **most common primary malignancy of the globe.** The step 1 question is **RB suppressor gene (chromosome 13).** That's the same chromosome osteosarcoma patients have issues with and why these guys are at **increased risk of facial osteosarcoma after radiation.** **If you see calcification in the globe of a child - this is the answer.** The globe should be normal in size (or bigger), where coats is usually smaller. It's **usually seen before age 3** (rare after age 6). The trivia is gonna be where else it occurs. They can be **bilateral** (both eyes - 30%), *trilateral* (both eyes, and the pineal gland), and *quadrilateral* (both eyes, pineal, and suprasellar).

Orbital Vascular Malformations:

Lymphangioma - These are actually a mix of venous and lymphatic malformations. They are ill-defined and lack a capsule. The usual distribution is infiltrative (multi-spatial) involving, pre septal, post septal, extraconal, and intraconal locations. Fluid-Fluid levels are the money shot, and the most likely finding to be shown by someone writing a multiple choice test question. They do NOT increase with valsalva.

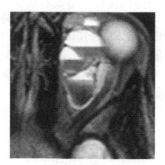

**Lymphangioma
– *Fluid Fluid Levels***

Varix - These occur secondary to weakness in the post capillary venous wall (gives you massive dilation of the valveless orbital veins). Most likely question is going to pertain to the fact that **they distend with provocative maneuvers** (valsalva, hanging head, etc...). Another piece of trivia is that they are the *most common cause of spontaneous orbital hemorrhage.* They can thrombose and present with pain.

Carotid-Cavernous Fistula: These come in two flavors: (1) Direct - which is secondary to trauma, and (2) Indirect - which just occurs randomly in post menopausal women. The direct kind is a communication between the intracavernous ICA and cavernous sinus. The indirect kind is usually a dural shunt between meningeal branches of the ECA and Cavernous Sinus.

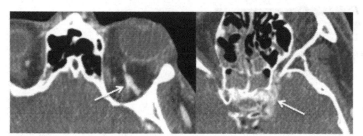

Carotid-cavernous Fistula – *Prominent left superior ophthalmic vein, prominent left cavernous sinus with proptosis.*

> **Pulsatile Exophthalmos**
> *The Buzzword*
>
> C-C Fistula is probably the most common cause.
>
> NF-1 can also cause it, from *sphenoid wing dysplasia.*

Orbital Infection:

Pre-Septal/ Post Septal Cellulitis - The location of orbital infections are described by their relationship to the orbital septum. The testable trivia is probably (1) that the orbital septum originates from the periosteum of the orbit and inserts in the palpebral tissue along the tarsal plate, (2) that pre-septal infections usually start in adjacent structures likely teeth and the face , and that (3) post-septal infections are usually from paranasal sinusitis.

Dacryocystitis - This is inflammation and dilation of the lacrimal sac. It has an Aunt Minnie look, with a well circumscribed round rim enhancing lesion centered in the lacrimal fossa. The etiology is typically obstruction then bacterial infection (staph and strep).

Orbital Subperiosteal Abscess: If you get inflammation under the periosteum it can progress to abscess formation. This is usually associated with ethmoid sinusitis. This also has a very classic look.

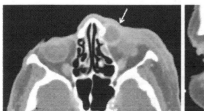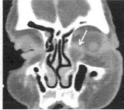

Dacroyocyctitis

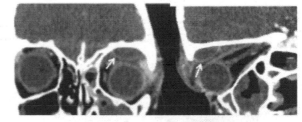

Orbital Subperiosteal Abscess

Misc:

Optic Neuritis: There will be **enhancement of the optic nerve**, *without enlargement* of the nerve/sheath complex. Usually (70%) unilateral, and painful. You will often see intracranial or spinal cord demyelination – in the setting of Devics (neuromyelitis optica). 50% of patient's with acute optic neuritis will develop MS.

Papilledema: This is really an eye exam thing. Having said that you can sometimes see dilation of the optic nerve sheath.

Thyroid Orbitopathy: This is seen in 1/4 of the Graves cases and is the most common cause of exophthalmos. The antibodies that activate TSH receptors also activate orbital fibroblasts and adipocytes.

Things to know:
- Risk of compressive optic neuropathy
- Enlargement of ONLY MUSCLE BELLY (spares tendon) - different than *pseudo tumor*
- NOT Painful - different than *pseudo tumor*
- Order of Involvement: IR > MR > SR > LR > SO "I'M SLOw"

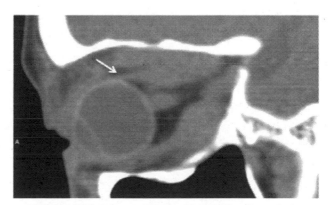

Thyroid Orbit – *Spares Tendon Insertion*

SECTION 3: SPINE

Anatomy Trivia

Cord Blood Supply: There is an anterior blood supply and a posterior blood supply to the cord. These guys get taken out with different clinical syndromes.

- *Anterior spinal artery* - arises bilaterally as two small branches at the level of the termination of the vertebral arteries. These two arteries join around the level of the foramen magnum.

- *Artery of Adamkiewicz* – This is the most notable reinforcer of the anterior spinal artery. In 75% of people is comes off the left side of the aorta between T8 and T1. It supplies the lower 2/3 of the cord. This thing can get covered with the placement of an endovascular stent graft for aneurysm or dissection repair leading to spine infarct.

- *Posterior Spinal Artery* – arises from either the vertebral arteries or the posterior inferior cerebellar artery. Unlike the anterior spinal artery this one is somewhat discontinuous and reinforced by multiple segmental or radiculopial branches.

Conus Medullaris: This is the terminal end of the spinal cord. It usually terminates at around L1. Below the inferior endplate of the L2 / L3 body should make you think tethered cord (especially if shown in a multiple choice setting).

Which nerve is compressed?

There are 31 pairs of spinal nerves, with each pair corresponding to the adjacent vertebra – the notable exception being the "C8" nerve. Cervical disc herniations are less common than lumbar ones.

The question is most likely to take place in the lumbar spine (the same spot most disc herniations occur). In fact more than 90% of herniations occur at L4-L5, and L5-S1.

A tale of two herniations. It was the best of times, it was the worst of times…

Scenario 1:

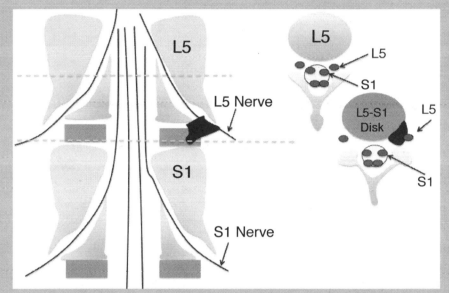

A Foraminal Disc Will Smash the Exiting Nerve.

In this case the L5 Nerve

Scenario 2:

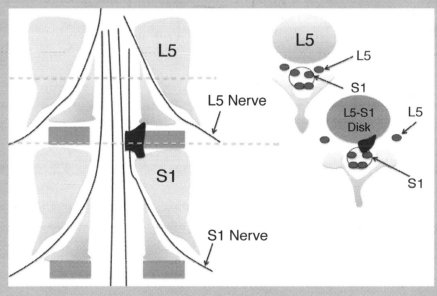

A Central or Paracentral Disc Will Smash the Descending Nerve.

In this case the S1 Nerve

Epidural Fat: The epidural fat is not evenly distributed. The epidural space in the cervical cord is predominantly filled with venous plexus (as apposed to fat). In the lumbar spine there is fat both anterior and posterior to the cord.

Degenerative Changes

Stenosis: Spinal stenosis can be congenital (associated with short pedicles) or be acquired. The Torg-Pavlov ratio can be used to call it (vertebral body width to cervical canal diameter < 0.85). Symptomatic stenosis is more common in the cervical spine (versus the thoracic spine or lumbar spine). You can get some congenital stenosis in the lumbar spine from short pedicles, but it's generally not symptomatic until middle age.

Disc Nomenclature: In order to "improve accuracy" with regard to the lumbar spine various administrative regulatory bodies have decided on the vocabulary you are allowed to use.

- *"Focal Herniation"* is a herniated disc less comprising than 90 degrees of the disc circumference.
- *"Broadbased Herniation"* is a herniated disc in between 90-180 degrees.
- *"Protrusion"* – is a term used when the distance between the edge of the disc herniation is less than the distance between the edges of the base.
- *"Extrusion"* is a term used when the edges of the disc are greater than the distance of the base.

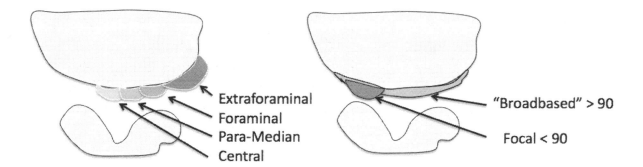

Schmorl Node: This is a herniation of disc material through a defect in the vertebral body endplate into the actual marrow.

Scheuermann's – This is multiple levels (at least 3) of Schmorl's nodes in the spine of a teenager, resulting in kyphotic deformity (40 degrees in thoracic or 30 degrees in thoracolumbar).

Limbus Vertebra – This is a fracture mimic, that is the result of herniated disc material between the non-fused apophysis and adjacent vertebral body.

Endplate Changes: Commonly referred to as "Modic Changes." There is a progression in the MRI signal characteristics that makes sense if you think about it. You start out with degenerative changes causing irritation / inflammation so there is edema (T2 bright). This progresses to chronic inflammation with leads to some fatty change – just like in the bowel of an IBD patient – causing T1 bright signal. Finally, the whole thing gets burned out and fibrotic and it's T1 and T2 dark. As a prominent factoid, Type 1 changes look a lot like Osteomyelitis (clinical correlation in recommended).

Modic – Endplate Marrow Changes Associated with Degenerative Disease	
Type 1 "Edema"	T1 Dark, T2 Bright
Type 2 "Fat"	T1 Bright, T2 Bright
Type 3 "Scar"	T 1 Dark, T2 Dark

Annular Tears: You can have tears in your dorsal annulus. They are usually bright on T2 and have a curvilinear look. They are so bright that some people call them "high intensity zones." They may be a source of pain (radial pain fibers - trigger "discogenic pain") but are also seen as incidentals.

Myelogram Technique

Big point: Contrast should flow freely away from the needle tip gradually filling the thecal sac. The outlining of the the cauda equine is another promising sign that you did it right. If contrast pools at the needle tip or along the posterior or lateral thecal sac without free-flow, a subdural injection or injection in the fat around the thecal sac should be suspected.

Prior to the LP *(per ACR-ASNR recommendations)*
- STOP Coumadin 4-5 days
- STOP Plavix for 7 days
- Hold LMW Heparin for 12 hours
- Hold Heparin for 2-4 hours - document normal PTT
- Aspirin and NSAIDs are fine (not contraindicated)

Post Operative Back Trivia:

"Failed Back Surgery Syndrome" –Another entity invented by NEJM to take down the surgical subspecialties. Per the NEJM these greedy surgeons generally go from a non-indicated spine surgery, to a non-indicated leg amputation, to a non-indicated tonsillectomy on an innocent child. Text books will define it as recurrent or residual low back pain in the patient after disk surgery. This occurs about 40% of the time (probably more), since most back surgery is not indicated and done on inappropriate candidates. Causes of FBSS are grouped into early and late for the purpose of multiple choice test question writing:

Complications of Spine Surgery	
Recurrent Residual Disk	Will lack enhancement (unlike a scar – which will enhance on delays)
Epidural Fibrosis	Scar, that is usually posterior, and enhance homogeneously
Arachnoiditis	Buzzwords are *"clumped nerve roots" and "empty thecal sac"*, Enhancement for 6 weeks post op is considered normal. After 6 weeks may be infectious or inflammatory.
Conjoined Nerve Roots	Two adjacent nerve roots sharing an enlarged common sleeve – at a point during their exit from the thecal sac
12,000 Square Foot Mansion Syndrome	As spine surgeons perform more and more unnecessary surgeries they need something to spend all that money on.

Scar vs Residual Disc:

T1 Pre Contrast they will look the same… like a bunch of mushy crap.
T1 Post Contrast they disc will still look like mushy crap, but the scar will enhance.

Trauma to the Spine:

Jefferson	Burst Fracture of C1	Axial Loading
Hangman	Bilateral Pedicle or Pars Fracture of C2	Hyperextension
Teardrop	Can be flexion or extension	Flexion (more common)
Clay-Shoveler's	Avulsion of spinous process at C7 or T1	Hyperflexion
Chance	Horizontal Fracture through thoracolumbar spine ("seatbelt").	

Jefferson Fracture: This is an axial loading injury (jumping into a shallow pool) – with the blow typically to the top of the head. The anterior and posterior arches blow out laterally. They would most likely show it on a plain film open mouth odontoid view (the CT would be too easy). Remember the C1 lateral masses shouldn't slide off laterally.

Important trivia to remember: **Neurologic (cord) damage is rare**, because all the force is directed into the bones.

Odontoid Fracture Classification:
- Type 1: Upper part of Odontoid (maybe stable) – this is actually rare
- Type 2: Fracture at the base – unstable - and by far the most common.
- Type 3: Fracture through dens into the body of C2. This is unstable, but has the best prognosis for healing.

Os Odontoideum: A mimic for a type 1 Odontoid fracture. This is an ossicle located at the position of the normal odontoid tip (the orthotopic position). The base of the dens is usually hypoplastic. The thing to know are that **this is prone to subluxation and instability**. It's association with Morquio's syndrome.

Orthotopic vs Dystopic: Orthotopic is the position right on top of the dens. Dystopic is when it's fused to the clivus.

Hangman's Fracture: Seen most commonly when the chin hits the dashboard in an MVA ("direct blow to the face"). The **fracture is through the bilateral pars at C2** (or the pedicles – which is less likely). You will have anterior subluxation of the C2 body. Cord damage is actually uncommon with these, as the acquired pars defect allows for canal widening. There is often an associated fracture of the anterior inferior corner at C2 – from avulsion of the anterior longitudinal ligament.

Flexion Teardrop: This represents a teardrop shaped fracture fragment at the anterior-inferior vertebral body. Flexion injury is bad because it is associated with anterior cord syndrome (85% of patients have deficits). This is an unstable fracture, associated with posterior subluxation of the vertebral body.

Anterior Cord Syndrome: The anterior portion of the cord is jacked. Motor function and anterior column sensations (pain and temperature) are history. The dorsal column sensations (proprioception and vibration) are still intact.

Extension Teardrop: Another anterior inferior teardrop shaped fragment with avulsion of the anterior longitudinal ligament. This is less serious than the flexion type.

Flexion Teardrop	Extension Teardrop
Impaction Injury	Distraction Injury
Unstable	Stable (maybe)
Hyperflexion	Hyperextension
Classic History: "Ran into wall"	Classic History" Hit from behind"

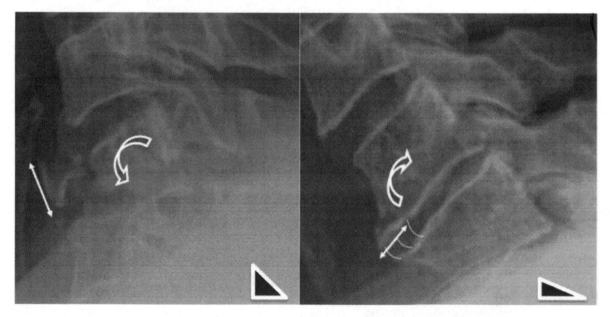

Flexion   Extension

Clay-Shoveler's Fracture: This is an avulsion injury of a lower cervical / upper thoracic spinous process (usually C7). It is the result of a forceful hyperflexion movement (like shoveling). The "ghost sign" describes a double spinous process at C6-C7.

Facet Dislocation: This is a spectrum: Subluxed facets -> Perched -> Locked.

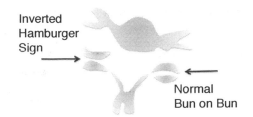

Inverted
Hamburger
Sign

Normal
Bun on Bun

- Unilateral: If you have a unilateral facet (usually from hyperflexion and rotation) the superior facet slides over the inferior facet and gets locked. The unilateral is a stable injury. You will have the inverted hamburger sign on axial imaging on the dislocated side.

- Bilateral: This is the result of severe hyperflexion. You are going to have disruption of the posterior ligament complex. When this is full on you are going to have the dislocated vertebra displaced forward one –half the AP diameter of the vertebral body. This is highly unstable, and strongly associated with cord injury.

Atlantoaxial Instability - The articulation between C1 and C2 allows for lateral movement (shaking your head no). The transverse cruciform ligament straps the dens to the anterior arch of C1. The distance between the anterior arch and dens shouldn't be more than 5mm. The thing to know is the association with Down syndrome and juvenile RA. Rotary subluxation can occur in children without a fracture, with the kid stuck in a "cock-robbin" position – which looks like torticollis. Actually differentiating from torticollis is difficult and may require dynamic maneuvers on the scanner. This never, ever, ever happens in the absence of a fracture in an adult (who doesn't have Downs or RA). Having said that people over call this all the time in adults who have their heads turned in the scanner.

Benign Vs Malignant Compression Fracture: This is a high yield distinction and practical in the real world.

Malignant	Benign
Convex posterior vertebral body cortex	Retropulsed fragment
Involves Posterior Elements	Transverse T1 and T2 dark band
Epidural / Paraspinal Mass	
Multiple Lesions	

Trauma to the Cord: There is a known correlation between spinal cord edema length and outcome. Having said that, you need to know the most important factor for outcome is the presence of a hemorrhagic spinal cord injury (these do very very badly).

Spinal Cord Syndromes		
Central Cord	Old lady with spondylosis or young person with bad extension injury.	Upper Extremity Deficit is worse than lower (corticospinal tracts are lateral in lower extremity)
Anterior Cord	Flexion Injury	Immediate Paralysis
Brown Sequard	Rotation injury or penetrating trauma	One half motor, other half sensory
Posterior Cord	Uncommon – but sometimes seen with hyperextension	Proprioception gone

Congenital / Developmental

Pars Interarticularis Defects: This is considered a fatigue or stress fracture, probably developing in childhood (they are more common in athletic kids). They are usually not symptomatic (only 25% are). The most common level is L5-S1 (90%), with all the rest at L4-L5. They tend to have more spondylolisthesis and associated degenerative change at L4-L5 than L5-S1. They can be seen on the oblique plain film as a "collar on the scottie dog."

Pars Defects with Anteriorlithesis will have neuroforaminal stensosis, with spinal canal widening (when severe will have spinal canal stenosis as well).

Terminal Ventricle (ventricularis terminalis): This is a developmental variant. Normally, a large portion of the distal cord involutes in a late stage of spinal cord embryology. Sometimes this process is not uniform and you get stuck with a stupid looking cyst at the end of your cord. These things are usually small (around 4mm), and cause no symptoms. Sometimes they can get very big (like this example) and cause some neurologic symptoms.

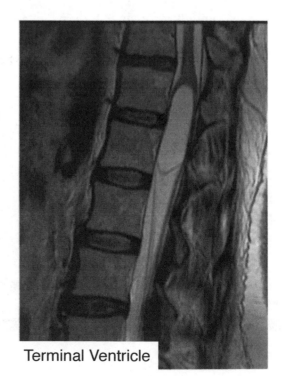

Terminal Ventricle

Spinal Dysraphism:

You can group these as open or closed (closed with and without a mass). Open means neural tissue exposed through a defect in bone and skin (spina bifida aperta). Closed means the defect is covered by skin (spina bifida occulta).

Open Spinal Dysraphisms: This is the result of a failure of the closure of the primary neural tube, with obvious exposure of the neural placode through a midline defect of the skin. You have a dorsal defect in the posterior elements. The **cord is going to be tethered.** There is an association with diastematomyelia and Chiari II malformations. Early surgery is the treatment / standard of care.

- *Myeloceles*: This is the more rare type where the neural placode is flush with the skin.

- *Myelomeningoceles:* This is the more common type (98%) where the neural placode protrudes above the skin. These are more common with Chiari II malformations.

Closed Spinal Dysraphisms with Subcutaneous Mass

- *Meningoceles*: This is herniation of a CSF filled sac through a defect in the posterior elements (spina bifida). It is most typical in the lumbar or sacral periods. Although they can occur in the cervical spine. They may be anterior (usually pre-sarcral). An important point is **that neural tissue is not present in the sac.**

- *Lipomyelocele / Lipomyelomeningoceles:* These are lipomas with a dural defect. On exam you are going to have a subcutaneous fatty mass above the gluteal crease. **These are 100% associated with tethered cord** (myelomeningocele may or may not).

- *Terminal Myelocystocele* – This is a herniation of the terminal syrinx into a posterior menigoccele via a posterior spinal defect.

Closed Spinal Dysraphisms without Subcutaneous Mass

- *Intradural lipomas* – Most common in the thoracic spine also the dorsal aspect. They don't need to be (but can be) associated with posterior element defects.

- *Fibrolipoma of the filum terminale* – This is often an incidental finding. There will be a linear T1 bright structure in the filum terminale. The filum is not going to be unusually thickened and the conus will be normally located.

- *Tight filum terminale* – This is a thickened filum terminale (> 2mm), with a low lying conus (below the inferior endplate of L2). You may have an associated terminal lipoma. The "**tethered cord syndrome**" is based on the clinical findings of low back pain and leg pain plus urinary bladder dysfunction. This is the result of stretching the cord with growth of the canal.

- *Dermal Sinus* – This is an epithelium lined tract that extends from the skin to deep soft tissues (sometimes the spinal canal, sometimes a dermoid or lipoma). These are T1 low signal (relative to the background high signal from fat).

Diastematomyelia – This describes a sagittal split in the spinal cord. They almost always occur between T9-S1, with normal cord both above and below the split. You can have two thecal sacs (or just one), and each hemicord has its own central canal and dorsal/ventral horns. Classification systems are based on the presence / absence of an osseous or fibrous spur and duplication or non-duplication of the thecal sac.

Caudal Regression: This is a spectrum of defect in the caudal region that ranges from partial agenesis of the coccyx to lumbosacral agenesis. The associations to know are VACTERL and Currarino triad. Think about this with maternal diabetes. "Blunted sharp" high terminating cord is classic, with a "shield sign" from the opposed iliac bones (no sacrum).

Currarino Triad:

Anterior Sacral Meningocele,

Anorectal malformation,

Sacrococcygeal osseous defect (simitar sacrum).

Spinal Vascular Disorders

AVFs / AVMs: There are 4 types. **Type 1 is by far the most common** (85%). **It is a Dural AVF**; the result of a fistula between the dorsal radiculomedullary arteries and radiculomedullary vein / coronal sinus – with the dural nerve sleeve. It is acquired and seen in older patients who present with progressive radiculomyelopathy. The most common location is the thoracic spine. If anyone asks the "gold standard for diagnosis is angiography", although CTA or MRA will get the job done. You will have T2 high signal in the central cord (which will be swollen), with serpentine perimedullary flow voids (which are usually dorsal).

Spinal AVM / AVFs	
Type 1	**Most Common Type** (85%). **Dural AVF** – with a single coiled vessel
Type 2	**Intramedullary Nidus** from anterior spinal artery or posterior spinal artery. Can have aneurysms, and can bleed. Most common presentation is SAH. Associated with HHT and KTS (other vascular syndromes).
Type 3	**Juvenile**, very rare, often complex and with a terrible prognosis
Type 4	Intradural **perimedullary** with subtypes depending on single vs multiple arterial supply. These tend to occur **near the conus.**

Foix Alajouanine Syndrome: This is a myelopathy association with a Dural AVF. The classic history is a 45 year old male with lower extremity weakness and sensory deficits. You have increased T2 signal (either at the conus, or lower thoracic spine), with associated prominent vessels. The underlying pathophysiology is venous hypertension – secondary to the vascular malformation.

Misc Disorders Affecting the Spine

Pagets – This is discussed in detail in the MSK chapter, but is such a high yield topic that it's worth touching on again. The incidence increases with age (around 8% at age 80). It's at increased risk for fracture, and has a 1% risk of sarcoma degeneration (usually high grade).

It's shown two ways in the spine:
- (1) An enlarged "ivory vertebrae",
- (2) Picture frame vertebrae (sclerotic border).

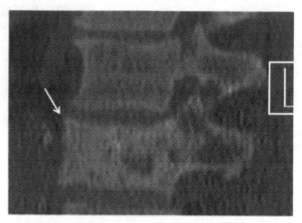

Ivory Vertebrae – Pagets *(or mets)*

Renal Osteodystrophy – Another high yield topic covered in depth in the MSK chapter. The way it's shown in the spine is the "Rugger Jersey Spine" – with sclerotic bands at the top and bottom of the vertebral body. You could also have paraspinous soft tissue calcifications

Osteopetrosis - Another high yield topic covered in depth in the MSK chapter. This is a genetic disease with impaired osteoclastic resorption. You have thick cortical bone, with diminished marrow. On plain film or CT it can look like a Rugger Jersey Spine or Sandwich vertebra. On MR you are going to have loss of the normal T1 bright marrow signal, so it will be T1 and T2 dark.

"H-Shaped Vertebra" – This is usually a **buzzword for sickle cell**, although it's only seen in about 10% of cases. It results from microvascular endplate infarct. If you see "H-Shaped vertebra" the answer is sickle cell. If sickle cell isn't a choice the answer is Gauchers. Another tricky way to ask this is to say which of the following causes **"widening of the disc space."** Widened disc space is another way of describing a "H Shape" without saying that.

Infectious

Discitis / Osteomyelitis:

Infection of the disc and infection of the vertebral body nearly always go together. The reason has to do with the route of seeding; which typically involves seeding of the vertebral endplate (which is vascular), subsequent eruption and crossing into the disc space, and eventual involvement of the adjacent vertebral body.

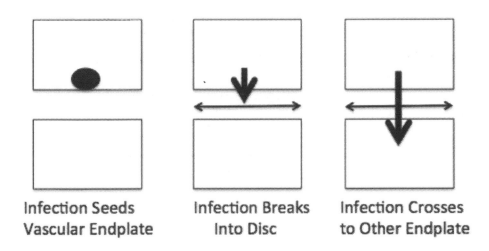

| Infection Seeds Vascular Endplate | Infection Breaks Into Disc | Infection Crosses to Other Endplate |

In adults, the source is usually from a recent surgery, procedure, or systemic infection. In children it's usually from hematogenous spread. For the Step 1 trivia: Staph A is the most common bug, and always think about an IV drug user. Almost always (80%) of the time the ESR and CRP are elevated.

Imaging: Early on it's very hard to see with plain films, you will need MRI. You are looking for paraspinal and epidural inflammation, T2 bright disc signal, disc enhancement

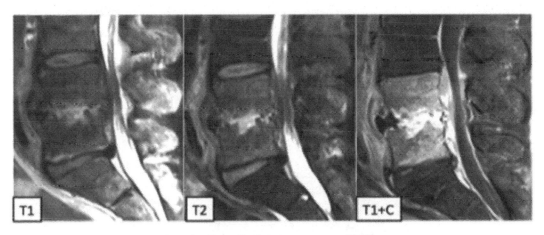

Vertebral Osteomyelitis

Pott's Disease: TB of the spine is more common in "developing" countries. It behaves in a few different ways, and that makes it easy to test on.

Things to know about TB in the spine:
- *It tends to spare the disc space*
- *It tends to have multi-level thoracic "skip" involvement*
- *Buzzword "Calcified Psoas Abscess"*
- *Buzzword "Gibbus Deformity" – which is a destructive focal kyphosis*

Brucellosis: This is uncommon in the USA. It's somewhat unique feature make it testable. Just know that it favors the lower lumbar spine & SI joints, and can spare the disk space (similar to TB). Vertebral destruction and paraspinal abscess are actually less common. Step 1 buzzword was "cow's milk" or "farm exposure."

Epidural Abscess: This is an infected collection between the dura and periostium. Its usually MRSA and the patient usually has HIV or is a bad diabetic. This is most likely to be shown with diffusion. A collection that restricts is going be an abscess (in the spine and in the brain) – most of the time. It should also be T1 dark, T2 bright, with peripheral enhancement.

Cord Pathology

Syrinx – Also known as *"a hole in the cord"*. People use the word "syrinx" for all those fancy French / Latin words (hydromyelia, syringomyelia, hydrosyringomyelia, syringohydromyelia, syringobulbia etc…). They do this because they don't know what those words mean. Here is the way I do it… if there is a perfectly central high signal dilation in the middle of the cord, surrounded by totally normal cord I call it "central cord dilation" or "benign central cord dilation" , if there is the same thing but the cord around it looks "sick" - its also got high signal, or the cord is atrophic, etc… then I use the word "myelia." Myelia is a word to use when you want to say it's pathologic.

Most (90%) cord dilations (healthy and sick ones) are congenital, and associated with Chiari I and II, as well as Dandy-Walker, Klippel-Feil, and Myelomeningoceles. The other 10% are acquired either by trauma, tumor, or vascular insufficiency.

Demyelinating:

Broadly you can think of cord pathology in 5 categories: Demyelinating, Tumor, Vascular, Inflammatory, and Infectious.

In the real world, the answer is almost always MS – which is by far the most common cause. The other three things it could be are Neuromyelitis Optica (NMO), acute disseminating encephalomyelitis (ADEM) or Transverse Myelitis (TM).

MS	Usually Short Segment	Usually Part of the Cord	Not swollen, or Less Swollen	Can Enhance / Restrict when Acute
TM	Usually Long Segment	Usually involves both sides of the cord	Expanded Swollen Cord	Can Enhance
NMO	Usually Long Segment	Usually involves both sides of the cord		Optic Nerves Involved
ADEM			Not swollen, or Less Swollen	
Infarct	Usually Long Segment			Restricted Diffusion
Tumor			Expanded Swollen Cord	Can Enhance

MS in the Cord: "Multiple lesions, over space and time." The lesions in the spine are typically short segment (< 2), usually only affect half / part of the cord. The cervical cord is the most common location. There are usually lesions in the brain, if you have lesions in the cord (isolated cord lesions occur about 10% of the time). The lesions can enhance when acute – but this is more common than in the brain. You can sometimes see cord atrophy if the lesion burden is large.

Transverse Myelitis: This is a focal inflammation of the cord. The causes are numerous (infectious, post vaccination – classic rabies, SLE, Sjogrens, Paraneolastic, AV-malformations). You typically have at least 2/3 of the cross sectional area of the cord involved, and focal enlargement of the cord. Spliters with use the terms "Acute partial" for lesions less than two segments, and "acute complete" for lesions more than two segments. The factoid to know is that the "Acute partials" are higher risk for developing MS.

ADEM: As described in the brain section, this is usually seen after a viral illness or infection typically in a child or young adult. The lesions favor the dorsal white matter (but can involve grey matter). As a pearl, the presence of cranial nerve enhancement is suggestive of ADEM. The step 1 trivia, is that the "anti-MOG IgG" test is positive in 50% of cases. Just like MS there are usually brain lesions (although ADEM lesions can occur in the basal ganglia and pons – which is unusual in MS).

NMO (Neuromyelitis Optica): This is also sometimes called Devics. It can be monophasic or relapsing, and favors the optic nerves and cervical cord. Tends to be longer segment than MS, and involve the full transverse diameter of the cord. Brain lesions can occur (more commonly in Asians) and are usually periventricular. If any PhDs ask the reason the periventricular location occurs is that the antibody (NMO IgG) attacks the Aquaporin 4 channels – which are found in highest concentration around the ventricles.

Subacute Combined Degeneration: This is a fancy way of describing the effects of a Vitamin B12 deficiency. The classic look is **bilateral symmetrically increased T2 signal in the dorsal columns**, without enhancement. The appearance has been described as an "inverted V sign." The signal change typically begins in the upper thoracic region with ascending or descending progression.

HIV Vacuolar Myelopathy: This has been described as a late finding in AIDS patients. You have spinal cord atrophy, and T2 high signal symmetrically involving the posterior columns. It looks like subacute combined degeneration.

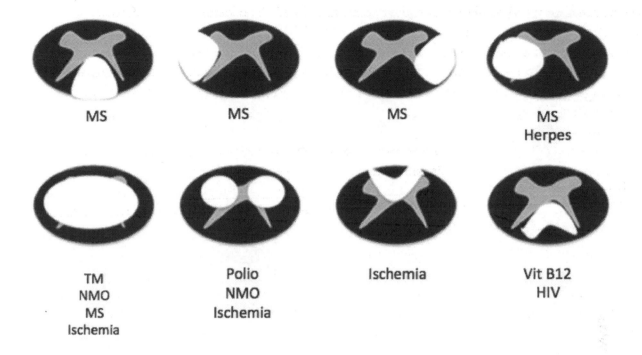

MS	MS	MS	MS Herpes
TM NMO MS Ischemia	Polio NMO Ischemia	Ischemia	Vit B12 HIV

Spinal Cord Infarct: Cord infarct /ischemia can have a variety of causes. The most common cause is "idiopathic," although I'd expect the most common multiple choice scenario to revolve around treating an aneurysm with a stent graft, or embolizing a bronchial artery. Impairment involving the anterior spinal artery distribution is most common. With anterior spinal artery involvement you are going to have central cord / anterior horn cell high signal on T2 (because gray matter is more vulnerable to ischemia).

The "owl eye appearance" of anterior spinal cord infarct is a buzzword.

It's usually a long segment, being more than 2 segments. Diffusion using single shot fast spin echo or line scan can be used with high sensitivity (to compensate for artifacts from spinal fluid movement).

Inflammatory / Infectious:

Arachnoiditis: This is a general term for inflammation of the subarachnoid space. It can be infectious but can also be post-surgical. **It actually occurs about 10-15% of the time after spine surgery, and can be a source of persistent pain / failed back.**

It's shown two ways:

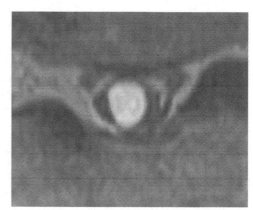

Empty Thecal Sac Sign

(1) **Empty Thecal Sac Sign** – Nerve roots are adherent peripherally, giving the appearance of an empty sac.

(2) *Central Nerve Root Clumping.* This can range in severity from a few nerves clumping together, to all of them fused into a single central scarred band.

Guillain Barre Syndrome (GBS) - One of those weird auto-immune disorders that causes ascending flaccid paralysis. The step 1 trivia was **Campylobacter**, but you can also see it after surgery, or in patients with lymphoma or SLE.

The thing to know is **enhancement of the nerve roots of the cauda equina**.

Other pieces of trivia that are less likely to be asked are that the facial nerve is the most common cranial nerve affected, and that the anterior spinal roots enhance more than the posterior ones.

Chronic Inflammatory Demylinating Polyneuropathy (CIDP) - The chronic counterpart to GBS. Clinically this has a gradual and protracted weakness (GBS improves in 8 weeks, CIDP does not). The buzzword is thickened, enhancing, "onion bulb" nerve roots.

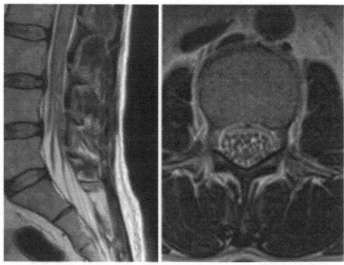

CIDP - Diffuse Thickening of the Nerve Roots

Tumor:

The classic teaching is to first describe the location of the tumor, as either (1) Intramedullary, (2) Extramedullary Intradural, or (3) Extradural. This is often easier said than done. Differentials are based on the location.

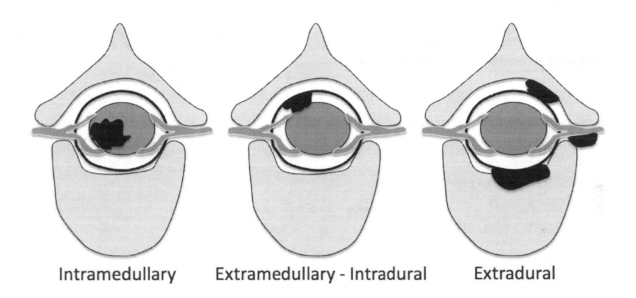

Intramedullary	Astrocytoma, Ependymoma, Hemangioblastoma
Extramedullary Intradural	Schwannoma, Meningioma, Neurofibroma, Drop Mets
Extradural	Disc Disease (most common), Bone Tumors, Mets, Lymphoma

Intramedullary:

- **Astrocytoma** – This is the most common intramedullary tumor in peds. It favors the upper thoracic spine. There will be fusiform dilation of the cord over multiple segments. They are dark on T1, bright on T2, and they enhance. They may be associated with rostral or caudal cysts which are usually benign syrinx formation.

Astrocytoma	Ependymoma
More in Cervical Cord	More in Lower Cord
Eccentric	Central
Longer Segment	Shorter Segment
	More Often Hemorrhagic
Most common intramedullary in PEDS	Most common intramedullary in Adults

- **Ependymoma** – This is the most common primary cord tumor of the lower spinal cord , conus / filum terminale. This is the **most common intramedullary mass in adults**. Although you can certainly see them in the cervical cord as well. The "**myxopapillary form**" is exclusively found in the conus /filum locations. They can be hemorrhagic, and have a **dark cap on T2.** They have tumoral cysts about ¼ of the time. They are a typically long segment (averaging 4 segments).

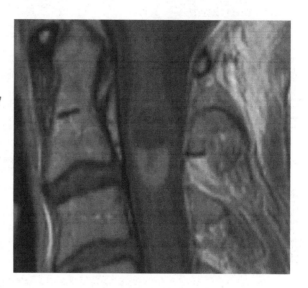

- **Hemangioblastoma** - These are associated with Von Hippel Lindau (30%). The thoracic level is favored (second most common is cervical). The classic look is a wide cord, with considerable edema. Adjacent serpinginous draining meningeal varicosities can be seen.

- **Intramedullary Mets:** This is very very rare, but when it does happen its usually lung (70%).

VHL Associations:

- Pheochromocytoma
- CNS Hemangioblastoma *(cerebellum 75%, spine 25%)*
- Endolymphatic Sac Tumor
- Pancreatic Cysts
- Pancreatic Islet Cell Tumors
- Clear Cell RCC

Extramedullary Intradural:

- **Schwannoma:** This is the most common tumor to occur in the Extramedullary Intradural location. The are benign, usually solitary, usually arising from the dorsal nerve roots. This can be multiple in the setting of NF-2 and the Carney Complex. The appearance is variable, but the classic look is a dumbbell with the skinny handle being the intraforaminal component. They are T1 dark, T2 bright, and will enhance. They look a lot like neurofibromas. If they have central necrosis or hemorrhage that favors a schwannoma.

- **Neurofibroma:** This is another benign nerve tumor *(composed of all parts of the nerve: nerve + sheath)*, that is also usually solitary. There are two flavors: solitary and plexiform. The plexiform is a multilevel bulky nerve enlargement that is pathognomonic for NF-1. Their lifetime risk for malignant degeneration is around 5-10%. Think about malignant degeneration in the setting of rapid growth. They look a lot like schwannomas. If they have a hyperintense T2 rim with a central area of low signal – "target sign" that makes you favor neurofibroma.

Schwannoma	Neurofibroma
Do NOT envelop the adjacent nerve root	Do envelop the adjacent nerve root (usually a dorsal sensory root)
Solitary	Solitary
Multiple makes you think NF-2	Associated with NF -1 (even when single)
Cystic change / Hemorrhage	T2 bright rim, T2 dark center "target sign"

- **Meningioma:** These guys adhere to but do not originate from the dura. They are more common in women (70%). They favor the posterior lateral thoracic spine, and the anterior cervical spine. They enhance brightly and homogeneously. They are often T1 iso to hypo, and slightly T2 bright. They can have calcifications.

- **Drop Mets:** Medulloblastoma is the most common primary tumor to drop. Breast cancer is the most common systemic tumor to drop (followed by lung and melanoma). The cancer may coat the cord or nerve root, leading to a fine layer of enhancement.

Extradural:

- **Vertebral Hemangioma:** These are very common – seen in about 10% of the population. They classically have thickening trabeculae appearing as parallel lineal densities "jail bar" or "corduroy" appearance. In the vertebral body they are T1 and T2 bright, although the extraosseuous components typically lack fat and are isointense on T1.

- **Osteoid Osteoma:** This is also covered in the MSK chapter, but as a brief review focusing on the spine they love to involve the posterior elements (75%), and are rare after age 30. They tend to have a nidus, and surrounding sclerosis. The nidus is T2 bright, and will enhance. The classic story is night pain, better with aspirin. Radiofrequency ablation can treat them (under certain conditions).

- **Osteoblastoma:** This is similar to an Osteoid osteoma but larger than 1.5cm. Again, very often in the posterior elements – usually of the cervical spine.

- **Aneursymal Bone Cyst:** These guys are also covered in the MSK chapter. They also like the posterior elements and are usually seen in the first two decades of life. They are expansile (as the name implies) and can have multiple fluid levels on T2. They can get big, and look aggressive.

- **Giant Cell Tumor:** These guys are also covered in the MSK chapter. These are common in the sacrum, although rare anywhere else in the spine. You don't see them in young kids. If they show this it's going to be a **lytic expansile lesion in the sacrum with no rim of sclerosis.**

- **Vertebral Plana -** The pancake flat vertebral body. Just say Eosinophilc Granuloma in a kid (could be neuroblastoma met), and Mets / Myeloma in an adult.

- **Chordoma:** This is **most common in the sacrum** (they will want you to say clivus – that is actually number 2). The thing to know is that vertebral primary tend to be more aggressive / malignant than their counter parts in the clivus and sacrum. The classic story in the vertebral column is "involvement of two or more adjacent vertebral bodies with the intervening disc." Most are **very T2 bright.**

- **Leukemia:** They love to show it in the spine. You have loss of the normal fatty marrow – so it's going to be homogeneously dark on T1. More on this in the MSK chapter.

- **Mets:** The classic offenders are prostate, breast, lung, lymphoma, and myeloma. Think **multiple lesions, with low T1 signal.** Cortical breakthrough or adjacent paravertebral components are also helpful.

Blank for Notes / Scribes

Blank for Notes / Scribes

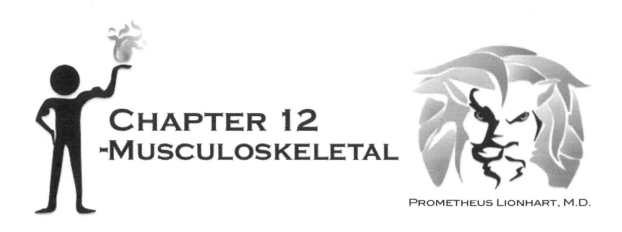

CHAPTER 12
-MUSCULOSKELETAL

PROMETHEUS LIONHART, M.D.

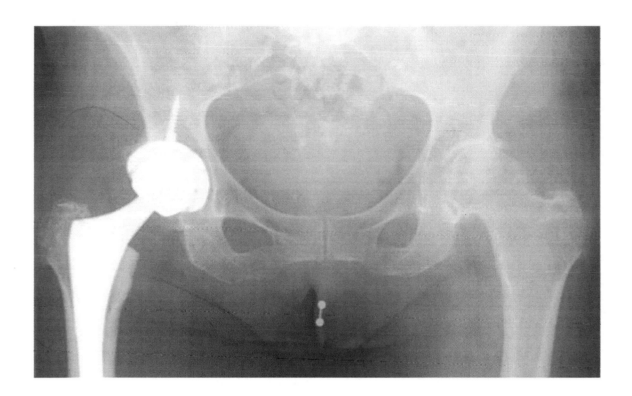

Highest Yield Tip:

In the real world MSK is full of differentials. However, for multiple choice test taking differential cases make terrible questions. So the test writers are left with three options: (1) Show a case with a differential but list 3 terrible distractors, (2) Show Aunt Minnies, or (3) Ask Trivia. As you read this chapter, I want you to focus on the testable trivia as this will make up the bulk of the more difficult questions.

Trauma / Acquired

Basic Fracture Trivia:

- *Stress fracture* is abnormal stress on normal bone.
- An *insufficiency fracture* is normal stress on abnormal bone.
- Bones heal in about 6-8 weeks (months for tibia), and remember that the osteolytic phase precedes new bone formation.

Hand / Wrist:

Scaphoid Fracture:
- Most common carpal bone fracture *May take 4-8 weeks for radiographic Δ of sclerosis to develop.*
- 70% at the waist
- Blood supply is distal to proximal; with the proximal pole most susceptible to AVN.
- The first sign of AVN = Sclerosis (the dead bone can't turn over / recycle)
- Proximal fractures are most susceptible to AVN and non-union
- Avulsion fractures occur at distal pole
- AVN on MRI - This is tricky stuff with lots of papers contradicting each other. Probably the most reliable is sign is DARK ON T1.

Scaphoid osteonecrosis in absence of trauma → Preiser's disease

---

SLAC and SNAC Wrists

Both are potential complications of trauma, with similar mechanisms.

SLAC Wrist (Scaphoid-Lunate Advanced Collapse) occurs with injury (or degeneration via CPPD) to the S-L ligament.

SNAC Wrist (Scaphoid Non-Union Advanced Collapse) occurs with a scaphoid fracture.

Just remember that the scaphoid always wants to rotate in flexion - the scaphoid-lunate ligament is the only thing holding it back. If this ligament breaks it will tilt into flexion, messing up the dynamics of the wrist. The radial scaphoid space will narrow, and the capitate will migrate proximally.

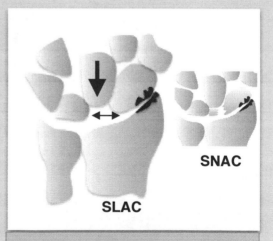

SNAC

SLAC

The things to know are;

- Radioscaphoid joint is first to develop degenerative changes

- Capitate will migrate proximally and there will eventually be a **DISI deformity**

Q: How do you Treat a SLAC Wrist ?

A: Depends on the patient's occupation and needs:

- o   Wrist Fusion = Maximum Strength, Loss of Motion
- o   Proximal Row Carpectomy = Maintain ROM, Lose Strength

Carpal Dislocations - *A spectrum of severity*

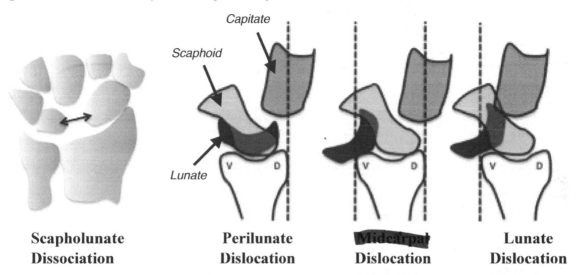

Scapholunate **Dissociation**	**Perilunate** **Dislocation**	~~**Midcarpal**~~ **Dislocation**	**Lunate** **Dislocation**
• SL- Wider Than 3mm • Clenched Fist View can worsen it (would make a good next step question) • Chronic SL dissociation can result in a SLAC wrist	Trivia to Know = 60% associated with Scaphoid Fractures	Trivia to Know = (1) Associated with ~~Triquetrolunate interosseous ligament disruption~~ (2) Associated with a Triquetral Fracture	Trivia to Know = It happens with a Dorsal radiolunate ligament injury

DISI vs VISI

This is a very confusing topic - thus high yield. If you have carpal ligament disruption the carpal bones will rotate the way they naturally want to. The reasons for their rotational desires are complex but basically have to do with the shape of the fossa they sit on. Just remember the scaphoid wants to flex (rock volar) and the lunate wants to extend (rock dorsal). The only thing holding them back is their ligamentous attachment to each other.

DISI (dorsal intercalated segmental instability) - I like to call this *dorsiflexion instability* because it helps me remember whats going on. After a "Radial sided injury" (scapholunate side) the lunate becomes free of the stabilizing force of the scaphoid and rocks dorsally. Remember SL ligament injury is common, so this is common.

VISI (volar intercalated segmental instability) - I like to call this *volar-flexion (palmar-flexion) instability* because it helps me remember whats going on. After a "Ulnar sided injury" (lunotriquetral side) the lunate no longer hast the stabilizing force of the lunotriquetral ligament and gets ripped volar with the scaphoid *(remember the scaphoid stays up late every night dreaming of tilting volar)*. Remember LT ligament injury is not common, so this is not common. It's so uncommon in fact that if you see it - it's probably a normal variant due to wrist laxity.

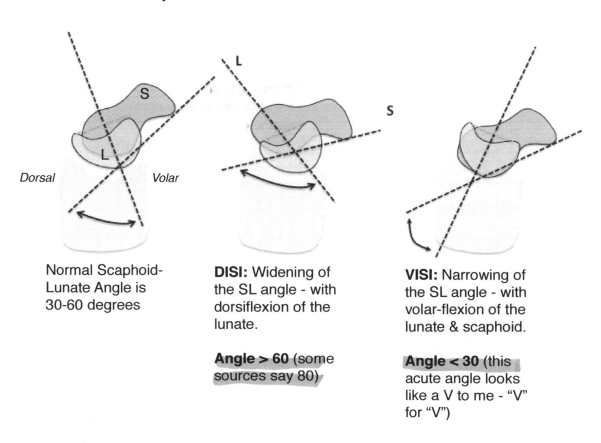

Normal Scaphoid-
Lunate Angle is
30-60 degrees

DISI: Widening of
the SL angle - with
dorsiflexion of the
lunate.

Angle > 60 (some
sources say 80)

VISI: Narrowing of
the SL angle - with
volar-flexion of the
lunate & scaphoid.

Angle < 30 (this
acute angle looks
like a V to me - "V"
for "V")

Bennett and Rolando Fractures

- They are both fractures at the base of the first metacarpal
- The Rolando fracture is comminuted (Bennett is not)
- *Trivia:* The pull of the **Abductor pollicis longus (APL)** tendon is what causes the dorsolateral dislocation in the Bennett Fracture

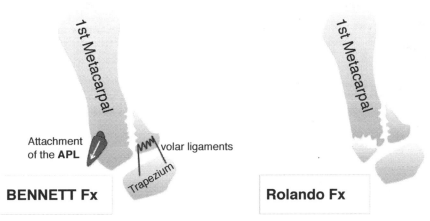

Attachment of the APL

volar ligaments

1st Metacarpal

Trapezium

BENNETT Fx

1st Metacarpal

Rolando Fx

Gamekeeper's Thumb

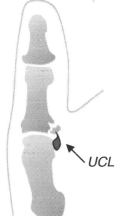

UCL

- Avulsion fracture at the base of the proximal first phalanx associated with **ulnar collateral ligament** disruption.
- The frequently tested association is that of a **"Stener Lesion."** A Stener Lesion is when the Adductor tendon gets caught in the torn edges of the UCL. The displaced ligament won't heal right, and will need surgery.
- It makes a "yo-yo" appearance on MRI - supposedly…

Carpal Tunnel Syndrome (CTS)

- Median Nerve Distribution (thumb-radial aspect of 4th digit), often bilateral, and may have thenar muscle atrophy.
- On Ultrasound, enlargement of the nerve is the main thing to look for
- It's usually from repetitive trauma,
- *Trivia* = **Association with dialysis**

Guyon's Canal Syndrome

- Entrapment of the ulnar nerve as it passes through Guyon's canal (formed by the pisiform and the hamate – and the crap that connects them). Classically caused by handle bars *"handle bar palsy."* Fracture of the hook of the hamate can also eat on that ulnar nerve.

Elbow / Forearm:

- Radial Head Fracture is most common in adults (supracondylar is most common in PEDs)
  - o Sail sign (posterior is positive)
- Capitellum fractures are associated with posterior dislocation

Eponyms:
- *Essex-Lopresti:* Fracture of the radial head + Anterior dislocation of the distal radial ulnar joint
- *Monteggia Fracture (MUGR):* Fracture of the proximal ulna, with anterior dislocation of the radial head.
- *Galeazzi Fracture (MUGR):* Radial shaft fracture, with anterior dislocation of the ulna at the DRUJ.

The Dreaded PEDs elbow *(Covered in the Peds chapter - see chapter 1, volume 1):*

Cubital Tunnel Syndrome
- The result of repetitive valgus stress
- *Anatomy Trivia:* the site where the ulnar nerve passes beneath the cubital tunnel retinaculum also known as the epicondylo-olecranon ligament or Osborne band
- Can occur from compression by any pathology (tumor, hematoma, etc…) , when it occurs from an **accessory muscle** it's classically the **anconeus epitrochlearis** - *also known as the "accessory anconeus."*

Shoulder (*MRI covered separately*)

Dislocation:
- *Anterior inferior* (subcoracoid) are by far the most common (like 90%).
  - Hill-Sachs is on the **Humerus**.
  - Hill-Sachs is on the posterior lateral humerus, and *best seen on internal rotation view.*
  - Bankart – anterior inferior labrum
  - Greater tuberosity avulsion fracture occurs in 10-15% of anterior dislocations in patient's over 40.
- *Posterior Dislocation*: uncommon – probably from seizure or electrocution
  - *Rim Sign* – no overlap glenoid and humeral head
  - *Trough Sign* – reverse Hill Sachs, impaction on anterior humerus
  - Arm may be locked in internal rotation on all views
- *Inferior Dislocation (luxatio erecta humeri)* – this is an uncommon form, where the arm is sticking straight over the head. The thing to know is 60% get neurologic injury (usually the axillary nerve).

Hill Sacs	Posterolateral humeral head impaction fracture (anterior dislocation)
Bankart	Anterior Glenoid Rim (anterior dislocation)
Trough Sign	Anterior humeral head impaction fracture (posterior dislocation)
Reverse Bankart	Posterior Glenoid Rim (posterior dislocation)

Memory Tool (works for me anyway)

I remember that hip dislocations are posterior - from the straight leg dashboard mechanism. Then I just remember that shoulders are the opposite of that (the other one, is the other one). **Shoulder = Usually Anterior**

Proximal Humerus Fracture: This is usually in an old lady falling on an out stretched arm. Orthopods use the Neer classifications (how many parts the humerus is in ?). Three or four part fractures tend to do worse.

The Post Op Shoulder (Prosthesis)

There are 4 Main Types: Humeral Head Resurfacing, Hemi-Arthroplasty, Total Shoulder Arthroplasty, and the Reverse Total Shoulder Arthroplasty.

Who gets what? - The surgical choice depends on two main factors: (1) is the cuff intact?, and (2) is the Glenoid Trashed ? Here is the breakdown:

	Cuff-Intact	Cuff- Deficient
Glenoid Intact	Resurfacing or Hemi	Hemi or Reverse
Glenoid Deficient	TSA	Reverse

Complications / Trivia:

—Total Shoulder Most Common Complication = Loosening of the Glenoid Component

—Total Shoulder Complication - *"Anterior Escape"* - This describes anterior migration of the humeral head after subscapularis failure.

—Reverse Total Shoulder Does NOT require an intact rotator cuff - patient rely heavily on the deltoid.

—Reverse Shoulder Complication - *Posterior Acromion Fracture* - from excessive deltoid tugging.

Hip / Femur

Femoral Neck Fractures:
- On the inside (**medial**) is the classic **stress** fracture location
- On the outside (**lateral)** is the classic **bisphosphonate** related fx location

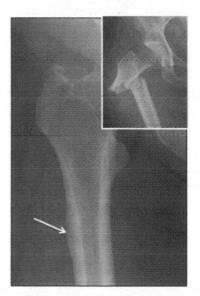

Bisphosphonate Fracture (Lateral Femur)
**Stress would be medial

Hip Fracture / Dislocation: You see these with dash board injuries. The **posterior dislocation** (almost always associated with a fracture as it's driven backwards) is much more common than the anterior dislocation.

> *Anterior Column vs Posterior Column* - the acetabulum is supported by two columns of bone that merge together to form an "inverted Y"
>
> o Iliopectineal Line = Anterior
> o Ilioischial Line = Posterior (remember you sit on your ischium)
> o The both column fracture by definition divides the ilium proximal to the hip joint, so you have no articular surface of the hip attached to the axial skeleton (that's a problem).
>
> *Corona Mortis:* The anastomosis of the inferior epigastric and obturator vessels sometimes rides on the superior pubic ramus. During a lateral dissection - sometimes used to repair a hip fracture this can be injured. I talk about this more in the vascular chapter.

Hip Fracture Leading to AVN: The location of the fracture may predispose to AVN. It's important to remember that since the femoral head gets vascular flow from the circumflex femorals a **displaced intracapsular fracture could disrupt this blood supply – leading to AVN.**

- ~~Testable Point:~~ *Degree of fracture displacement corresponds with risk of AVN.*

Avulsion Injury: This is seen more in kids than adults. Adult bones are stronger than their tendons. In kids it's the other way around. One pearl is that if you see an **isolated "avulsion" of the lesser trochanter in a seemingly mild trauma / injury in an adult - query a pathologic fracture.** Now, to discuss what I believe is the highest yield topic in MSK for the CORE, "where did the avulsion come from?" The easiest way to show this is a plain film pelvis (or MRI) with a tug/avulsion injury to one of the muscular attachment sites. The question will most likely be *"what attaches there?"* or *"which muscle got avulsed?"*

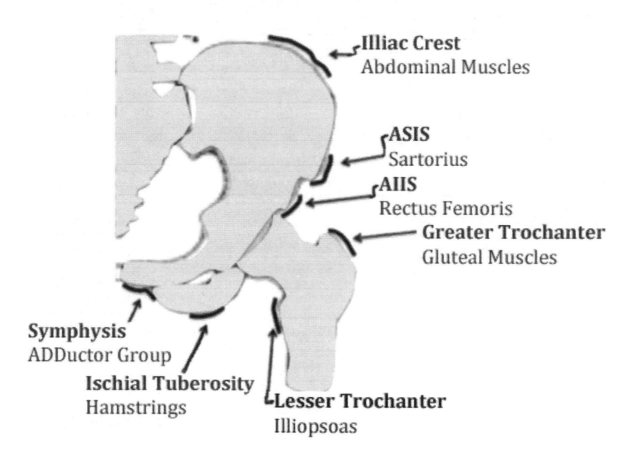

Illiac Crest
Abdominal Muscles

ASIS
Sartorius

AIIS
Rectus Femoris

Greater Trochanter
Gluteal Muscles

Symphysis
ADDuctor Group

Ischial Tuberosity
Hamstrings

Lesser Trochanter
Illiopsoas

Snapping Hip Syndrome: The clinical sensation of "snapping" or "clicking" with hip flexion and extension. For a multiple choice testing standpoint all you need to know is (1) that it exists, (2) there are three types, and (3) what muscle each type involves.

Snapping Hip Syndrome	
External (most common)	Iliotibial Band over Greater Trochanter
Internal	Iliopsoas over Iliopectineal eminence or femoral head
Intra-Articular	Labral tears / joint bodies

Femoroacetabular Impingement (FAI): This is a syndrome of painful hip movement. It's based on hip / femoral deformities, and honestly might be total BS. Supposedly it can lead to early degenerative changes. There are two described subtypes:

Pincer Impingement	Cam Impingement
Middle Aged Women	Young Man
Over Coverage of the femoral head by the acetabulum	Bony protrusion on the antero-superior femoral head-neck junction
"Cross Over Sign" *anterior acetabular rim "crossing over" the posterior rim.	*"Pistol Grip Deformity"* Describes the appearance of the femur

Femoroacetabular Impingement

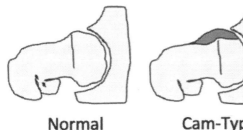
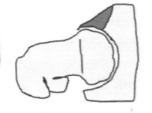

Normal   Cam-Type   Pincer-Type

Memory Aid

I remember that the femoral one (cam-type) is more common in men because the femoral head kinda looks like a penis.

Be honest, you were thinking that too.

"Cross Over Sign" – A sign of pincer type FAI. This refers to the anterior and posterior rims of the acetabulum forming a "figure of eight" on AP pelvis. It is extremely unreliable, and heavily based on positioning.

Trivia - Most common location for an acetabular labral tear = Anterior Superior

Sacrum:

You can get fractures of the sacrum in the setting of trauma, but if you get shown or asked anything about the sacrum it's going to be either (a) SI degenerative change - discussed later, (b) unilateral SI infection, (c) a chordoma - discussed later, (d) sacral agenesis, or (e) an insufficiency fracture. Out of these 5 things the insufficiency fracture is probably the most likely.

Sacral Insufficiency Fracture - The most common cause is postmenopausal **osteoporosis.** You can also see this in patients with renal failure, patients with RA, **pelvic radiation, mechanical changes after hip arthroplasty**, or extended steroid use. They are often (usually) occult on plain films. They will have to show this either with a bone scan, or MRI.

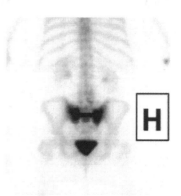

"Honda Sign"
Sacral Insufficiency Fx

The classic "**Honda Sign**" from the "H" shaped appearance is probably the most likely presentation on a multiple choice test.

Knee / Tibia / Fibula:

Segond Fracture: This is a fracture of the **Lateral** Tibial Plateau (*common distractor is medial tibia*). The thing to know is that it is **associated with ACL tear (75%),** and occurs with **internal rotation.**

Reverse Segond Fracture: This is a fracture of the **Medial** Tibial Plateau. The thing to know is that it is **associated with a PCL tear,** and occurs with **external rotation.** There is also an associated **medial meniscus** injury.

Arcuate Sign This is an avulsion of **proximal fibula** (insertion of arcuate ligament complex). The thing to know is that **90% are associated with cruciate ligament injury (usually PCL)**

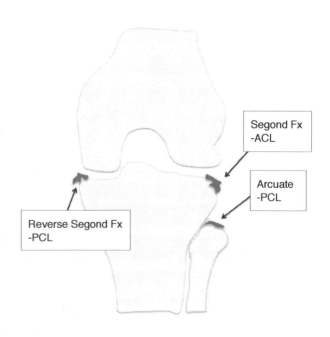

Segond Fx
-ACL

Arcuate
-PCL

Reverse Segond Fx
-PCL

Deep Intercondylar Notch Sign: This is a depression of the lateral femoral condyle (terminal sulcus) that occurs secondary to an impaction injury. This is **associated with ACL tears.**

Patella Dislocation: Basically **always lateral,** and the Medial Patello-Femoral Ligament is injured. There is a characteristic appearance on MRI, which will be shown and discussed later in this chapter.

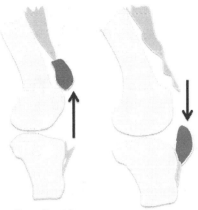

Patella Alta   Patella Baja

Patella Alta / Baja: The patella will move up or down in certain traumatic situations. If the quadricep tendon tears you will get unopposed pull from the patellar tendon resulting in a low patella (Baja). If the patella tendon tears you will get unopposed quadriceps tendon pull resulting in a high patella (Alta).

The "classic" association with patellar tendon tear (Alta) is **SLE,** (also can see in elderly, trauma, athletics, or RA). "Bilateral patellar rupture" is a buzzword for chronic steroids.

Tibial Plateau Fracture: This injury most commonly occurs from axial loading (falling and landing on a straight leg). The **lateral plateau is way more common than the medial**. If you see medial, it's usually with lateral. Some dude named Schatzker managed to get the classification system named after him, of which type 2 is the most common (split and depressed lateral plateau).

[handwritten margin notes: 1 - split; III depression; IV - med + lat; V metaphysis]

Pilon Fracture (Tibial plafond fracture): This injury also most commonly occurs from axial loading, with the talus being driven into the tibial plafond. The fracture is characterized by comminution and articular impaction. About 75% of the time you are going to have fracture of the distal fibula.

Tibial Shaft Fracture: This is the most common long bone fracture. It was also *listed as the most highly tested subject in orthopedic OITE exam (with regard to trauma)*, over the last 8 years. Apparently there are a bunch of ways to put a nail or plate in it. It doesn't seem like it could be that high yield for the CORE compared to other fractures with French or Latin sounding names.

Tillaux Fractures: This a **salter-harris 3**, through the anterolateral aspect of the distal tibial epiphysis.

Triplane Fracture: This is a **salter-harris 4**, with a vertical component through the epiphysis, horizontal component through the physis, and oblique through the metaphysis.

Maisonneuve Fracture: This is an unstable fracture involving the medial tibial malleolus and/or **disruption of the distal tibiofibular syndesmosis.** The most common way to show this is to first show you the ankle with the widened mortis, and *"next step?"* get you to ask for the proximal fibula - which will show the **fracture of the proximal fibular shaft.** This fracture pattern is unique as the forces begin distally in the tibiotalar joint and ride up the syndesmosis to the proximal fibula. For some reason knowing that the fracture **does not extend into the hindfoot** is a piece of valuable trivia.

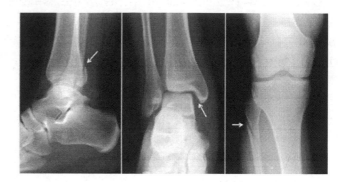

Maisonneuve Fracture:

Foot / Ankle

Casanova Fracture – If you see bilateral calcaneal fractures, you should *"next step?"* look at the spine for a compression or burst fracture. These tend to occur in axial loading patterns (possibly from jumping out a window to avoid an angry husband).

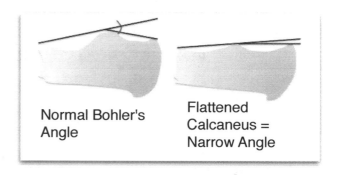

Normal Bohler's Angle

Flattened Calcaneus = Narrow Angle

also known as Lover's fracture

Trivia: Peroneal tendons can become entrapped with lateral calcaneal fractures.

Bohler's Angle – The line drawn between the anterior and posterior borders of the calcaneus on a lateral view. An angle less than (20) is concerning for a fracture.

Jones Fracture: This is a fracture at the base of the fifth metatarsal, 1.5cm distal to the tuberosity. These are placed in a non-weight bearing cast (may require internal fixation- because of risk of non-union. .

Avulsion Fracture of the 5ᵗʰ Metatarsal: This is more common than a jones fracture. The classic history is a dancer. It may be **secondary to tug from the lateral cord of the plantar aponeurosis or peroneus brevis** (this is controversial).

Stress Fracture of the 5th Metatarsal: This is considered a high risk fracture (hard to heal).

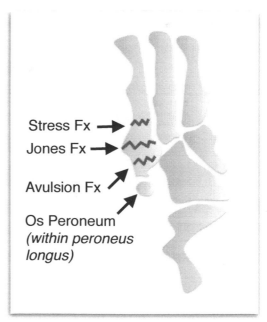

Stress Fx →

Jones Fx →

Avulsion Fx

Os Peroneum
(within peroneus longus)

LisFranc Injury: This is the **most common dislocation of the foot**. The Lisfranc joint is the articulation of the tarsals and metatarsal heads. This joint would make a good place to amputate if you were a surgeon assisting in the Napoleonic invasion of Russia. The LisFranc ligament connects the medial cuneiform to the 2nd metatarsal base on the plantar aspect. If the ligament goes out you can see two patterns: (1) "Homo-lateral" - everyone moves lateral, (2) "Divergent" - the 1st MT goes medial, the 2nd-5th MT goes lateral.

What you need to know:
- Can't exclude it on a non-weight bearing film
- Associated fractures are most common at the base of the 2nd MT - *"Fleck Sign"*
- Fracture non-union and post traumatic arthritis are gonna occur if you miss it (plus a lawsuit).

"Fleck Sign" - This is a small bony fragment in the LisFranc Space (between 1st MT and 2nd MT) - that is associated with an avulsion of the LF ligament.

Spine: *Fractures and other acquired pathologies of the spine are discussed in detail in the spine section of the neuro chapter.*

Divergent Lisfranc - associated common c̄ Charcot joint.

Stress / Insufficiency Fractures:

Stress Fracture vs Insufficiency Fracture: A stress fracture is the result of abnormal stress on normal bone. An insufficiency fracture is the result of normal stress on abnormal bone.

Compressive Side vs Tensile Side: This comes up in two main areas - the femoral neck and the tibia. Fractures of the compressive side are constantly getting pushed back together - these do well. Fractures of the tensile side are constantly getting pulled apart - these are a pain in the ass to heal.

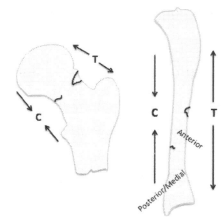

Compressive vs Tensile Forces
-Femoral Neck and Tibia

- **Femoral Stress Fracture:** Fractures along the compressive (medial) side are more common, typically seen in a younger person along the inferior femoral neck. Fractures along the tensile (lateral) side are more common in old people.

- **Tibial Stress Fracture:** This is the *most common site of a stress fracture in young athletes*. These are most common on the compressive side (posterior medial) in either the proximal or distal third. Less common are the tensile side (anterior) fractures, and these favor the mid shaft. They are bad news and don't heal - often called "*dreaded black lines.*"

SONK (Spontaneous Osteonecrosis of the Knee): This is totally named wrong, as it is another type of insufficiency fracture. You see this in old ladies with the classic history of "sudden pain after rising from a seated position." Young people can get it too (much less common), usually seen after a meniscal surgery.

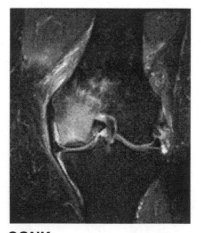

SONK-
-Diffuse Increased Signal (edema)

Things to know about SONK:
- *It's an insufficiency fracture (NOT osteonecrosis) think SINK not SONK*
- *Favors the medial femoral condyle (area of maximum weight bearing) -*
- *Usually unilateral in an old lady without history of trauma*
- *Associated with meniscal injury*

Navicular Stress Fracture – You see these in runners who run on hard surfaces. The thing to know is that just like in the wrist, the navicular is high risk for AVN.

March Fracture: This is a metatarsal stress fracture, which is fairly common. Classically seen in military recruits that are marching all day long.

Calcaneal Stress Fracture – The calcaneus is actually the most fractured tarsal bone. The fractures are usually intra-articular (75%). The stress fracture will be seen, with the fracture line perpendicular to the trabecular lines.

High Risk vs Low Risk Stress Fractures: You can sort these based on the likelihood of uncomplicated healing when treated conservatively.

High Risk	Low Risk
Femoral Neck (tensile side)	Femoral Neck (compressive side)
Transverse Patellar Fracture	Longitudinal Patellar Fracture
Anterior Tibial Fracture (midshaft)	Posterior Medial Tibial Fracture
5th Metatarsal	2nd and 3rd Metatarsal
Talus	Calcaneus
Tarsal Navicular	
Sesamoid Great Toe	

Osteoporosis / Osteopenia & Complications:

Osteopenia: This just means increased lucency of bones. Although this is most commonly caused by osteoporosis that is not always the case.

Osteomalacia: This is a soft bone from excessive uncalcified osteoid. This is typically related to vitamin D issues (either renal causes, liver causes, or other misc causes). It generally looks just like diffuse osteopenia. For the purpose of multiple choice you should think about 4 things; Ill-defined trabeculae, Ill-defined corticomedullary junction, bowing, and "Looser's Zones."

Looser Zones: These things are wide lucent bands that transverse bone at right angles to the cortex. You should think two things: **osteomalacia** and **rickets.** Less common is OI. The other piece of trivia is to understand **they are a type of insufficiency fracture.**

Osteoporosis: The idea is that you have low bone density. Bone density peaks around 30 and then decreases. It decreases faster in women during menopause. The imaging findings are a thin sharp cortex, prominent trabecular bars, lucent metaphyseal bands, and spotty lucencies.

Causes: Age is the big one. Medications (steroids, heparin, dilantin), Endocrine issues (cushings, hyperthryoidism), Anorexia, and Osteogenesis Imperfecta.

Complications: Fractures – Most commonly of the spine (2nd most common is the hip, 3rd most common is the wrist).

DEXA: This is a bone mineral density test and an excellent source of multiple choice trivia.

General Things to know about DEXA
- T score = Density relative to young adult
- T score defines osteopenia vs osteoporosis
- T score > 1.0 = Normal, -1.0 to -2.5 = Osteopenia, < **-2.5 Osteoporosis**
- Z score = Density relative to aged match control "to **Za Za**me Age"
- False negative / positives (see below)

False Positive / Negative on DEXA: DEXA works by measuring the density. Anything that makes that higher or lower than normal can fool the machine.

False Positive:
- Absent Normal Structures: Status post laminectomy

False Negative:
- Including excessive Osteophytes, dermal calcifications, or metal
- Including too much of the femoral shaft when doing a hip - can elevate the number as the shaft normally has denser bone.
- Compression Fx in the area measured

Reflex Sympathetic Dystrophy (RSD):

Can cause severe osteopenia (like disuse osteopenia). Some people say it **looks like unilateral RA, with preserved joint spaces**. Hand and shoulder are most common sites of involvement. May occur after trauma or infection resulting in an overactive sympathetic system. It's one of the many causes of a 3 phase hot bone scan. In fact, *intra-articular uptake* of tracer on bone scan in patients with RSD (secondary to the increased vascularity of the synovial membrane), and this is somewhat characteristic.

Transient Osteoporosis:

There are two types of presentations.:

Transient osteoporosis of the hip: For the purpose of multiple choice tests by far you should expect to see the **female in the 3rd trimester of pregnancy** with involvement of the left hip. Having said that, it's actually more common in men in whom it's usually bilateral. The joint space should remain normal. It's self limiting (hence the word transient) and resolves in a few months. *Plain film shows osteopenia, MRI shows Edema, Bone scan shows increased uptake focally.*

Regional migratory osteoporosis - This is an idiopathic disorder which has a very classic history of **pain** in a joint, which gets better then shows up in another joint. It's associated with osteoporosis – which is also self limiting. It's more common in men.

Osteoporotic Compression Fracture: Super Common. On MR you want to see a *"band like"* fracture line - which is typically T1 dark (T2 is more variable). The non-deformed portions of the vertebral body should have normal signal.

Neoplastic Compression Fracture: Most vertebral mets don't result in compression fracture until nearly the entire vertebral body is replaced with tumor. If you see abnormal marrow signal (not band like) with involvement of the posterior margin you should think about cancer. *Next step ?* - look at the rest of the spine - mets are often multiple.

OCDs/ OCLs

Osteochondritis Dissecans (OCD): The new terminology is actually to call these "OCLs" (the "L" is for Lesion). This a spectrum of aseptic separation of an osteochondral fragment which can lead to gradual fragmentation of the articular surface and secondary OA. Most of the time it is secondary to trauma, although it could also be secondary to AVN.

Where it happens: Classic locations include the femoral condyle (most common site in the knee), patella, talus, and capitellum.

Staging: There is a staging system, which you probably need to know exists.

- Stage 1: Stable – Covered by intact cartilage, Intact with Host Bone
- Stage 2: Stable on Probing, Partially not intact with host bone.
- Stage 3: Unstable on Probing, Complete discontinuity of lesion.
- Stage 4: Dislocated fragment

Treatment / Who cares? If the fragment is unstable you can get secondary OA. You want to **look for high T2 signal undercutting the fragment from the bone to call it unstable** (edema can force a false positive). Thus, the absence of high T2 signal at the bone fragment interface is a good indicator of osseous bridging and stability. Granulation tissue at the interface (which will enhance with Gd), does not mean it's stable.

Osteochondroses: These are a group of conditions (usually seen in childhood) that are characterized by involvement of the epiphysis, or apophysis with findings of collapse, sclerosis, and fragmentation – suggesting osteonecrosis.

bone infarct – double line sign on MR.

Kohlers	Tarsal Navicular	Male 4-6. Treatment is not surgical.
Freiberg Infraction	Second Metatarsal Head	Adolescent Girls – can lead to secondary OA
Severs	Calcaneal Apophysis	Some say this is a normal "growing pain"
Panners	Capitellum	Kid 5-10 "Thrower" ; does not have loose bodies.
Perthes	Femoral Head	White kid; 4-8.
Kienbock	Carpal Lunate	Associated with negative ulnar variance. Seen in person 20-40. *men ages* *Rare under 15*

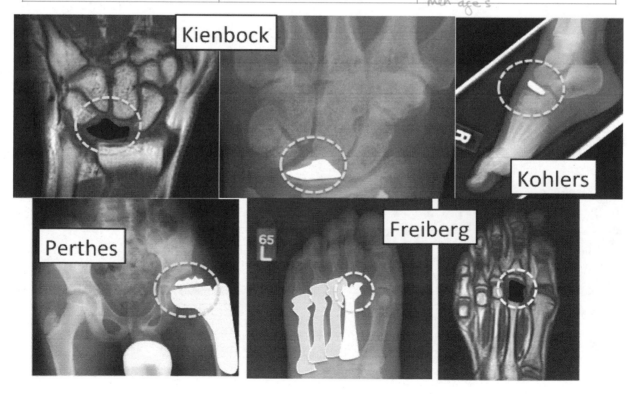

Soft Tissue Injury / Acquired *(stuff likely shown with MRI)*

MRI of the Wrist / Hand:

Don't panic if you are shown a MRI of the wrist, there are only a few things that they can show you. First let's briefly review the anatomy. With regard to the extensor tendons there are four things to know:

- There are 6 extensor compartments (5 fingers + 1 for good luck).

- First compartment (APL and EPB) are the ones affected in de Quervain's

- Third compartment has the EPL which courses beside Lister's Tubercle.

- The sixth compartment (Extensor Carpi Ulnaris) – can get an early tenosynovitis in rheumatoid arthritis.

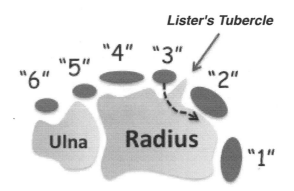

Carpal Tunnel: They could show you the carpal tunnel, but only to ask you about anatomy.

What goes through the carpal tunnel (more easily asked as what does NOT go through)?

Knowing what is in (and not in) the carpal tunnel is high yield for multiple choice testing. The tunnel lies deep to the palmaris longus, and is defined by 4 bony prominences (pisiform, scaphoid tubercle, hook of hamate, trapezium tubercle), with the transverse carpal ligament wrapping the contents in a fibrous sheath.

The tunnel contains 10 things (4 Flexor Profudus, 4 Flexor Superficials, 1 Flexor Pollicis Longus, and 1 Median Nerve). The Flexor Carpi Radialis is not truly in the tunnel. The extensor tendons are on the other side of the hand. Note that flexor pollicis longus goes through the tunnel, but flexor pollicis brevis does not (it's an intrinsic handle muscle). Palmaris longus (if you have one) does NOT go through the tunnel.

Does NOT go through the tunnel
-Flexor Carpi Radialis
-Flexor Carpi Ulnaris
-Palmaris Longus (if you have one)
-Flexor Pollicis BREVIS

Anatomic Trivia Regarding the Spaces of the Wrist:

Which synovial spaces normally communicate ? The answer is **pisiform recess and radiocarpal joint**. I can think of two ways to ask this (1) related to fluid – the bottom line is that excessive fluid in the pisiform recess should not be considered abnormal if there is a radiocarpal effusion, and (2) that either space can be used for wrist arthrography.

Other joint spaces in the body, easily lending to multiple choice testing:

Glenohumeral Joint and Subacromial Bursa	Should NOT communicate. Implies the presence of a full thickness rotator cuff tear.
Ankle Joint and Common (lateral) Peroneal Tendon Sheath	Should NOT communicate. Implies a tear of the calcaneofibular Ligament.
Achilles Tendon and Posterior Subtalar Joint	Should NOT communicate. The Achilles tendon does NOT have a true tendon sheath.
Pisifrom Recess and Radiocarpal Joint	Should normally communicate.

Common Pathology Seen on MRI of the Wrist / Hand:

Triangular Fibrocartilage Tears: These can be acute or chronic. The acute one is going to be a young person with a tear on the ulnar side. The chronic one is more likely to be shown with ulnar abutment syndrome (positive ulnar variance with cystic change in the lunate). Degeneration of this cartilage is common (50% at age 60).

Scapholunate Ligament Tear: The Terry Thomas look (gap between the scaphoid and lunate) on plain film. There are actually 3 parts (volar, dorsal, and middle), with the dorsal band being the most important for carpal stability. Predisposed for DISI deformity and all that crap I talked about earlier.

Kienbocks: AVN of the lunate, seen in people in their 20s-40s. *The most likely testable trivia is the association with negative ulnar variance.* It's going to show signal drop out on T1.

De Quervain's Tenosynovitis: This is the so called "Washer Woman's Sprain" or "Mommy Thumb" from repetitive activity / overuse. The classic history is "new mom - holding a baby." The affected area is the **first dorsal (extensor) compartment** (extensor pollicis brevis and abductor pollicis longus). This is way more common in women. The presence or absence of an intratendinous septum is a prognostic factor.

How it's shown:

- *This can be shown with ultrasound, as increased fluid within the first extensor tendon compartment*
- *This can be shown with MRI, as increased T2 signal in the tendon sheath*

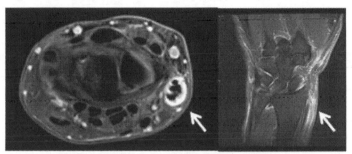

DeQuervain's Syndrome

Intersection Syndrome: A repetitive use issue (classically *seen in rowers*), where the first extensor compartment, cross over those of the second extensor compartment. The result is extensor carpi radialis brevis and longus tenosynovitis .

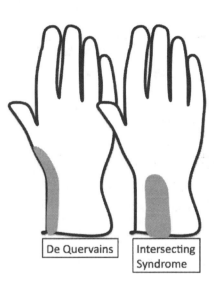

De Quervains | Intersecting Syndrome

Tenosynovitis : This is an inflammation of the tendon, with increased fluid seen around the tendon. This will be shown on MRI.

Diffuse:

- **Nontuberculous Mycobacterial Infection** – The hand and the wrist are the most common areas affected. This is a diffuse exuberant tenosynovitis that spares the muscles. It usually occurs in patients who are immunocompromised.

- **Rheumatoid Arthritis:** A nice trick is to show that multiple flexor tendons , or extensor carpi ulnaris - tenosynovitis can present as an early RA (before bone findings).

Focal:

- **Overuse:** This is going to be classic locations like 1st extensor compartment for De Quervains.

- **Infection:** The hard rule is that tenosynovitis of any flexor tendon is a surgical emergency as it can spread rapidly to the common flexors of the wrist. You can get increased pressures and necrosis of the tendons. Delayed treatment tend to do terrible.

Gamesmanship Wrist Compartments	
Isolated 1st	De Quervains
1st + 2nd	Intersecting
Isolated 6th	Early RA
Multiple Flexors	RA

Dupuytren Contracture: This is the most common of the fibromatoses. The classic scenario is a white person from North Europe with alcoholic liver disease. It's a nodular mass on the palmar aspect of the aponeurosis that progresses to cord–like thickening and eventual contracture (usually involving the 4th finger). It's bilateral about half the time.

Finger Tumor: They can show scalloping on a plain film of the finger, but if they want a single diagnosis they need to show a MRI. There is a long differential, but the only things they are going to show are:

- **Glomus Tumor:** This is a benign vascular tumor seen at the tips of fingers (75% in hand). It will be T1 low, **T2 bright**, and **enhance avidly**.

- **Giant Cell Tumor of the Tendon Sheath:** This is **basically PVNS of the tendon**. Typically found in the hand (palmar tendons). Can cause erosions on the underlying bone. Will be soft tissue density, and be **T1 and T2 dark** (contrasted to a glomus tumor which is T1 dark, T2 bright, and will enhance uniformly). **Will bloom on gradient.**

- **Fibroma:** This is a benign overgrowth of the tendon collagen. It's going to be low on T1 and low on T2. **Will NOT bloom like a GCT will.**

Finger Tip Tumors / Masses		
Glomus	T1 Dark, T2 Bright, Enhances avidly.	T2 Bright, Enhance Avidly.
Giant Cell Tumor Tendon	T1 Dark, T2 Dark, Variable Enhancement, Bloom on Gradient	Bloom on Gradient
Fibroma	T1 Dark, T2 Dark. No Blooming	Does NOT Bloom on Gradient.

Common Pathology Seen on MRI of the Elbow:

If you are shown an MRI of the Elbow don't panic, there are only a few things they can show you.

Cubital Tunnel Syndrome

- The result of repetitive valgus stress
- *Anatomy Trivia:* the site where the ulnar nerve passes beneath the cubital tunnel retinaculum also known as the epicondylo-olecranon ligament or Osborne band
- Can occur from compression by any pathology (tumor, hematoma, etc…) , when it occurs from an **accessory muscle** it's classically the **anconeus epitrochlearis**

Partial Ulnar Collateral Ligament Tear:

For the exam all you really need to know is that throwers (people who valgus over load) hurt their ulnar collateral ligament (which attaches on the medial coronoid - *sublime tubercle*). The ligament has three bundles, and the **anterior bundle is by far the most important**. If you get any images it is most likely going to be of the partial UCL tear, described as the **"T sign,"** with contrast material extending medial to the tubercle.

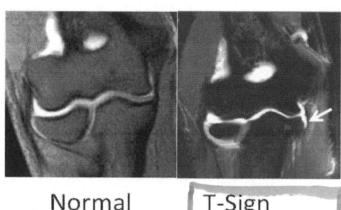

Normal

T-Sign
"UCL Partial Tear"

Panner Disease: This is one of the osteochondroses of the capitellum. It's seen in kids 5-10, and thought to be related to trauma from throwing (baseball playing). It looks a lot like an OCD lesion of the elbow (which also favors the capitellum).

Panner	Osteochondritis Dissecans
Affects the Capitellum	Also favors the Capitellum
Age 5-10	Teenager
Low T1, High T2	Low T1, High T2
No Loose Bodies	Loose Bodies

Lateral Epicondylitis *(more common than medial) – seen in Tennis Players -*
- Extensor Tendon Injury (classically extensor carpi radialis brevis)
- Radial Collateral Ligament Complex – Tears due to varus stress

Medial Epicondylitis *(less common than lateral) – seen in golfers*
- Common flexor tendon and ulnar nerve may enlarge from chronic injury

Epitrochlear Lymphadenopathy – This is a classic look for cat-scratch disease.

Dialysis Elbow: This is the result of olecranon bursitis from constant pressure on the area, related to positioning of the arm during treatment.

—

Common Pathology Seen on MRI of the Shoulder:

Impingement / Rotator Cuff Tears: This is a high yield / confusing subject that is worth talking about in a little more detail. In general, rotator cuff pathology is the result of overuse activity (sports) or impingement mechanisms. There are two types of impingement with two major sub-divisions within those types. Like many things in Radiology if you get the vocabulary down, the pathology is easy to understand.

External: This refers to impingement of the rotator cuff overlying the bursal surfaces (superficial surfaces) that are adjacent to the coracoacromial arch. As a reminder the arch is made up of the coracoid process, acromion, and coracoacromial ligament.

Primary External Causes (Abnormal Coracoacromial Arch) :

• The **hooked acromion** (type III Bigliani) is more associated with external impingement than the curved or flat types.

• **Subacromial osteophyte formation** or thickening of the coracoacromial ligament

• **Subcoracoid impingement**: Impingement of the subscapularis between the coracoid process and lesser tuberosity. This can be secondary to congenital configuration, or a configuration developed post traumatically after fracture of the coracoid or lesser tuberosity.

Secondary External Causes (Normal Coracoacromial Arch):

• **"Multidirectional Glenohumeral Instability"** – resulting in micro-subluxation of the humeral head in the glenoid, resulting in repeated microtrauma. The important thing to know is this is *typically seen in patients with generalized joint laxity,* often involving both shoulders.

Internal: This refers to impingement of the rotator cuff on the undersurface (deep surface) along the glenoid labrum and humeral head.

• **Posterior Superior:** This is a type of impingement that occurs when the posterior superior rotator cuff (junction of the supra and infraspinatus tendons) comes into contact with the posterior superior glenoid. Best seen in the ABER position, where these tendons get pinched between the labrum and greater tuberosity. This is seen in athletes who make overhead movements (throwers, tennis, swimming).

• **Anterior Superior:** This is internal impingement that occurs when the arm is in horizontal adduction and internal rotation. In this position, the undersurface of the biceps and subscapularis tendon may impinge against the anterior superior glenoid rim.

High Yield Trivia Points on Impingement	
Subacromial Impingement – most common form, resulting from attrition of the coracoacromial arch.	Damages **Supraspinatus Tendon**.
Subcoracoid Impingement – Lesser tuberosity and coracoid do the pinching.	Damages **Subscapularis**
Posterior Superior Internal Impingement – Athletes who make overhead movements. Greater tuberosity and posterior inferior labrum do the pinching.	Damage **Infraspinatus** (and posterior fibers of the supraspinatus).

Rotator Cuff Tears: A tear of the articular surface is more common (3x more) than the bursal surface. The underlying mechanism is usually degenerative, although trauma can certainly play a role. The **most common of the four muscles to tear is the Supraspinatus.** The teres minor is the least common to tear. **A partial tear that is > 50% is what the surgeon wants to know**.

"Massive rotator cuff tear" - refers to at least 2 out of the 4 rotator cuff muscles.

A final general piece of trivia is that a tear of the fibrous rotator cuff interval (junction between anterior fibers of the Supraspinatus and superior fibers of the subscapularis), is still considered a rotator cuff tear.

How do you know it's a full thickness tear? You will have high T2 signal in the expected location of the tendon. On T1 you will have **Gad in the bursa.**

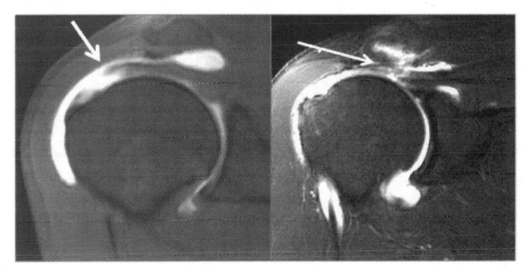

Full Thickness Tear

- With Gad crossing over the cuff into the bursa.

Injury to the Labrum:

SLAP: Labral tears favor the <u>superior</u> margin and track anterior to posterior. As this tear involves the labrum at the insertion of the long head of the biceps ,injury to this tendon is associated and part of the grading system (type 4).

Things to know about SLAP tears:

- When the SLAP extends into the biceps anchor (type 4) the surgical management changes from a debridement to a debridement + biceps tenodesis.

- The mechanism is usually an over-head movement (classic = swimmer)

- People over 40 usually have associated Rotator Cuff Tears injury

- **NOT associated with Instability** *(usually)*

SLAP Mimic - The Sublabral Recess. This is essentially a normal variant where you have incomplete attachment of the labrum at 12 o'clock. The 12 o'clock position on the labrum has the shittiest blood flow - that's why you see injury there and all these development variants.

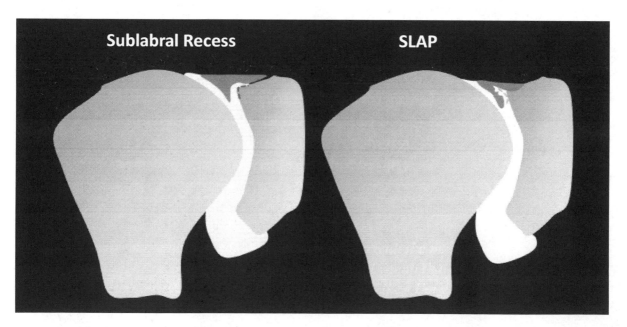

Sublabral Recess	SLAP
Follows Contour of Glenoid	Extends Laterally
SMOOTH Margin	Ratty Margin
Located at Biceps Anchor	Located at Biceps Anchor & Posteriorly

Labral Tear Mimic - The Sublabral Foramen -
The is an unattached (but present) portion of the
labrum - located at the anterior-superior labrum
(1 o'clock to 3 o'clock).

As a rule it should NOT extend below the equator
(3 o'clock position).

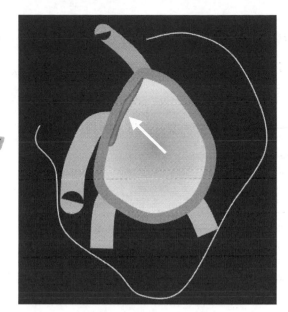

Labral Tear Mimic - The Buford Complex - A commonly tested (and not infrequently
seen) variant is the Buford Complex. It's present in about 1% of the general population. This
consists of an **absent anterior/superior labrum** (1 o'clock to 3 o'clock)**, along with a
thickened middle glenohumeral ligament**.

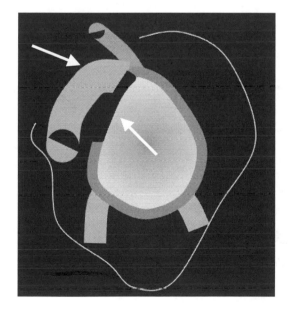

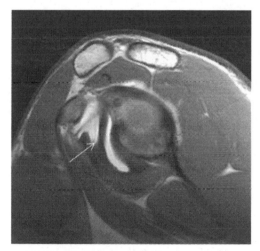

Buford Complex
-Thick Middle GH Ligament

Bankart Lesions: There is an alphabet soup of Bankart (anterior dislocation) related injuries.

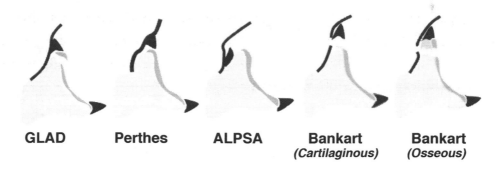

| GLAD | Perthes | ALPSA | Bankart *(Cartilaginous)* | Bankart *(Osseous)* |

GLAD = Glenolabral Articular Disruption. It's the most mild version, and it's basically a superficial anterior inferior labral tear with associated articular cartilage damage ("impaction injury with cartilage defect"). Not typically seen in patient's with underlying laxity. It's common in sports. **No instability** *(aren't you GLAD there is no instability)*

Perthes = Detachment of the anteroinferior labrum (3-6 o'clock) with medially stripped but *intact periosteum*.

ALPSA = Anterior Labral Periosteal Sleeve Avulsion. Medially displaced labroligamentous complex with absence of the labrum on the glenoid rim. *Intact periosteum*. It scars down to glenoid.

True Bankart: Can be cartilaginous or osseous. *The periosteum is disrupted*. There is often an associated Hill Sach's fracture.

GLAD	Perthes	ALPSA	True Bankart
Superficial partial labral injury with cartilage defect	Avulsed anterior labrum (only minimally displaced). Inferior GH complex still attached to periosteum	Similar to perthes but with "bunched up" medially displaced inferior GH complex	Torn labrum
No instability	Intact Periosteum (lifted up)	Intact Periosteum	*Periosteum Disrupted*

Misc - Shoulder

HAGL: A non Bankart lesion that is frequently tested is the **HAGL** (Humeral avulsion glenohumeral ligament). This is an **avulsion of the inferior glenohumeral ligament**, and is most often the result of an anterior shoulder dislocation (just like all the above bankarts). The "J Sign" occurs when the normal U-shaped inferior glenohumeral recess is retracted away from the humerus appearing as a J.

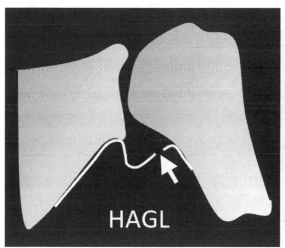 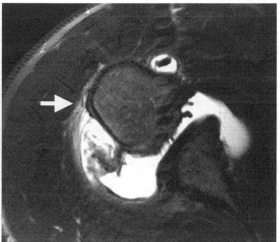

Subluxation of the Biceps Tendon: The subscapularis attaches to the lesser tuberosity. It sends a few fibers across the bicipital groove to the greater tuberosity ,which is called the "transverse ligament". A tear of the subscapularis opens these fibers up and allows the biceps to dislocate (usually medial). **Subscapularis Tear = Medial Dislocation of the Long Head of the Biceps Tendon.**

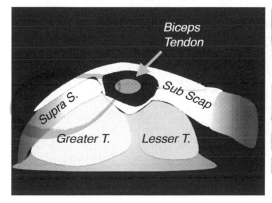 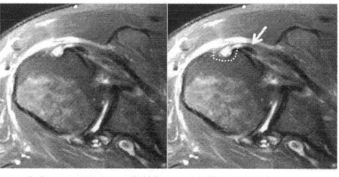

Sub Scap Tendon - Forming portions of the *"Transverse Ligament"* that holds the biceps tendon in the grove

Subluxation of Biceps Tendon
Occurs with Tear of the Subscapularis

Nerve Entrapment: *High Yield Trivia:*

Suprascapular Notch vs Spinoglenoid Notch: A cyst at the level of the suprascapular notch will affect the supraspinatus and the infraspinatus. At the level of the spinoglenoid notch it will only affect the infraspinatus.

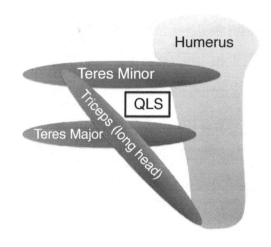

***Dotted Line = Suprascapular Nerve

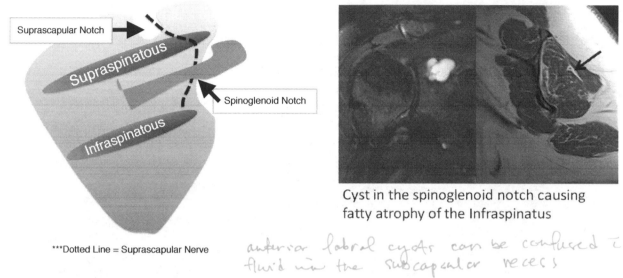

Cyst in the spinoglenoid notch causing fatty atrophy of the Infraspinatus

anterior labral cysts can be confused c̄ fluid in the subcapular recess

Quadrilateral Space Syndrome: Compression of the Axillary Nerve in the Quadrilateral Space (usually from fibrotic bands). They will likely show this with **atrophy of the teres minor**. Another classic question is to name the borders of the quadrilateral space: Teres Minor Above, Teres Major Below, Humeral neck lateral, and Triceps medial.

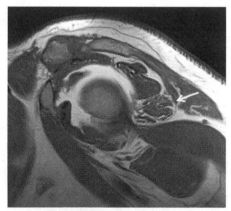

Quadrilateral Space Syndrome – Atrophy of Teres Minor

Parsonage-Turner Syndrome: Think about this when you see muscles affected by pathology in two or more nerve distributions (suprascapular and axillary etc..). The condition is an idiopathic involvement of the brachial plexus.

MRI of the Knee

I want to focus on how the ABR is likely to ask the questions with two main pathways: (1) Total Trivia (2) Aunt Minnie Images

Anatomy:

Ligaments: The ACL has two bundles. The long one (anteromedial) tightens the knee in flexion. The short one (posterior lateral) tightens the knee in extension. The PCL is the strongest ligament in the knee (you don't want a posterior dislocation of your knee resulting in dissection of your popliteal artery).

Meniscus: The meniscus is "C shaped", thick along the periphery and thin centrally. There are two main things to know about the meniscus:

- Medial meniscus is thicker posteriorly. Lateral meniscus has equal thickness between anterior and posterior portion.

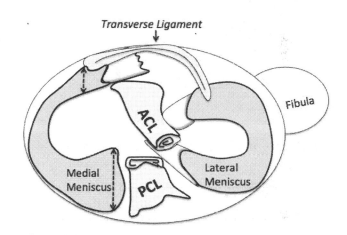

- The Peripheral "Red Zone" is vascular and might heal. The Central "white zone" is avascular and will not heal.

- The blood supply comes from the geniculate arteries (which enter peripherally).

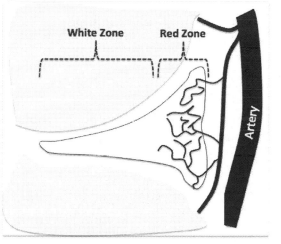

- There are two meniscofemoral ligaments (Wrisberg, Humphry) which can be mimics of meniscal tears. Wrisberg is in the back (*"humping Humphry"*). You could also remember that "H" comes before "W" in the alphabet.

Tendons:

- The conjoint tendon is formed by the biceps femoris tendon and the LCL.

- The PCL and Patellar tendon may have foci of intermediate signal intensity on sagittal images with short echo time (TE) sequences where the tendon forms an angle of 55 degrees with the main magnetic field (***magic angle phenomenon***). This will NOT be seen on T2 sequences (with long TE). This phenomenon is reduced at higher field strengths due to greater shortening of T2 relaxation times.

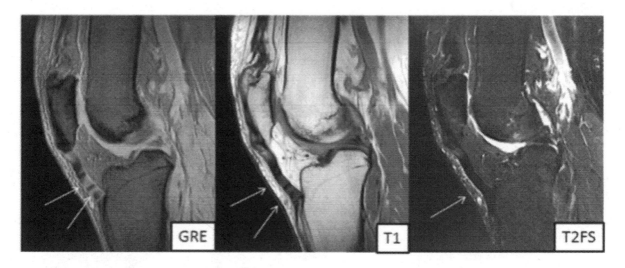

Magic Angle: You see it on short TE sequences (T1, PD, GRE). It goes away on T2.

Pathology:

Meniscal Tears: The peripheral meniscus (red zone) has better vasculature than the inner 2/3s (white zone) and might heal on its own. Broadly you can think about tears as either vertical or horizontal. Vertical tears can be sub divided into radial and longitudinal.

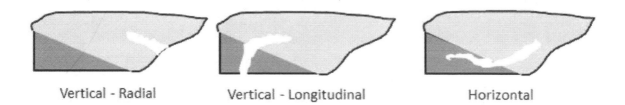

Vertical - Radial   Vertical - Longitudinal   Horizontal

Meniscal cysts are most often seen near the lateral meniscus and are often associated with horizontal cleavage tears.

Meniscocapsular Separation: The deepest layer of the **MCL** complex (capsular ligament) is relatively weak and is the first to tear; therefore there is an association with meniscocapsular separation.

Bakers Cyst:

Occurs between the semimembranosus and the MEDIAL head of the gastric

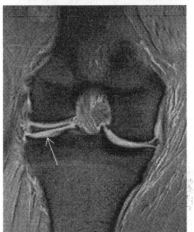

Discoid Meniscus: This is a normal variant of the **lateral meniscus** that is **prone to tear.** It's not C-shaped, but instead shaped like a disc. In other words, it's too big (too many bow-ties!).

There are three types, with the most rare and most prone to injury being the *Wrisberg Variant*.

Discoid Meniscus

Bucket Handle Tear: This is a torn meniscus (usually **medial** - 80%), that flips medially to lie anterior to the PCL. The classic Aunt Minnie appearance is that of a "**double PCL.**" Another piece of trivia is that a double PCL can **only occur in the setting of an intact ACL**, otherwise it won't flip that way. Just know it sorta indirectly proves the ACL is intact (I can just see some knucklehead asking that).

vertical tear
presents c locking of the knee

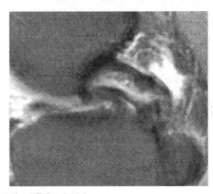

Double PCL
-Bucket Handle Meniscal Tear

Meniscal Ossicle: This is a focal ossification of the posterior horn of the medial meniscus, that can be secondary to trauma or simply developmental. They are often associated with radial root tears.

ACL Tear: ACL tears happen all the time, usually in people who are stopping and pivoting.

Things to know about ACL tears:
- Associated with Segond Fracture
- ACL Angle lesser than Blumensaat's Line
- **O'donoghue's Unhappy Triad: ACL Tear, MCL Tear, Medial Meniscal**
- *Classic Kissing Contusion Pattern:* The lateral femoral condyle (sulcus terminals) bangs into the posterior lateral tibial plateau. This is 95% specific in adults.

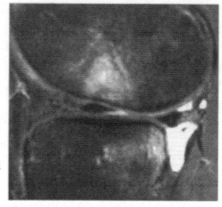

ACL Tear
"Kissing Contusion Pattern"

ACL Mucoid Degeneration: This can mimic acute or chronic partial tear of the ACL. There will be no secondary signs of injury (contusion etc..). It predisposes to ACL **ganglion cysts,** and they are usually seen together. The **T2/STIR buzzword is "celery stalk"** because of the striated look. The T1 **buzzword is "drumstick"** because it looks like a drum stick.

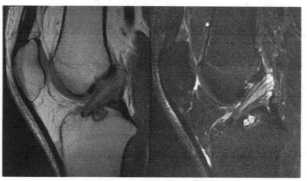

Mucoid Degeneration of ACL
-"Drumstick / Celery Stick"

ACL Repair:

- Method 1: Using the middle one-third of the patellar tendon, with the patella bone plug attached to one end and tibial bone plug attached at the other.

- Method 2: Use a four-strand hamstring graft often made of semitendinosus or gracilis tendon, or both. Then fold and braid the segment to form a quadruple-thickness structure. The graft is then attached with interference screws, endobuttons, or staples. There is a lower reported morbidity related to harvest site using this method.

Posterior Lateral Corner (PLC)- The most complicated anatomy in the entire body. My God this posterior lateral corner! Just think about the LCL, the IT band, the biceps femoris, and the popliteus tendon. If you see injury to any of those (or edema in the fibular head), you need to question PLC injury (instability).

Who cares? *Missed PLC injury is a very common cause of ACL reconstruction failure.*

Complications:

"Roof Impingement" – If the tibial tunnel is placed too far anterior (partially or completely anterior to the intersection of the Blumensaat line), the graft may bump up against the anterior inferior margin of the intercondylar roof. The **positioning of the tibial tunnel is the primary factor in preventing impingement**.

"Maintaining Isometry" – *"Isometry"* is a word Orthopods use to define constant length and tension of the graft during full range of motion. Positioning of the **femoral tunnel** is the primary factor in maintaining isometry.

"Arthrofibrosis" Can be focal or diffuse (focal is more common). The focal form is the so called **"Cyclops" lesion** – so named because of its arthroscopic appearance. It's gonna be a low signal speculated mass-like scar in Hoffa's fat pad. It's bad because it limits extension.

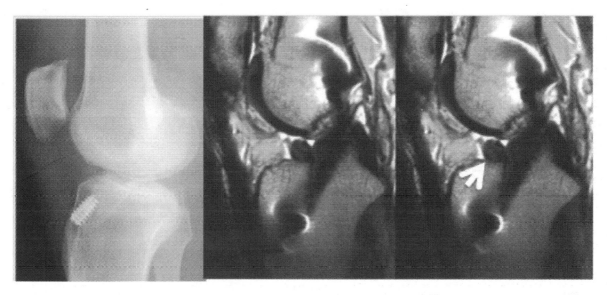

Cyclops Lesion – Scar associated with ventral graft

"Graft Tear" The graft is most susceptible to tear in the remodeling process (4-8 months post op). Signs of graft tear are increased T2 signal, and fiber discontinuity. Uncovering of the posterior horn of the lateral meniscus, and anterior tibial translation are considered good secondary signs.

PCL Tear: The posterior collateral ligament is the strongest ligament in the knee. A tear is actually uncommon, but you should think about it with a posterior dislocation.

Patella Dislocation - Dislocation of the patella is usually lateral because of the shape of the patella and femur. The contusion pattern is classic.

Things to know about Patella Dislocation:
- It's Lateral
- Contusion Pattern - Classic
- Associated tear of the MPFL (medial patellar femoral ligament)

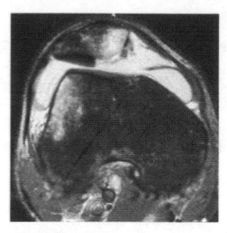

Patella Dislocation
Classic Contusion Pattern

—

The Foot / Ankle:

I'll lead with the most likely anatomic trivia, which is the tendons at the medial and lateral ankle.

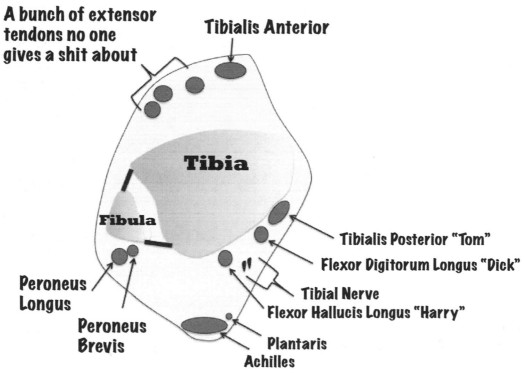

The Mythical **Master Knot of Henry** - This has a funny sounding name, therefore it's high yield. This is where Dick (FDL) crosses over Harry (FHL) at the medial ankle.

Whats the Master Knot of Henry? It's a "Harry Dick"

Common Pathology Seen on MRI of the Ankle / Foot:

Ligamentous Injury: The highest yield fact is that the **anterior talofibular ligament is the weakest ligament and the most frequently injured** (usually from inversion).

Posterior Tibial Tendon Injury / Dysfunction: This results in a progressive flat foot deformity, as the PTT is the primary stabilizer of the longitudinal arch. When chronic, the tear is most common behind the medial malleolus (this is where the most friction is). When acute, the tear is most common at the insertion into the navicular bone. **Acute Flat Arch should make you think of PTT tear.** You will also have a hindfoot valgus deformity (from unopposed peroneal brevis action). The other point of trivia to know is that the spring ligament is a secondary supporter of the arch (it holds up the talar head), and it will thicken and degenerate without the help of the PTT. Don't get it twisted though, the spring ligament is very thick and strong and almost never ruptures in a foot/ankle trauma.

I Say Acute Flat Foot, You Say Posterior Tibial Tendon Injury

Classic Progression - *PTT out then Spring Ligament Out, Then Sinus Tarsi gets jacked, then you heel strike on a painful flat foot and get plantar fasciitis*

Split Peroneus Brevis: You can see longitudinal splits in the peroneus in people with inversion injuries. The history is usually "chronic ankle pain". The tendon will be C shaped or **boomerang shaped** with central thinning and partial envelopment of the peroneus longus. Alternatively, there may be 3 instead of 2 tendons. The tear occurs at the lateral malleolus. There is a strong (80%) association with lateral ligament injury.

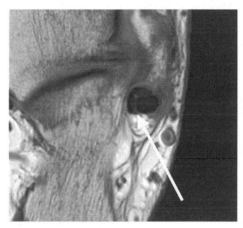

Split Peroneus Brevis
-Boomerang

Anterolateral Impingement Syndrome: Injury to the anterior talofibular ligaments and tibiofibular ligaments (usually from an inversion injury) can cause lateral instability, and chronic synovial inflammation. You can eventually produce a "mass" of hypertrophic synovial tissue in the lateral gutter. The **MRI finding is a "meniscoid mass" in the lateral gutter of the ankle**, which is a balled up scar (**T1 and T2 dark**).

Sinus Tarsi Syndrome: The space between the lateral talus and calcaneus. The syndrome is caused by hemorrhage or inflammation of the synovial recess with or without tears of the associated ligaments (talocalcaneal ligaments, inferior extensor retinaculum). There are associations with rheumatologic disorders and abnormal loading (flat foot in the setting of a posterior tibial tendon tear). The **MRI finding is obliteration of fat in the sinus tarsi space**, and replacement with scar.

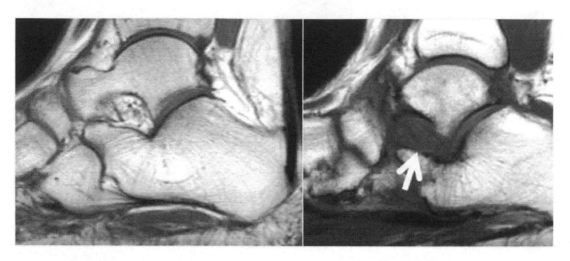

Normal Sinus Tarsi -Full of Fat
Sinus Tarsi Syndrome -Full of Scar

Tarsal Tunnel Syndrome: Pain in the distribution of the tibial nerve (first 3 toes), from compression as it passes through the tarsal tunnel (behind the medial malleolus). It's usually unilateral (unlike carpal tunnel which is usually bilateral).

Achilles Tendon Injury: Acute rupture is usually obvious. The ability to plantar flex should be lost on exam (*unless a plantaris muscle is intact - a common trick question*).

Xanthoma: Think about a xanthoma if the Achilles tendon is really enlarged / fusiform thickened. This can be seen in people with familial hypercholesterolemia, and is often bilateral.

Plantar Fasciitis: This is an inflammation of the fascia secondary to repetitive trauma. The pain is localized to the origin of the plantar fascia, and worsened by dorsiflexion of the toes. Buzzword is "***most severe in the morning.***" Plain film might show heel spurs, MRI may show a thickened fascia (> 4mm) , with increased T2 signal, most significant near its insertion at the heel. A bone scan may show increased tracer in the region of the calcaneus (from periosteal inflammation).

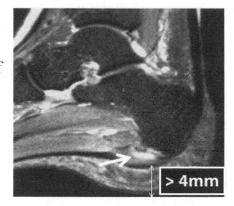

Plantar Fasciitis

Morton's Neuroma: Soft tissue mass shown between the 3rd and 4th metatarsal heads is most likely a Morton's Neuroma (especially on multiple choice tests). They classically show it on short axis, T1 (it will be dark). The proposed pathology results from compression / entrapment of the plantar digital nerve in this location by the intermetatarsal ligament. Over time this results in thickening and development of perineural fibrosis.

It's a big stupid scar, that looks like a dumbbell between the 3rd and 4th metatarsals. It's usually unilateral in a women.

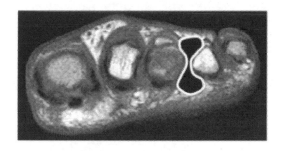

Morton's Neuroma
-Dumbbell Scar Between 3rd and 4th Metatarsals

Infection

Infection

With regard to osteomyelitis, radiographs will be normal for 7-10 days. Essentially, osteomyelitis can have any appearance , occur in any location, and at any age. Children have hematogenous spread usually hitting the long bones (metaphysis). Adults are more likely to have direct spread (in diabetic). However, you can have hematogenous spread in certain situations as well. General rule is that septic joins are more common in adults, osteomyeltitis is more common in kids.

Knee Jerks:
- *Osteomyelitis in Spine = IV Drug User*
- *Osteomyelitis in Spine with Kyphosis = Gibbus Deformity = TB*
- *Unilateral SI joint = IV Drug User*
- *Psoas Muscle Abscess = TB*

Hallmarks are destruction of bone and periosteal new bone formation.

Brodie's Abscess is a chronic infection (bone abscess). It's usually well circumscribed. It may have an osseous sequestrum (piece of necrotic bone surrounded by granulation tissue). As mentioned above, a sequestration has a DDx (Osetomyelitis, EG, Lymphoma, Fibrosarcoma).

Some frequently tested vocabulary:
- *Sequestrum = Piece of necrotic bone surround by granulation tissue*
- *Involucrum = Thick sheath of periosteal bone around sequestrum*
- *Cloaca = The space /tract where there dead bone lives*

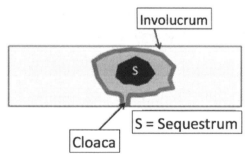

Acute bacterial osteomyelitis can be thought of in three different categories: 1) hematogenous seeding (*most common in child*), 2) contiguous spread, and 3) direct inoculation of the bone either from surgery or trauma.

Acute hematogenous osteomyelitis has a predilection for the long bones of the body, specifically the metaphysis, which has the best blood flow and allows for spreading of the infection via small channels in the bone that lead to the subperiosteal space.

More Trivia that Multiple Choice Writers Love:
- *Age < 1 month = Multicentric involvement, **often with joint involvement***
  - *Bone scan often negative (75%) at this age*
- *Age < 18 months = Spread to epiphysis through blood*
- *Age 2-16 years = Trans-physeal vessels are closed (primary focus is metaphysis).*

In the slightly older baby (<18 months) these vessels from the metaphysis to the epiphysis atrophy and the growth plate stops the spread (although spread can still occur). This creates a "septic tank" effect. This same thing happens with certain cancers (leukemia); the garbage gets stuck in the septic tank (metaphysis). Once the growth plates fuse, this obstruction is no longer present.

MRI findings of osteomyelitis: Low signal in the bone marrow on T1 imaging adjacent to an ulcer or cellulitis is diagnostic.

The Ghost Sign: *Neuropathic Bone vs Osteomyelitis in a Neuropathic Bone*
A bone that becomes a ghost (poor definition of margins) on T1 imaging, but then re-appears (more morphologically distinct) on T2, or after giving IV contrast is more likely to have osteomyelitis.

Discitis/ Osteomyelitis:

Infection of the disc and infection of the vertebral body nearly always go together. The reason has to do with the route of seeding; which typically involves seeding of the vertebral endplate (which is vascular), with subsequent eruption and crossing into the disc space, and eventual involvement of the adjacent vertebral body.

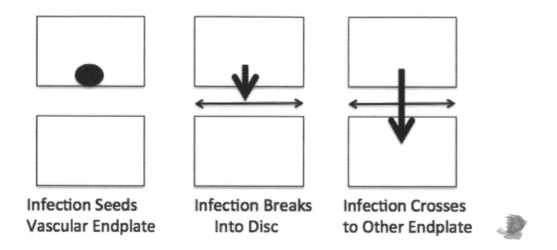

Infection Seeds Vascular Endplate   **Infection Breaks Into Disc**   **Infection Crosses to Other Endplate**

In adults, the source is usually from a recent surgery, procedure, or systemic infection. In children it's usually from hematogenous spread. For the Step 1 trivia: Staph A is the most common bug, and think gram negatives with an IV drug user. Almost always (80% of the time) the ESR and CRP are elevated.

Imaging: Early on it's very hard to see with plain films, you will need MRI. You are looking for paraspinal and epidural inflammation, T2 bright disc signal, and disc enhancement. Remember Gallium is superior to WBC scan in the spine. *This is discussed in the neuro chapter - spine section.*

Pott's Disease: TB of the spine is more common in "developing" countries. It behaves in a few different ways, and that makes it easy to test on.

Things to know about TB in the spine:
- *It tends to **spare the disc space***
- *It tends to have multi-level thoracic "skip" involvement*
- *Buzzword "Large paraspinal abscess*
- *Buzzword "Calcified Psoas Abscess"*
- *Buzzword "Gibbus Deformity" – which is a destructive focal kyphosis*

Mimic - Brucellosis (unpasteurized milk from an Amish Person) , can also have some disc space preservation.

Septic Arthritis You see this the most in large joints which have an abundant blood supply to the metaphysis (shoulder, hip, knee). *IV drug users will get it in the SI joint, and sternoclavicular joint.* Conventional risk factors include being old, having AIDS, RA, and prosthetic joints. On plain film you might see a joint effusion, or MRI will show synovial enhancement. If untreated this will jack your joint in less than 48hours.

> *Pneumoarthrogram Sign*
> - If you can demonstrate air within a joint - you can exclude a joint effusion. No joint effusion = No septic joint.

Necrotizing Fasciitis: This is a very bad actor that kills very quickly. The good news is that it's pretty rare, typically only seen in HIVers, Transplant patients, diabetics, and alcoholics. It's usually polymicrobial (the second form is Group A Strep). **Gas is only seen in a minority of cases, but if you see gas in soft tissue this is what they want.** Diffuse fascial enhancement is what you'd see if the ER is dumb enough to order cross sectional imaging (they often are). Fournier Gangrene is what they call it in the scrotum.

TB: This is a special topic (high yield) with regard to MSK infection. It's not that common, with <5% of patients with TB having MSK involvement. Although on multiple choice tests, I think you'll find it appears with a high frequency.

Key Points to know:
- The vertebral body is involved with sparing of the disc space until late in the disease (very different than more common bacterial infections).
- *"Gibbus Deformity"* is a focal kyphosis seen in "Potts Disease", among many other things.
- *"Rice Bodies"* – These are sloughed, infarcted synovium seen with end stage RA, and TB infection of joints.
- *Tuberculosis Dactylitis (Spina Ventosa)* – Typically affects kids more than adults with involvement of the short tubular bones of the hands and feet. It is often a smoldering infection without periosteal reaction. Classic look is a **diaphyseal expansile lesion** with soft tissue swelling.

Aggressive Lesions

There are tons of primary osseous malignancies, the most common are myeloma/ plasmacytoma (27%), Osteosarcoma (20%) and Chondrosarcoma (20%). According to Helms, the **wide zone of transition is the best sign that a lesion is aggressive**. This is actually a useful pearl.

Myeloma / Plasmacytoma / Mets - *Discussed in the cystic bone lesion section*

Osteosarcoma: There are a bunch of subtypes, but for the purpose of this discussion there are 4. Conventional Intramedullary (85%), Parosteal (4%), Periosteal (1%), Telangiectatic (rare). All the subtypes produce bone or osteoid from neoplastic cells. Most are idiopathic but you can have secondary causes (*usually seen in elderly*) XRT, Pagets, Infarcts, etc…

Conventional Intramedullary: More common, and higher grade than the surface subtypes (periosteal, and parosteal). Primary subtypes typically occur in young patients (10-20). The most common location is the femur (40%), and proximal tibia (15%).

Buzzwords include various types of aggressive periosteal reactions:

- *"Sunburst"-* periosteal reaction that is aggressive and looks like a sunburst
- *Codman triangle -* With aggressive lesions, the periosteum does not have time to ossify completely with new bone (e.g. as seen in single layer and multi-layered periosteal reaction), so only the edge of the raised periosteum will ossify – creating the appearance of a triangle.
- *Lamellated* (onion skin reaction) – multi layers of parallel periosteum, looks like an onion's skin.

High Yield Trivia:
- *Osteosarcoma met to the lung is a "classic" (frequently tested) cause of occult pneumothorax.*
- **"Reverse Zoning Phenomenon"** – more dense mature matrix in the center, less peripherally (*opposite of myositis ossificans*).

Pathologic Fracture - At risk ?

Reasons to be concerned include:

(1) Lytic lesions,
(2) Lesions > 3cm in size,
(3) Lesions involving more than 50% of the cortex.

These measurements are CT or Plain film… NOT MRI.

Parosteal Osteosarcoma: Generally low grade, **BULKY** parosteal bone formation. Think Big… just say Big. This guy loves the posterior distal femur (*because of this location it can mimic a cortical desmoid early on*). The lesion is metaphyseal 90% of the time. The buzzword is "***string sign***" – which refers to a radiolucent line separating the bulky tumor from the cortex.

Periosteal Osteosarcoma
Worse prognosis than parosteal but better than conventional osteosarcoma. Tends to occur in the diaphyseal regions, classic medial distal femur.

This vs That: **Parosteal vs Periosteal Osteosarcoma**	
Parosteal	**Periosteal**
Early Adult / Middle Age	Age Group (15-25)
Metaphysis (90%)	Diaphyseal
Likes Posterior Distal Femur	Likes Medial Distal Femur
Marrow extension (50%)	Usually no marrow extension
Low Grade	Intermediate Grade

Telangiectatic Osteosarcoma: About 15% have a narrow zone of transition. Fluid-Fluid levels on MRI is classic. They are High on T1 (from methemoglobin). Can be differentiated from ABC or GCT (maybe) by tumor nodularity and enhancement.

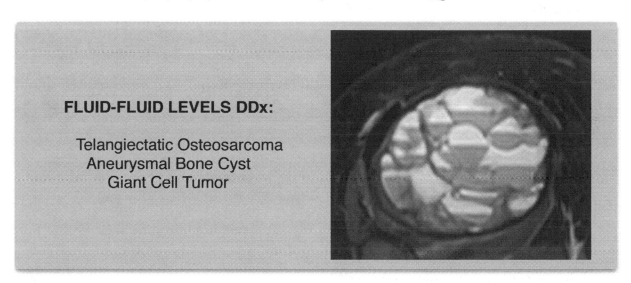

FLUID-FLUID LEVELS DDx:

Telangiectatic Osteosarcoma
Aneurysmal Bone Cyst
Giant Cell Tumor

Chondrosarcoma: Usually seen in older adults (M>F). Likes flat bones, limb girdles, proximal tubular bones. Can be central (intramedullary) or peripheral (at the end of an osteochondroma). Most are low grade.

Risk Factors: Pagets, and anything cartilaginous (osteochondromas, maffucci's etc…)

If you want to say chondroblastoma but it's an adult think clear cell chondrosarcoma

Ewings: *Permeative lesion in the diaphysis of a child = Ewings (could also be infection, or EG).* Extremely rare in African-Americans. Likes to met bone to bone. Does NOT form osteoid from tumor cells, but can mimic osteosarcoma because of its marked sclerosis (*sclerosis occurs in the bone only, not in the soft tissue – which is NOT the case in osteosarcoma*).

Chordoma Usually seen in adults (30-60), usually slightly younger in the clivus and slightly older in the sacrum. Most likely questions regarding the chordoma include location (**most common sacrum**, second most common clivus, third most common vertebral body), and the fact that they are **very T2 bright**.

Chordoma Most Commons:
* Most common primary malignancy of the spine.
* Most common primary malignancy of the sacrum.
* When involving the spine, most common at C2.
* Midline, Midline, Midline!

Aggressive Soft Tissue Lesions

Fibrosarcoma / Malignant Fibrous Histiocytoma (MFH)

* **Fibrosarcoma:** Just like osteosarcoma can be primary or secondary (from Pagets, infarct etc..) These are lytic malignant tumors that DO NOT produce osteoid or chondroid matrix. They are almost **"Always Lytic",** and may be permeative or moth eaten. Also **"NOT T2 Bright"** – which most tumors are.

* **MFH: Now called Pleomorphic Undifferentiated Sarcoma "PUS."** This actually used to be lumped in with Fibrosarcoma – but now they are separate. MFHs are way more common than Fibrosarcomas (*most common soft tissue sarcoma in adults*). From a radiology perspective, they look the same. So when you say one you should say the other.

   Trivia: Bone infarcts can turn into MFH - *"sarcomatous transformation of infarct"*

   Pearl: I like the old name "Fibrous" - because it reminds me that parts of the tumor will be dark on MR.

Synovial Sarcoma: Seen most commonly in the lower extremities of patients aged 20-40. They occur close to the joint (but **not in the joint**). To confuse the issue they may have secondary invasion into the joint (10%), however for the purpose of multiple choice tests they "never involve the joint."

They could show this tumor in 3 different ways: (1) as the "**triple sign**", which is high, medium, and low signal all in the same mass (probably in the knee) on T2, (2) as the "**bowl of grapes**" which is a bunch of fluid –fluid levels in a mass (probably in the knee), or (3) as a plain x-ray with a soft tissue component and calcifications – this would be the least likely way to show it.

Synovial Sarcoma Trivia:
- Most sarcomas don't attack bones; Synovial Sarcoma Can
- Most sarcomas present as painless mass; Synovial Sarcomas Hurt
- Soft tissue calcifications + Bone Erosions are highly suggestive
- They are slow growing and small in size often leading to people thinking they are B9.
- 90% have a translocation of X-18.
- Most common malignancy in teens/young adults of the **foot**, ankle, and lower extremity

When I say "Ball like tumor" in the extremity of a young adult, you say Synovial Sarcoma.

Liposarcoma - This is the second most common soft tissue sarcoma. You see it in middle aged people (40-60), with the classic location being the **retroperitoneum** (can also happen in the extremities). The most common type (well-differentiated) is also the least aggressive.

When I say "Fatty Mass in the retroperitoneum," you say Liposarcoma

Things that make you think it is a liposarcoma (and not a lipoma)
- Inhomogenous attenuation - soft tissues masses in the fat
- Infiltration of adjacent structures
- "Deep and Big"

Trivia: Myxoid Liposarcoma is the MC liposarcoma in patients < 20. - They can be T2 Bright (expected), but T1 dark (confusing) - don't call it a cyst. Don't call it a comeback (I've been here for years). They'll need gad+

Lymphoma - *Discussed in the peds chapter.*

Treatment High Yields

- *Osteosarcoma:* Chemo first (to kill micro mets) , followed by wide excision
- *Ewings:* Both Chemo and Radiation, followed by wide excision.
- *Chondrosarcoma:* usually just wide excision (they are usually low grade, and main concern is local recurrence).
- *Giant Cell Tumor:* Because it extends to the articular surface usually requires arthroplasty.

"Don't Touch Lesions" – Characteristically Benign Lesions, that look Aggressive but are NOT – and should NOT be biopsied because of possibly misleading pathology.		
Myositis Ossificans	Circumferential calcifications with a lucent center	Can look scary on MRI if imaged early because of edema, and avid enhancement
Avulsion Injury	Typical location near the pelvis	Can have an aggressive periosteal reaction
Cortical Desmoid	Characteristic location on the posterior medial epicondyle of the distal femur	Can be hot on bone scan.
Synovial Herniation Pit "Pitt's Pit"	Characteristic location in the femoral neck	Lytic appearing lesion

Bone Biopsy - The route of biopsy should be discussed with the orthopedic surgeon, to avoid contaminating compartments not involved by the tumor (or not going to be used in the resection process).

Special considerations:
- Pelvis: Avoid crossing gluteal muscles (may be needed for reconstruction).
- Knee: Avoid the joint space via crossing suprapatellar bursa or other communicating bursae. Avoid crossing the quadriceps tendon unless it is involved.
- Shoulder: Avoid the posterior 2/3rd (axillary nerve courses post -> anterior, therefore a posterior resection will denervate the anterior 1/3).

B9 Lesions

FEGNOMASHIC is the mnemonic for cystic bone lesions made popular by Clyde Helms. As it turns out, you can rearrange the letters of FEGNOMASHIC to form a word FOGMACHINES. I find it a lot easier to remember a mnemonic if it actually forms a real word. Having said that the whole idea of memorizing a list of 11 or 12 things is really stupid. You would never give a differential that included all of those, they occur in different places, in different ages, and often look very different. Differentials (for people who know what they are looking at) are usually never deeper than 3 or 4 things. If you are giving a differential of 12 things, just say you don't know what it is.

First a brief discussion of location & Age

> **Age:**
>
> The key to remember is that
> - < 30 = EG, ABC, NOF, Chondroblastoma, and Solitary Bone Cysts
> - Any Age = Infection
> - > 40 = Mets and Myeloma (unless it's neuroblastoma mets).

Epiphysis:

In general, only a few lesions tend to arise in the epiphysis. The "four horseman of the (e)apophysis" is the mnemonic I like to use, and I think about the company AIG that was involved in some scandal a few years ago. **AIG** "the evil" Company.

> **Epiphyseal Equivalents:**
>
> Big ones to remember are the carpals, the patella, the greater trochanter, and the calcaneus

ABC, Infection, Giant Cell, and Chondroblastoma.
The caveat is that ABC is usually metaphyseal but after the growth plate closes it can extend into the epiphysis.

For the purpose of multiple choice tests it is important to not forget about the malignant tumor at the end of the bone (epiphysis) – Clear Cell Chondrosarcoma. This guy is slow growing, with a variable appearance (lytic, calcified, lobulated, ill defined, etc…). Just remember **if they say malignant epiphyseal you say Clear Cell Chondrosarcoma.**

Metaphysis

The metaphysis is the fastest growing area of a bone, with the best blood supply. This excellent blood supply results in an increased predilection for Mets and Infection. Most of the cystic bone lesions can occur in the metaphysis.

Diaphysis

Just like the metaphysis, most entities can occur in the diaphysis (they just do it less).

Now a discussion on the pathology:

Fibrous Dysplasia: Fibrous dysplasia is a skeletal developmental anomaly of osteoblasts – failure of normal maturation and differentiation. The disorder can occur at any age . It can be monostotic (20s & 30s) or polyostotic (< 10 year old).

Famously has a very variably appearance, with phases like pagets (lytic, mixed, blastic). The buzzword is "**ground glass**." The catch phrase is "**long lesion in a long bone**." The textbook appearance "lytic lesion with a hazy matrix" The discriminator used by Helms is "**no periosteal reaction or pain**."

Likes the ribs and long bones. If it occurs in the pelvis, it also hits the ipsilateral femur (**Shepherd Crook deformity**). If it's multiple it likes the skull and face (Lion-like faces).

This vs That: **McCune Albright vs Mazabraud Syndrome**	
McCune Albright	**Mazabraud**
Polyostotic Fibrous Dysplasia	Polyostotic Fibrous Dysplasia
Girl	Woman (*middle aged*)
Café au lait spots	Soft Tissue Myxomas
Precocious Puberty	Increased Risk Osseous Malignant Transformation

Adamantinoma: A total zebra (*probably a unicorn*). A tibial lesion that **resembles fibrous dysplasia** (mixed lytic and sclerotic). It is potentially malignant.

Enchondroma: This guy is a tumor of the medullary cavity composed of hyaline cartilage. It appears as a lytic lesion with irregularly speckled calcification of chondroid matrix, classically described as **ARCS AND RINGS.** Having said that the **chondroid matrix is not found in the fingers or toes** *** *this is a high yield factoid for the purpose of multiple choice tests.* The enchondroma is actually the most common cystic lesion in the hands and feet. Just like fibrous dysplasia this lesion does not have periostitis.

The trick to differentiating enchondroma vs a low grade chondrosarcoma is the history of pain.

This vs That: **Ollier's vs Maffucci's**	
Ollier's	Maffucci's
ONLY Enchondromas	**M**ORE than just Enchondromas (also Hemangiomas) **Look for those *phleboliths!*
	Malignant potential (20% turn into chondrosarcoma, and other cancers GI, Ovary)

Eosinophilic Granuloma (EG): This is typically included in every differential for people less than 30. It can be solitary (usually) or multiple.

There are 3 classic appearances - for the purpose of multiple choice:
(1) Vertebra plana in a kid
(2) Skull with lucent "beveled edge" lesions (also in a kid).
(3) "Floating Tooth" with lytic lesion in alveolar ridge --- this would be a differential case

The appearance is highly variable and can be lytic or blastic, with or without a sclerotic border, and with or without a periosteal response. Can even have an osseous sequestrum.

Classic DDx for Vertebra Plana (MELT)
- Mets / Myeloma
- EG
- Lymphoma
- Trauma / TB

Classic DDx for Osseous Sequestrum:
- Osteomyelitis
- Lymphoma
- Fibrosarcoma
- EG
- *Osteoid Osteoma can mimic a sequestrum

Giant Cell Tumor (GCT): This guy has some key criteria (which lend themselves well to multiple choice tests). They include:
- Physis MUST be closed
- Non Sclerotic Border
- Abuts the articular surface

Another trick is to show you a pulmonary met, and ask if it could be GCT? The answer is yes (although this is rare) GCT is considered "quasi-malignant" because they can be locally invasive and about 5% will have pulmonary mets (which are still curable by resection). As a result of this, they should be resected with wide margins.

Things to know about GCTs:
- Most common in the knee - abutting the articular surface
- Most common at age 20-30 * physis must be closed
- There is an association with ABCs (they can turn into them)
- They are "quasi-malignant" - 5% have lung mets
- Fluid levels on MRI

Nonossifying Fibroma (NOF): These are very common. They are seen in children, and will spontaneously regress (becoming more sclerotic before disappearing). They are *rare in children not yet walking.* Just like GCTs they like to occur around the knee. They are classically described as eccentric with a thin sclerotic border (remember GCTs don't have a sclerotic border). They are called fibrous cortical defects when smaller than 2cm.

Vocab: NOFs are the larger version (>3cm) of a fibrous cortical defect (FCD). A wastebasket term for the both of them is simply "fibroxanthoma."

 Jaffe-Campanacci Syndrome: Syndrome of multiple NOFs, café-au-lait spots, mental retardation, hypogonadism, and cardiac malformations.

Osteoid Osteoma *"Pain at night, relieved by aspirin."* It's classically found in two spots (1) meta/diaphysis of long bones and (2) the posterior elements of the spine. One way to test this is to show a plain film that is probably an osteoid osteoma then follow it with an MRI showing "lots of edema." I'll say that again ***large amount of edema for the size of the lesion.***

Another piece of trivia is that when you have them in the spine (most common in the lumbar spine), you frequently have an associated **painful scoliosis** with the **convexity pointed away from the lesion.** These can be treated with percutaneous radiofrequency ablation (as long as it's not within 1cm of a nerve or other vital structure – *typically avoided in hands, spine, and pregnant patients*).

Association of Osteoid Osteoma
Painful Scoliosis
Growth Deformity: Increased length and girth of long bones
Synovitis: Can be seen if intra-articular, leading to early onset arthritis
Arthritis: Can occur from primary synovitis, or secondarily from altered joint mechanics.

Osteoblastoma: Basically it's an osteoid osteoma that is larger than 2cm. It's seen in patients < 30years old. They are most likely to show this in the posterior elements. It also occurs in the long bones (35%) and when it does it is usually diaphyseal (75%).

Metastatic Disease: Should be on the differential for any patient over 40 with a lytic lesion. As a piece of trivia renal cancer is ALWAYS lytic (usually).

> *Classic Blastic Lesions:* Prostate, Carcinoid, Medulloblastoma
> *Classic Lytic Lesions:* Renal and Thyroid

Multiple Myeloma (MM): Plasma cell proliferation increases surrounding osteolytic activity (in case someone asks you the mechanism). Usually in older patient (40s-80s). Plasmacytomas can precede clinical or hematologic evidence of myeloma by 3 years.

They usually have discrete margins, and can be solitary or multiple. Vertebral body destruction with sparing of the posterior elements is classic. Bone Scan is often negative, *skeletal survey is better* (but horrible pain to read), and MRI is the most sensitive.

Additional classic (testable) scenario: *MM manifesting as Diffuse Osteopenia*

Myeloma Related Conditions:

> ***Plasmacytoma*** *(usually under 40):* This is a discrete, solitary mass of neoplastic monoclonal plasma cells in either bone or soft tissue (*extramedullary sub type*). It is associated with latent systemic disease in the majority of affected patients. It can be considered as a singular counterpart multiple myeloma. The lesions look like a geographic lytic area, sometimes with **expansile** remodeling.

> *"Mini Brain Appearance"* – Plasmacytoma in vertebral body

> ***POEMS:*** This is basically "*Myeloma with Sclerotic Mets.*" It's a rare medical syndrome with plasma cell proliferation (typically myeloma) with neuropathy, and organomegaly.

Aneurysmal Bone Cyst (ABC): Aneurysmal bone cysts are aneurysmal lesions of bone with thin-walled, blood-filled spaces (fluid-fluid level on MRI). Patients are usually < 30. They may develop following trauma.

Location: Tibia > Vert > Femur > Humerus

They can be described as primary ABC, presumably arising denovo or secondary ABC, associated with another tumor (classic GCT). They are commonly associated with other benign lesions.

> **Classic DDx for Lucent Lesion in Posterior Elements**
> * Osteoblastoma
> * ABC
> * TB

Things to know about ABC:
- Up to 40% of secondary ABC's are associated with giant cell tumor of bone.
- It's on the DDx for Fluid - Fluid Level on MRI
- Patient < 30
- Tibia is the most common site

Solitary (Unicameral) Bone Cyst: It would be unusual to see one of these in a patient older than 30. Most common in the tubular bones (90-95)% usually humerus or femur. Unique feature: "Always located centrally."

It's going to be shown one of two ways: (1) With a fracture through it in the humerus (probably with a fallen fragment sign) or (2) As a lucent lesion in the calcaneus (probably with a fallen fragment sign).

The *fallen fragment sign* (bone fragment in the dependent portion of a lucent bone lesion) is pathognomonic of solitary bone cyst.

Brown Tumor (Hyperparathyroidism): The "brown tumor" represents localized accumulations of giant cells and fibrous tissue (in case someone asks). They appear as lytic or sclerotic lesions with other findings of hyperparathyroidism (subperiosteal bone resorption). In other words, they need to tell you he/she has hyperparathyroidism first. They may just straight up tell you, or they will show you some bone resorption first (classically on the side of a finger, edge of a clavicle, or under a rib).

These things have different stages of healing / sclerosis. They resorb and can become totally sclerotic /healed, when the Hyper PTH is treated.

Chondroblastoma: This is seen in kids (90% age 5-25). They classically show it in two ways (1) In the epiphysis of the tibia on a 15 year old, or (2) in an epiphyseal equivalent.

[handwritten: 2nd + 3rd decade.]

So what are the epiphyseal equivalents???
- *Patella*
- *Calcaneus*
- *Carpal Bones*
- *And all the Apophyses (greater and less trochanter, tuberosities, etc...)*

Features of the tumor include; A thin sclerotic rim, extension across the physeal plate (25-50%), periostitis (30%). Actual location: femur > humerus > tibia . This may show bone marrow edema, and soft tissue edema on MRI (MRI can mislead you into thinking it's a bad thing). This is one of the only bone lesions that is often **NOT T2 bright**. They tend to reoccur after resection (like 30% of the time).

Gamesmanship Hip: When you have a chondroblastoma in the hip, it tends to *favor the greater trochanter (more than the femoral epiphysis).*

Chondromyxoid fibroma: This is the least common benign lesion of cartilage. It is usually in patients younger than 30. The typical appearance is osteolytic, elongated in shape, eccentrically located, metaphyseal lesion, with cortical expansion and a "bite" like configuration. Sorta looks like a NOF.

The Hip

Greater Trochanter - Remember this is also an *epiphyseal equivalent* and the chrondroblastomas prefer it to the femoral epiphysis. You can get all the other DDxs (ABC, Infection, GCT here as well). Plus, you can have avulsions of the gluteus medius and minimus.

Lesser Trochanter - An avulsion here - without significant clinical history should make you think pathologic fracture.

The Intertrochanteric Region: Classic DDx here : Lipoma, Solitary Bone Cyst, and Monostotic Fibrous Dysplasia.

The Calcaneus

There are several classic lesions that can be shown in the calcaneus. There are also several non-classic lesions that can be shown (sneaky things).

The classic 3:

> **Solitary Bone Cyst:** This will have sharp edges. A thick sclerotic edge with a multiloculated appearance is helpful. The "fallen fragment" will be more in the bottom if shown – although fractures in the calcaneus are much less common than in the arm.

> **Pseudo-cyst** – This is a variation on the normal trabecular pattern, which creates a central triangular radiolucent area. Supposedly the persistence of thin trabeculae, and visible nutrient foramen, along with the classic location are helpful in telling it from the other benign entities.

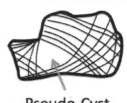

Pseudo-Cyst

> **Interosseous Lipoma:** If they show you this, it will either have to have (a) fat density on CT or MRI, or (b) a **central fragment** – stuck within the middle of the fat. This calcification / fat necrosis occurs about 50% of the time in the real world

Sneaky things:

Just remember that the calcaneus is an *epiphyseal equivalent* so **ABC, Infection, GCT, and Chondroblastoma** can all occur there - think about these when the lesion is more posterior.

In the setting of subtalar degenerative change you can get a **geode** that mimics a cystic lesion (think about this in older patients – 60s with obvious arthritis).

Some Random Benign Lesion Differentials

No Periostitis or Pain	Multiple (FEEMHI)
• Fibrous Dysplasia • Enchondroma • NF • Solitary Bone Cyst (unless fractured)	• Fibrous Dysplasia • EG • Enchondroma • Mets / Myeloma • Hyperparathyroidism

Misc Conditions:

Liposclerosing Myxofibroma: *Very characteristic location – at the intertrochanteric region of the femur.* Looks like a geographic lytic lesion with a sclerotic margin. Despite non-aggressive appearance, 10% undergo malignant degeneration so they need to be followed.

Osteochondroma: Some people think of this as more of a developmental anomaly (although they still always make the tumor chapter). Actually, it's usually listed as the most common benign tumor. They can be radiation induced, making them the *only benign skeletal tumor associated with radiation.*

They have a very small risk of malignant transformation (which supposedly can be estimated based on size of cartilage cap). Supposedly a cap >1.5cm is concerning.

Key Points:
- They point away from the joint
- The bone marrow flows freely into the lesion

Multiple Hereditary Exostosis: AD condition with multiple osteochondromas. They have an **increased risk of malignant transformation**.

Trevor Disease (Dysplasia Epiphysealis Hemimelica - DEH): Osteochondromas develop in an epiphyses causing significant joint deformity (**most common in ankle** and knee). You see this is young children. The osteochondroma looks more like an irregular mass. They tend to be treated with surgical excision.

Supracondylar Spur (Avian Spur): This is an Aunt Minne, and normal variant. This is an osseous process, that usually does nothing, but can compress the median nerve if the **Ligament of Struthers** smashes it.

This vs That: Osteochonroma vs Supracondylar Spur	
Osteochondroma	**Supracondylar Spur**
Points AWAY from joint	Points TOWARD the joint

Periosteal Chondroma (Juxta-Cortical Chondroma): When you see a lesion in the finger of a kid think this. It's a rare entity, or cartilaginous origin. "Saucerization" of the adjacent cortex with sclerotic periosteal reaction can be seen.

Osteofibrous Dysplasia: This is a benign lesion found exclusively in the tibia or fibula in children (10 and under – usually). It looks like an NOF , but centered in the anterior tibia, with associated anterior tibial bowing. It can occur with Adamantinoma, and the two cannot be differentiated with imaging.

When I say looks like NOF in the anterior tibia with anterior bowing, you say Osteofibrous Dysplasia.

Tibial Bowing

Most likely shown as an Aunt Minnie - NF-1 anterior with a fibular pseudoarthrosis, Rickets with wide growth plates, or Blounts tibia vara.

The most likely pure trivia question is that physiology bowing is smooth, lateral, and occurs from 18months - 2 years.

NF-1	**Anterior Lateral** - Unilateral	May be unilateral. May have hypoplastic fibula with pseudarthrosis.
Foot Deformities	Posterior	
Physiologic Bowing	Lateral – Bilateral Symmetric	Self limiting **between 18 months and 2 years**.
Hypophosphatasia	Lateral	"Rickets in a newborn"
Rickets	Lateral	Widening and irregularity of the growth plates.
Blount	Tibial Vara – Often asymmetric	Early walking, Fat, black kid.
Osteogenesis Imperfecta	Involves all long bones	
Dwarfs	Short Limbs	

Arthritis

Arthritis is tricky. Anne Brower wrote a book *called Arthritis in Black and White*, which is probably the best book on the subject. The problem is that book is 415 pages. So, I'm going to try and offer the 10 page version.

Epidemiology

Although there are over 90 different rheumatic diseases recognized by the American College of Rheumatology, only a few tend to show up on multiple choice tests (and at the view box).

You can broadly categorize arthritis into 3 categories:
- Degenerative (OA, Neuropathic)
- Inflammatory (RA, and Variants)
- Metabolic (Gout, CPPD)

Degenerative:

Osteoarthritis is the most common cause. The pathogenesis is that you have mechanical breakdown (hard work) which leads to cartilage degeneration (fissures, micro-fractures) and fragmentation of subchondral bone (sclerosis, and subchondral cysts). You get all the classic stuff, joint space narrowing (NOT symmetric), subchondral cysts, endplate changes, vacuum phenomenon, etc… The poster boy is the osteophyte.

Neuropathic Joint. The way the case is classically shown is a bad joint followed by the reason for a bad joint (syringomyelia, spinal cord injury, etc…). A way to think about this is "*osteoarthritis with a vengeance*." The buzzword is "Surgical Like Margins." Basically nothing else causes this kind of destruction. I like to describe the joints as a deformity, with debris, and dislocation, having dense subchondral bone, and destruction of the articular cortex. The classic scenario is a shoulder that looks like it's been amputated, and then they show you a syrinx.

Inflammatory:

Erosive Osteoarthritis *(Inflammatory Osteoarthritis)*. The buzzword is "gull wing", which describes the central erosions. It is seen in postmenopausal women and favors the DIP joints.

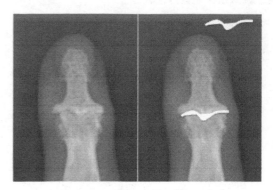

Erosive OA - Gullwing

Rheumatoid Arthritis: There is a ton of trivia related to this disease. It's not a disease of bone production. Instead it is characterized by osteoporosis, soft tissue swelling, marginal erosions and <u>uniform joint space narrowing</u>. It's often bilateral and symmetric. Classically spares the DIP joints (opposite of erosive OA).

Trivia: The 5th Metatarsal head is the first spot in the foot, 2nd + 3rd MCPs + 3rd PIP in the hand.

RA in the Hand Pearls - Expect the IP joints (PIP) to be involved AFTER the MCP joints. The First CMC is classically spared (or is the last carpal to be involved). The first CMC should NOT be first. Obviously OA loves the first CMC so this is helpful in separating them. Psoriasis on the other hand, also tends to make the first CMC go last.

- **Felty Syndrome:** RA > 10 years + Splenomegaly + Neutropenia

- **Caplan Syndrome:** RA + Pneumoconiosis

The distribution of RA vs OA in the hip is a classic teaching point:

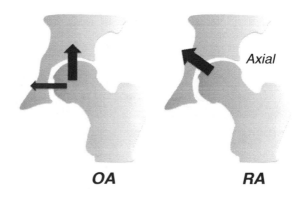

OA   RA

Rheumatoid Variants
- Psoriatic Arthritis
- Reiter's syndrome *(Reactive arthritis)*
- Ankylosing Spondylitis
- Inflammatory Bowel Disease

Psoriatic Arthritis: This is seen in 30% of patients with psoriasis. In almost all cases (90%) the skin findings come first, then you get the arthritis. As a point of trivia, there is a strong correlation between involvement of the nail and involvement of the DIP joint. The classic description is "erosive change with bone proliferation (IP joints > MCP joints). The erosions start in the margins of the joint and progress to involve the central portions (can lead to a "pencil sharpening" effect). The hands are the most commonly affected (second most common is the feet). Up to 40% of cases will have SI joint involvement (asymmetric).

Additional Buzzwords
- "Fuzzy Appearance" to the bone around the joint (bone proliferation)
- Sausage Digit – whole digit has soft tissue swelling
- Ivory Phalanx – sclerosis and/or bone proliferation (most commonly the great toe)
- Pencil in Cup Deformities
- Ankylosis in Finger
- "Mouse Ears"
- Acral osteolysis

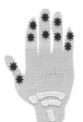 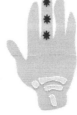  

IP Joints   Ray Pattern   Pencil in Cup   Mouse Ears

When I say Ankylosis in the Hand, You Say (1) Erosive OA or (2) Psoriasis

RA	Psoriasis
Symmetric	Asymmetric
Proximal (favors MCP, carpals)	Distal (favors IP joints)
Osteoporosis	No Osteoporosis
No Bone Proliferation	Bone Proliferation - the form of periostitis
Can Cause "Mutilans" When Severe	Can Cause "Mutilans" When Severe

Reiter's (Reactive arthritis): Apparently Reiter was a Nazi (killed a bunch of people with typhus vaccine experiments). So, people try not to give him any credit for things (hence the name change to Reactive arthritis). Regardless of what you call it, it's **a very similar situation to Psoriatic arthritis** – both have bone proliferation and erosions, and asymmetric SI joint involvement. The difference is that **Reiter's is rare in the hands** (tends to affect the feet more). Just remember Reiters below the waist.

Ankylosing Spondylitis: This disease favors the spine and SI joints. The classic buzzword is **"bamboo spine"** from the syndesmophytes flowing from adjacent vertebral bodies. Shiny corners is a buzzword, for early involvement. As you might imagine these spines are susceptible to fracture in trauma. **SI joint involvement is usually the first site (symmetric).** The joint actually widens a little before it narrows. As a point of trivia, these guys can have an upper lobe predominant interstitial lung disease, with small cystic spaces.

Next Step - Any significant Ank Spon / DISH + Even Minor Trauma = Whole Spine CT

Random High Yield Topic: Ankylosing Spondylitis in the Hip
When the peripheral skeleton is involved in patient's with Ank Spond, think about the shoulders and hips (hips more common). Hip involvement can be very disabling.
Heterotopic Ossification tends to occur post hip replacement or revision. It occurs so much that they often get postoperative low dose radiation and NSAIDs to try as prophylactic therapy.
If they show you normal SI joints - then show you anything in the spine it's not AS. It has to hit the SI joints first (especially on multiple choice).

Inflammatory Bowel Disease – This occurs in two distinct flavors.

> (A): Axial Arthritis (favors SI joints and spine) – often unrelated to bowel disease
> (B): Peripheral Arthritis – this one varies depending on the severity of the bowel disease.

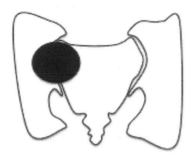

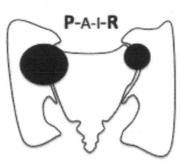

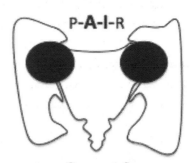

Unilateral = Infection   Asymmetric =   Symmetric =
Psoriasis, Reiters   Inflammatory Bowel, AS

Psoriatic Arthritis	Reiters (Reactive)	Ankylosing Spondylitis
M = F	M > F	M>F
Asymmetric SI Joint	Asymmetric SI Joint	Symmetric SI Joint
Hands, Feet, Thoracolumbar Spine	Feet, Lumbar Spine, SI joint	SI joint, Spine (whole thing)

Metabolic:

Gout: This is a crystal arthropathy from the deposition of uric acid crystals in and around the joints. It's almost always in a man over 40. The big toe is the classic location.

Buzzwords / Things to Know:
* Earliest Sign = Joint Effusion
* Spares the Joint Space (until late in the disease); Juxta-articular Erosions - away from the joint.
* "Punched out lytic lesions"
* "Overhanging Edges"
* Soft tissue tophi

Gout on MR

* Juxta-articular soft tissue masse (LOW ON T2).
* The tophus will typically enhance.

Gout Mimickers: There are 5 entities that can give a similar appearance to a gouty arthritis, although they are much less common. The way I remember them is

"**A**merican **R**oentgen **R**ay **S**ociety **H**ooray"
* *Amyloid*
* *RA (cystic)*
* *Reticular Histocytosis (the most rare)*
* *Sarcoid*
* *Hyperlipidemia*

CPPD: Calcium Pyrophosphate Dihydrate Disease is super common in old people. It often causes chondocalcinosis (although there are other causes). Synovitis + CPPD = "Pseudogout." CPPD loves the triangular fibrocartilage of the wrist, the peri odontoid tissue, and intervertbral disks. Another important phrase is **"degenerative change in an uncommon joint"** – shoulder, elbow, patellofemoral joint, radiocarpal joint. Having said that **pyrophosphate arthropathy is most common at the knee.**

- *If you see isolated disease in the patellofemoral, radiocarpal, or talonavicular joint think CPPD.*
- *Hooked MCP Osteophytes with chondrocalcinosis in the TFCC is a classic look (although hemochromatosis can also look that way).*

Remember - CPPD can (and does commonly) cause SLAC wrist by degenerating the SL Ligament.

"Milwaukee Shoulder" This is a destruction of the shoulder (**almost looks neuropathic**) but is secondary to **hydroxyapatite**. The articular surface changes will be very advanced, and you have a lot of intra-articular loose bodies. It's classically seen in an old women with a history of trauma to that joint.

> ### OA vs CPPD?
> There are many overlapping features including joint space narrowing, subchondral sclerosis, subchondral cyst, and osteophyte formation. However, CPPD has some unique features such as an "atypical joint distribution" – favoring compartments like the patellofemoral or radiocarpal. Subchondral cyst formation can be bigger than expected.

Hemochromatosis – This iron overload disease also is known for calcium pyrophosphate deposition and resulting chondrocalcinosis. It has a similar distribution to CPPD (MCP joints). Both CPPD and Hemochromatosis will have "hooked osteophytes" at the MCP joint. As a point of trivia, therapy for the systemic disease does NOT affect the arthritis.

Hyperparathyroidism - As you may remember from medical school this can be primary or secondary, and its effects on calcium metabolism typically manifest in the bones. Here are your buzzwords: "Subperiosteal bone resorption" of the radial aspect 2nd and 3rd fingers, rugger-jersey spine, brown tumors, terminal tuft erosions.

The classic ways this is shown:
- *Superior and inferior rib notching – bone resorption*
- *Resorption along the radial aspect of the fingers with brown tumors*
- *Tuft Resorption*
- *Rugger Jersey Spine*
- *Pelvis with Narrowing or "Constricting" of the femoral necks, and wide SI joints.*

Hyperparathyroidism

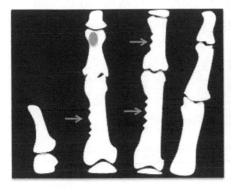 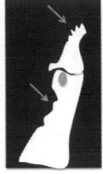 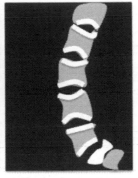 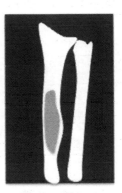

Subperiosteal Resorption, Tuft Resorption and brown tumors   **Rugger Jersey Spine**   **Brown Tumor**

Problem Solving: If you are given a picture of a hand or foot and asked what the arthritis is, it will probably be obvious (they show a gullwing for erosive OA, or bad carpals for RA, or the pencil in cup for psoriasis, or the 5th metatarsal for RA). If it's not made obvious with an "Aunt Minnie" appearance I like to use this approach to figure it out (I also use this in the real world).

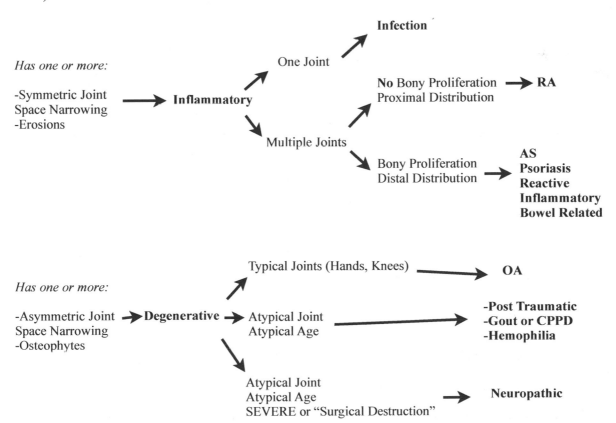

Has one or more:

-Symmetric Joint Space Narrowing
-Erosions → **Inflammatory**

One Joint → **Infection**

Multiple Joints → **No Bony Proliferation** Proximal Distribution → **RA**

Multiple Joints → **Bony Proliferation** Distal Distribution → **AS Psoriasis Reactive Inflammatory Bowel Related**

Has one or more:

-Asymmetric Joint Space Narrowing
-Osteophytes → **Degenerative**

Typical Joints (Hands, Knees) → **OA**

Atypical Joint Atypical Age → **-Post Traumatic -Gout or CPPD -Hemophilia**

Atypical Joint Atypical Age SEVERE or "Surgical Destruction" → **Neuropathic**

Spine Degenerative Change: In the real world it's usually just multilevel degenerative change. But in multiple choice world you should be thinking about other things. Shiny corners with early AS, or flowing syndesmophytes with later AS. DISH with the bulky osteophytes sparing the disc space. The big bridging lateral osteophyte is classically shown for psoriatic arthritis.

Vertebral Osteophytes	
"Flowing Syndesmophytes"	Ankylosing Spondylitis
Diffuse Paravertebral Ossifications	DISH
Focal Lateral Paravertebral Ossification	Psoriatic Arthritis

Cervical Spine: *Gamesmanship*
• **Fusion:** Either congenital (Klippel-Feil) or Juvenile RA.
• **Erosions of the Dens:** CPPD and RA famously do this.
• **Bad Kyphosis** = NF1

Misc Stuff That's Sorta in the Arthritis Category:

Systemic Lupus Erthematous: The Aunt Minnie Look is **reducible deformity of joints without articular erosions**. *Joint space narrowing and erosions are uncommon findings.* They can show you the hands with ulnar subluxations at the MCPs on Norgaard view, then they reduce on AP (because the hands are flat).

This ligamentous laxity also increases risk of **patellar dislocations**.

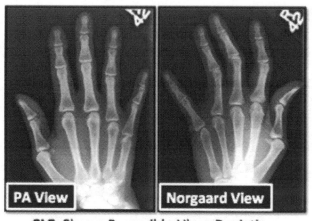

SLE: Shows Reversible Ulnar Deviation

Jaccoud's Arthropathy: This is **very similar to SLE** in the hand (people often say them together). You have non erosive arthropathy with ulnar deviation of the 2nd-5th fingers at the MCP joint. The **history is post rheumatic fever**.

DISH (Diffuse Idiopathic Skeletal Hyperostosis) : You see ossification of the anterior longitudinal ligament involving more than 4 levels with **sparing of the disc spaces**, you say DISH. The **thoracic spine is most commonly used**. These guys often have bony proliferation at pelvis, ischial tuberosities, at the trochanters, and iliac crests. There is **no sacroiliitis** (helps you differentiate from AS).

OPPL (Ossification of the Posterior Longitudinal Ligament): This is an ossification of the posterior longitudinal ligament. It is associated with DISH, ossification of the ligamentum flavum, and Ankylosing Spondylitis. It favors the cervical spine of old Asian men. It **can cause spinal canal stenosis, and lead to cord injury after minor trauma**. A key point is that it's bad news in the cervical spine (where it is most common), in the thoracic spine it is usually asymptomatic.

Destructive Spondyloarthropathy.: This is associated with patients on renal dialysis (for at least 2 years), and it most commonly affects the C-spine. It looks like bad degenerative changes or CPPD. Amyloid deposition is supposedly why it happens.

Mixed Connective Tissue Disease: One unique feature is that it is positive for some antibody – Ribonucleoprotein (RNP), and therefore *serology is essential to the diagnosis.*

Juvenile Idiopathic Arthritis: This occurs before age 16 (by definition). What you see is a washed out hand that has a proximal distribution (**carpals are jacked**), and ankylosed (**premature fusion of growth plates**). Serology is often negative (85%). In the knees, you see enlargement of the epiphyses and widened intercondylar notch – similar to findings in hemophilia.

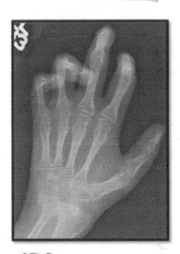

JRA
– Note the effect on the carpals

Amyloid Arthropathy: This is seen with patients on dialysis (less commonly in patients with chronic inflammation such as RA). The pattern of destruction can be severe – similar to septic arthritis or neuropathic spondyloarthropathy. The distribution is key, the **bilateral involvement of the shoulders, hips, carpals, and knees** being typical. **Carpal tunnel syndrome is a common clinical manifestation**. The **joint space is typically preserved** until later in the disease. When associated with dialysis it's rare before 5 years of treatment, but very common after 10 years (80%).

Congenital

Dwarfs, Coalitions, and Feet are discussed in detail in the PEDs chapter

Total Hip Arthroplasty Complications:

Loosening: This is the most common indication for revision. The criteria on x-ray is **>2mm at the interface** (suggestive). If you see **migration of the component** you can call it *(migration includes varus tilting of the femoral stem)*.

Particle Disease: Any component of the device that sheds will cause an inflammatory response. Macrophages will try and eat the particles and spew enzymes all over the place.

Things to know about particle disease (in THA):

- Most commonly seen in non-cemented hips
- Tends to occur 1-5 years after surgery
- X-ray shows "smooth" endosteal scalloping (distinguishes from infection)
- Produces no secondary bone response
- Can be seen around screw holes (particles are transmitted around screws)

Stress Shielding: The stress is transferred through the metallic stem, so the bone around it is not loaded. Orthopods call this "Wolff's Law" – where the unloaded bone just gets resorbed. The trivia to know is that it (1) happens more with uncemented arthroplasty and (2) increases the risk of fracture.

Wear Patterns: It is normal to have a little bit of thinning is the area of weight bearing – this is called "Creep." It is not normal to see wear along the superior lateral aspect.

Polyethylene Wear	Creep
Superior – Lateral	Axial Direction
Pathologic	Normal

Heterotopic Ossifications: This is very common (15-50%). It's usually asymptomatic. The trivia regarding multiple choice tests is that "hip stiffness" is the most common complaint. Also in Ank Spon patients, because they are so prone to heterotopic ossifications, they sometimes give them low dose prophylactic radiation prior to THA.

Marrow

This is a confusing topic and there are entire books on the subject. I'm going to attempt to hit the main points, and simplify the subject.

Bone marrow consists of three components: (1) Trabecular Bone – the support structure, (2) Red Marrow – for making blood, and (3) Yellow Marrow – fat for a purpose unknown at this time.

Marrow Conversion: The basic rules are that yellow marrow increases with age, in a predictable and progressive way. This is usually completed by the mid 20s. You are born with all red marrow, and the conversion of red to yellow occurs from the extremities to the axial skeleton (feet and hands first). Within each long bone the progression occurs epiphyses / apophyses first -> diaphysis -> followed by the distal metaphysis , and finally the proximal metaphysis. **Red marrow can be found in the humeral heads and femoral heads as a normal variant in adults.**

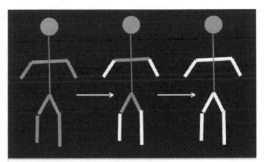

Red Marrow Converts to Yellow Marrow from Distal to Proximal

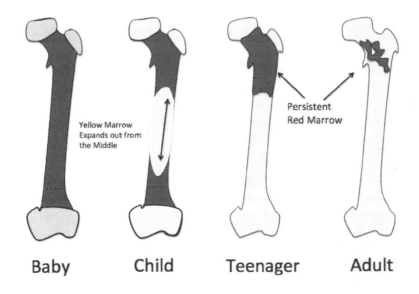

Yellow Marrow Expands out from the Middle

Persistent Red Marrow

Baby   Child   Teenager   Adult

So as a child you have diffuse red marrow except for ossified epiphyses and apophyses. As an adult you have yellow marrow everywhere except in the axial skeleton, and proximal metaphyses of proximal long bones.

Few Pearls on Marrow:

- Yellow marrow increases with age (as trabecular bone decreases with osteoporosis, yellow marrow replaces it).
- T1 is your money sequence: Yellow is bright, Red is darker than yellow (near iso-intense to muscle).
- Red marrow should never be darker than a normal disk or muscle on T1 (think about muscle as your internal control).
- Red marrow increases if there is a need for more hematopoiesis (reconversion – occurs in exact reverse order of normal conversion)
- Marrow turns yellow with stress / degenerative change in the spine

This question can be asked in 3 main ways:

    (1) What is the normal pattern of conversion?
    (2) What is the normal pattern of reconversion?
    (3) What areas are spared / normal variants?

(1) The epiphyses convert to fatty marrow almost immediately after ossification. Distal then proceeds medial (diaphysis first, then metaphysis).

(2) The pattern of reconversion: This occurs in the reverse order of normal marrow conversion, beginning in the axial skeleton and heading peripheral. The last to go are the more distal long bones. Typically the epiphyses are spared unless the hematopoietic demand is very high.

Spine -> Flat Bones -> Long Bone Metaphysis -> Long Bone Diaphysis -> Long Bone Epiphyses

(3) Patchy areas of red marrow may be seen in the proximal femoral metaphysis of teenagers. The **distal femoral sparring is especially true in teenagers and menstruating women.**

Leukemia: Proliferation of leukemic cells results in replacement of red marrow. **Marrow will look darker than muscle (and normal disks) on T1**. On STIR maybe higher than muscle because of the increased water content. T2 is variable often looking like diffuse red marrow.

Gamesmanship: They can show leukemia in two main ways
  (1) *Lucent metaphyseal bands in a kid*
  (2) *T1 weighted MRI showing marrow darker than adjacent disks, and muscle. Remember that Red Marrow is still 40% fat, and should be brighter than muscle on T1.*

Most infiltrative conditions affect the marrow diffusely. The exceptions are *multiple myeloma which has a predilection for focal deposits, and Waldenstrom's macroglobulinemia which causes infarcts.*

Chloroma (Granulocytic Sarcoma) - Just say "destructive mass in a bone of a leukemia patient." It's some kind of colloid tumor.

Metabolic / Misc

Calcium Hydroxyapatite: Most pathologic calcification in the body is calcium hydroxyapatite, which is also the most abundant form of calcium in bone.

Calcium hydroxyapatite deposition disease = **calcific tendinitis***.*

The calcium is deposited in tendons around the joint. The most common location for hydroxyapatite deposition is the shoulder. Specifically, the **supraspinatus tendon is the most frequent site of calcification**, usually at the insertion near the greater tuberosity. *The longus coli muscle is also a favorite location for multiple choice test writers.* It may be primary (idiopathic) or secondary. Secondary causes worth knowing are: chronic renal disease, collagen-vascular disease, **tumoral calciniosis** and hypervitaminosis D.

Osteopoikilosis: It's just a bunch of bone islands. Usually in epiphyses (different from blastic mets or osteosarcoma mets). It can be inherited or sporadic but if you are forced to pick a pattern - I'd go with *autosomal dominant.*

Mets vs Osteopoikilosis - Osteopoikilosis tends to joint centered. Sclerotic mets will be all over the place. Sclerotic mets believe in nothing Lebowski.

Osteopathia Striata: Linear, parallel, and longitudinal lines in metaphysis of long bones. Doesn't mean shit (usually - but can in some situations cause pain).

Engelmann's Disease: This is also known as progressive diaphyseal dysplasia or PDD. What you see is *fusiform bony enlargement* with sclerosis of the long bones. This is a total zebra that begins in childhood.

Things to know:

- *It's Bilateral and Symmetric*
- *It likes the long bones - usually shown in the tibia*
- *It's hot on bone scan*
- *It can involve the skull – and can cause optic nerve compression*

Pituitary Gigantism: If they happen to show you x-rays of Andre the Giant, look for **"widening of the joint space in an adult hip"** – can be a classic buzzword. Late in the game the cartilage will actually outgrow its blood supply, and collapse leading to **early onset osteoarthritis.** The formation of endochondral bone at existing chondro-osseous junctions results in widening of osseous structure.

Pigmented Villonodular Synovitis (PVNS) : PVNS is an uncommon benign neoplastic process that may involve the synovium of the joint diffusely or focally It can also affect the tendon sheath.

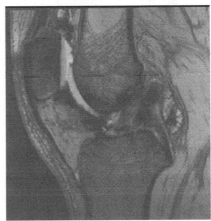

PVNS – Diffuse Blooming

Intra-Articular Disease : Basically it's **Synovial Proliferation + Hemosiderin Deposition**. The knee is by far the most common joint affected (65-80%). On plain film, features you will probably see are a joint effusion with or without marginal erosions. Osseous erosions with preservation of the joint space, and normal mineralization is typical. It is not possible to distinguish PVNS from *synovial chondromatosis (see below)* on plain film. MRI will be obvious with **blooming on gradient echo**, and this is the most likely way they will show this. Treatment is with complete synovectomy, although recurrence rate is 20-50%.

Trivia: Unusual in kids, but when present is typically polyarticular.

Giant Cell Tumor of the Tendon Sheath (PVNS of the tendon): Typically found in the hand (palmar tendons). Can cause erosions on the underlying bone. Will be soft tissue density, and be T1 and T2 dark *(contrasted to a **glomus tumor** which is T1 dark, **T2 bright,** and will enhance uniformly).*

Primary Synovial Chondromatosis: There are both primary and secondary types; secondary being the result of degenerative changes in the joint. The primary type is an extremely high yield topic. It is a metaplastic / true neoplastic process (not inflammatory) that results in the formation of multiple cartilaginous nodules in the synovium of joints, tendon sheaths, and bursea. These nodules will eventually progress to loose bodies. It usually affects one joint, and that one joint is usually the knee (70%). The popular are is usually a person in their 40s or 50s.

Joint bodies (which are usually multiple and uniform in size) may demonstrate the ring and arc calcification characteristic of chondroid calcification. Treatment involves removal of the loose bodies with or without synovectomy.

PVNS	Synovial Chondromatosis
Benign Neoplasia	Benign Neoplasia
Associated with Hemarthrosis	NOT Associated with Hemarthrosis
Never Calcifies	May Calcify

Secondary Synovial Chondromatosis: A lower yield topic than the primary type. This is secondary to degenerative change, and typically seen in an older patient. There will be extensive degenerative changes, and the fragments are usually fewer and larger when compared to the primary subtype.

Diabetic Myonecrosis: This is basically infarction of the muscle seen in poorly controlled type 1 diabetics. It **almost always involves the thigh (80%)**, or calf (20%). MRI will show marked edema with enhancement and irregular regions of muscle necrosis. You **should NOT biopsy this**, it delays recovery time and has a high complication rate.

Soft Tissue Hemangioma: This is a benign vascular tumor, that comes in several varieties (capillary being the most common type). They are more common in women, and *can enlarge during pregnancy*. They can look like a **bunch of phleboliths on plain film** (characteristic of the cavernous subtype). On CT you can see **intralesional fat**. On MR they are going to be T1 and T2 bright, again with intralesional fat. They are typically well defined with a lobulated border, and heterogenous features. They enhance avidly and may have blooming on gradient from the pheboliths.

Next Step - Suspecting hemangioma? think you see intralesional fat ? Plain film can be helpful to look for phleboliths.

Lipoma Arborescens: This is a zebra that affects the synovial lining of the joins and bursa.

The buzzword is "**frond – like**" depositions of fatty tissue.

It's seen in late adulthood (50s-70s), with the most common location being the suprapatellar bursa of the knee. Although it **can develop in a normal knee, it's often associated with OA, Chronic RA, or prior trauma**. It's usually unilateral. On MRI it's going to behave like fat – T1 and T2 bright with response to fat saturation.

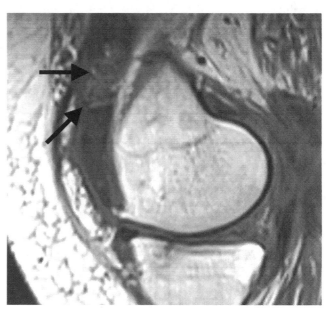

Lipoma Arborescens

 A sneaky trick is to show this on gradient – and how you pick up the chemical shift artifact at the fat-fluid interface.

This could also be shown on ultrasound with a "frond-like hyperechoic mass" and associated joint effusions.

AVN of the Hip: Variety of causes including Perthes in kids, sickle cell, gaucher's, steroid use etc.... It can also be traumatic with femoral neck fractures (*degree of risk is related to degree of displacement* / disruption of the retinacular vessels). AVN of the hip typically affects the superior articular surface, beginning more anteriorly.

Double Line Sign: Best seen on T2; inner bright line (granulation tissue), with outer dark line (sclerotic bone) . Seen in 80% of cases

Rim Sign: Best seen on T2; high T2 signal line sandwiched between two low signal lines. This represents *fluid between sclerotic borders of an osteochondral fragment*, and **implies instability**. (Stage III).

Crescent Sign: Seen on X-ray (optimally frog leg); Refers to a subchondral lucency seen most frequently anterolateral aspect of the proximal femoral head. It indicates imminent collapse.

Stages of Osteonecrosis:
- o   Zero = Normal
- o   One = Normal x-ray, edema on MR
- o   Two = Mixed Lytic / Sclerotic
- o   Three = Crescent Sign, Articular Collapse, Joint Space Preserved
- o   Four = Secondary Osteoarthritis

Thalassemia : This is a defect in the hemoglobin chain (can be alpha or beta – major or minor). From the MSK Radiologist prospective we are talking about "hair-on-end" skulls, expansion of the facial bones, "rodent faces" , expanded ribs "jail-bars". It is frequently associated with extramedullary hematopoiesis.

Thalassemia	Sickle Cell
Will Obliterate Sinuses	Will Not Obliterate Sinuses

Pagets
(High Yield Topic)

A relatively common condition that affects 4% of people at 40, and 8% at 80 *(actually 10%, but easier to remember 8%)*. M > F. Most people are asymptomatic. The pathophysiology of Pagets is not well understood.

The bones **go through three phases which progress from lytic to mixed to sclerotic** *(the latent inactive phase)*. The phrase **"Wide Bones with Thick Trabecula"** make you immediately say Pagets (nothing else really does that).

Lytic	Usually Asymptomatic
Mixed	Elevated Alkaline Phosphate. Fractures
Sclerotic	Elevated Hydroxyproline. More fractures. Sarcomas may develop.

Comes in two flavors: (1) Monostotic and (2) Polyostotic – with the poly subtype being much more common (80-90%).

Paget's Buzzwords / Signs:
- *Blade of Grass Sign:* Lucent leading edge in a long bone
- *Osteoporosis Circumscripta:* Blade of Grass in the Skull
- *Picture Frame Vertebra:* Cortex is thickened on all sides (Rugger Jersey is only superior and inferior endplates)
- *Cotton Wool Bone:* Thick disorganized trabeculae
- *Banana Fracture:* Insufficiency fracture of a bowed soft bone (femur or tibia).
- *Tam O'Shanter Sign:* Thick Skull
- *Saber Shin:* Bowing of the tibia
- *Ivory Vertebra:* This is a differential finding, including mets. Pagets tends to be expansile.

Complications: **Deafness is the most common complication.** Spinal stenosis from cortical thickening is very characteristic. Additional complications, cortical stress fracture, cranial nerves paresis, CHF (high output), secondary hyperparathyroidism (10%), **Secondary development of osteosarcoma (1%) – which is often highly resistant to treatment.** *As a piece of ridiculous trivia - giant cell tumor can arise from pagets.*

Trivia: Of all the tumors to which Paget may devolve to, Osteosarcoma is the Most Common.

Total Trivia: Pagets bone is hypervascular and may be 5 degrees hotter than other bone (get your thermometer ready). Alk Phos will be elevated (up to 20x) in the reparative phase.

Skull	Large Areas of Osteolysis in the Frontal and Occipital Bones "Osteoporosis Circumscripta", in the lytic phase. The skull will look "cotton wool" in the mixed phase. Favors the outer table.
Spine	Cortical Thickening can cause a "picture frame sign" (same as osteopetrosis). Also can give you an ivory vertebral body.
Pelvis	Most common bone affected. "Always" involves the iliopectineal line on the pelvic brim.
Long Bones	Advancing margin of lucency from one end to the other is the so called "blade of grass" or "flame." Will often spare the fibula, even in diffuse disease.

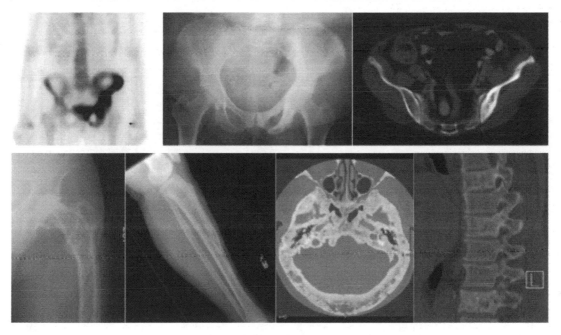

Pagets
-- Femur / Tibia, -- Expanded Bones, -- Coarsened Trabecula, -- Ivory Vertebrae

Other Imaging Modalities:

MRI: There are three marrow patterns that closely (but not exactly) follow the phases on x-ray.

Lytic / Early Mixed	Heterogenous T2, T1 is isointense to muscle, with a "speckled appearance"
Late Mixed	Maintained fatty high T1 and T2 signals
Sclerotic	Low signal on T1 and T2

Nuclear Medicine: The primary utility of a bone scan is in defining the extent of disease and to help assess response to treatment. The characteristic look for Pagets is "Whole Bone Involvement." For example, the **entire vertebral body including the posterior elements**, or the entire pelvis. The classic teaching is that Pagets is hot on all three phases (although often decreased or normal in the sclerotic phase).

Tendon Ultrasound:

It's absolutely incredible that I even need to go over this, but dinosaur radiologist's love this stuff.

Anisotropy: The most common and most problematic issues with ultrasounding tendons is this thing called "anisotropy." The tendon is normally hyperechoic, but if you look at it when it's NOT perpendicular to the sound beam it can look hypoechoic (injured?).

It's the biggest pain in the ass:

- Supraspinatus tendon – as it curves along the contours of the humeral head
- Long Head of the Biceps – In the bicipital groove

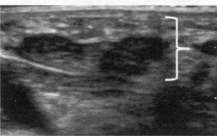

Normal Appearing Hyperechoic Tendon

Exact same tendon – now appearing Hypoechoic – when scanned non-parallel

Anisotropy

Tears: The tendon is usually hyperechoic. Focal hypoechoic areas are tears. It can be really tricky to tell if it's partial or complete (that's what MRI is for).

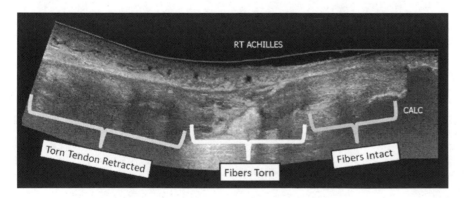

RT ACHILLES

CALC

Torn Tendon Retracted

Fibers Torn

Fibers Intact

Tenosynovitis: As discussed above there are a variety of causes. If they show it on ultrasound you are looking for increased fluid within the tendon sheath. You could also see associated peritendinous subcutaneous hyperemia on Doppler.

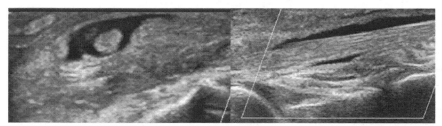

Tenosynovitis – Increased fluid in the tendon sheath

Plantar Fasciitis: This is another pathology that lends itself to a "what is it ?" type of ultrasound question. Hopefully, they at least tell you this is the foot (they could label the calcaneus). The finding will be thickening of the plantar fascia (greater than 4mm), with loss of the normal fibrillar pattern. If you see calipers on the plantar fascia – this is going to be the answer.

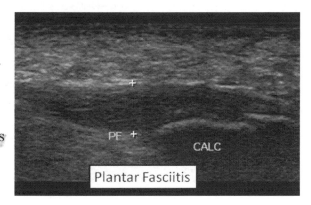

Trivia - Most commonly involves the central band (there are 3 bands - people who don't know anatomy think there are two).

Calcific Tendonitis: As described above, this is very common and related to hydroxyapatite. The most common site is the supraspinatus tendon, near its insertion. It will shadow just like a stone in the GB.

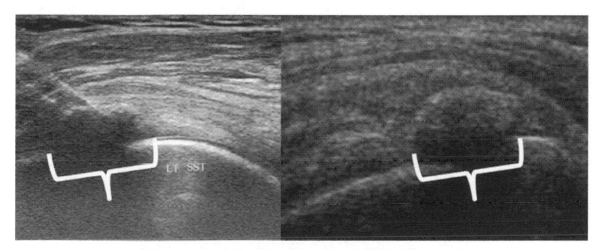

Calcific Tendonitis – Shadowing calcification in the classic location (supraspinatus)

Basic Procedural Trivia - The Arthrogram

An important point to remember is that the target is not actually the joint. The target is the capsule. In other words, you just need the needle to touch a bone within the capsule. The trick is to do this without causing contamination or damaging an adjacent structure (like an artery). *General Tip* - Avoid putting air in the joint, this will cause susceptibility artifact.

Hip: The general steps are as follows: (1) Mark the femoral artery. (2) Internally rotate the hip (slightly) to localize the femoral head-neck junction (your target). (3) Clean and numb the skin. (4) Advance a 20-22 gauge spinal needle into the joint - straight down on the superior head neck junction. (5) Inject a small amount of contrast to confirm position. Contrast should flow away from the tip. If the contrast just stays there it's not in a space. (6) Put the rest of the contrast in.

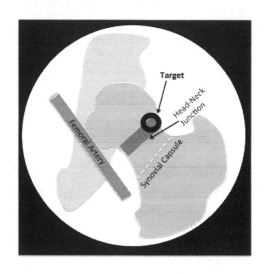

Trivia: The capsule is widest at the head-neck junction.

Trivia: The cocktail injected is around 14cc total (4cc Lidocaine, 10cc Visipaque, and only about 0.1cc Gd).

Shoulder: The general steps are as follows: (1) Supinate the hand (externally rotate the shoulder) (2) Clean and numb the skin. (3) Advance a 20-22 gauge spinal needle into the joint - straight down on the junction between the middle and inferior thirds of the humeral head - 2mm inside the cortex. (4) Once you strike bone, pull back 1mm and turn the bevel towards the humeral head - this should drop into the joint (5) Inject a small amount of contrast to confirm position. Contrast should flow away from the tip. If the contrast just stays there it's not in a space. (6) Put the rest of the contrast in.

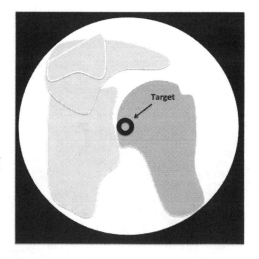

Trivia: The cocktail injected is around 12cc total (4cc Lidocaine, 8cc Visipaque, and only about 0.1cc Gd).

Blank for Notes / Scribbles

Blank for Notes / Scribbles

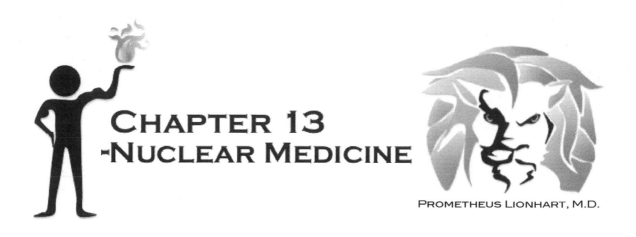

CHAPTER 13 -NUCLEAR MEDICINE

PROMETHEUS LIONHART, M.D.

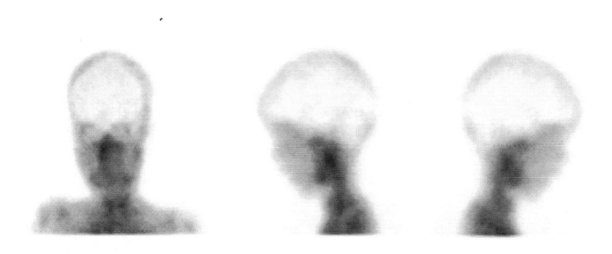

Highest Yield Tip:

Nuclear medicine is probably the most challenging section on the Exam (maybe second to physics). The reason it's so difficult is that there is a seemingly unending amount of trivia, very little of which is necessary to understanding or interpreting the exam, but nonetheless lends itself easily to multiple choice test writing. The more meaningless the trivia seems, the more likely it will be tested.

What Scan Is That?

Ok, here is the scenario that I want you to be prepared for:

The plane has crashed. All the nuclear techs are dead. Prior to the plane crashing, they completed several studies, but forgot to label them or give indications. The bean counter (non-MD) who is running the hospital is breathing down your neck to read these studies now, because the metrics he set up are gonna look bad at the next QA/QC meeting. So now you have to interpret nuclear studies, and you don't know why they did it or even what tracer was given.

Fortunately, you trained for this as part of your preparation for the Exam.

Seriously, this is famously one of the most common ways nuclear medicine is tested. It was like that on the old oral boards, and probably still like that now (same knuckle heads writing the questions). It's such a ridiculous thing to ask. My primary advice: *Don't Fight It... Embrace the Ridiculous Nature of the Test.*

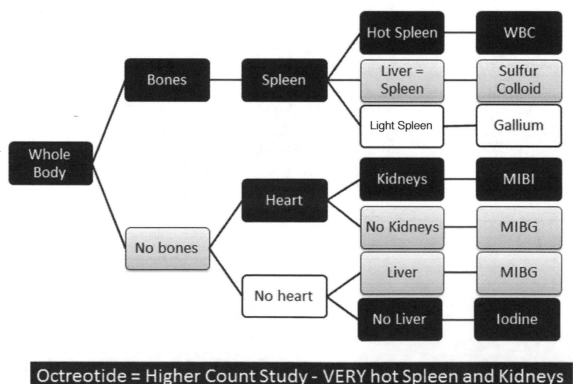

(* Note the MIBG is under both heart and no heart - this is because it's variable. MIBG with I-123 is more likely to have heart than I-131.

This is an alternative pathway that some people prefer. This one focuses more on photon output (how light or dark stuff is), and liver and spleen. It removes the confusion of heart "maybe" for MIBG.

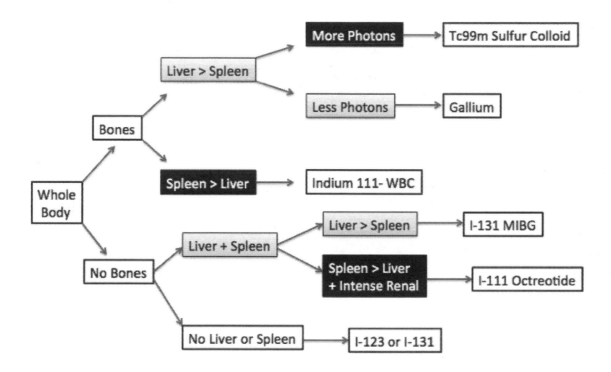

Another alternative way to work the bones pathway is to ask Lacrimal Glands? Gallium will have them, WBC scans and Sulfur Colloid will NOT. The trick on Lacrimal Glands is free Tc (but bones will be real weak on that one). MIBG can have lacrimal activity , but again no bones.

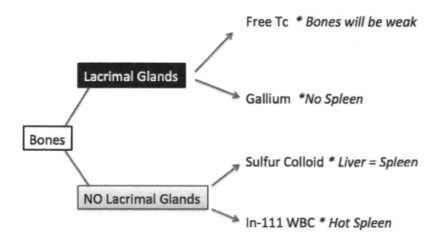

HOT Spleen: You should think Octreotide, and WBC Scans. Sulfur Colloid will have tracer in the spleen, but not as much as the liver.

MIBG: It has variable cardiac uptake, so it finds itself on multiple branch points. Cardiac activity is more often seen on an I-123 MIBG scan (as opposed to 1-131 MIBG). Another thing that helps me remember this stuff: when you do a MIBG you are often looking for neuroblastoma. If the kidney was also hot it would be hard to tell a mass near the kidney from the kidney – so part of the reason the study works is that the kidney does NOT take up MIBG.

Octreotide: This is a high count study, images should be cleaner. You can go down the "no bones" pathway. But the trigger should be **no bones + liver + dark spleen + dark kidneys**.

Tc WBC: The trick here can be imaging at 4 hours vs imaging at 24 hours. At 4 hours you can see lung uptake. At 24 hours the lungs are clearing up, but you start to get some bowel uptake. Just like an In-WBC the spleen is still darker than the Liver.

In WBC vs Tc WBC: Both will have hot spleens. Additionally, Tc is a higher count study and will typically look cleaner.

Tc WBC	In WBC
Renal	NO Renal
GI	NO GI

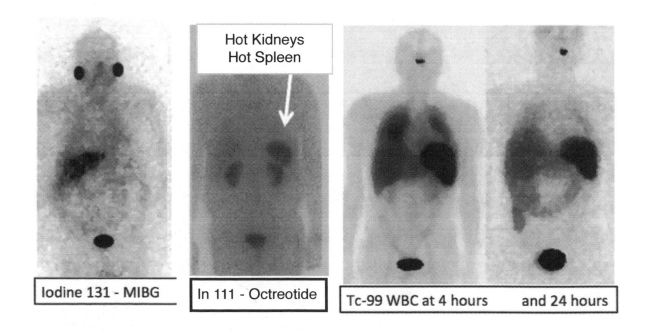

Iodine 131 - MIBG   In 111 - Octreotide

Hot Kidneys
Hot Spleen

Tc-99 WBC at 4 hours   and 24 hours

Skeletal Nuclear Medicine

The workhorse of skeletal imaging is methylene diphosphonate (MDP) tagged with Tc-99m. This is prepared from a kit which has MDP and stannous ion. You add free pertechnetate and the stannous ion reduces it so it will bind to the MDP. If you don't have enough stannous ion (*or you get air into the vial or syringe – that can cause oxidation*) you might get *free Tc* (salivary gland, thyroid, stomach uptake). After you inject the tracer (15-25mCi) you wait 2-4 hours to let the tracer clear from the soft tissues (so you can seem them bones).

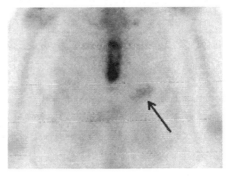

Free Tc: Gastric Uptake on Bone Scan
*incidental note of sternal met from breast CA

Mechanism: Phosphonate binding to bone (chemisorption). Distribution is based on blood flow and osteoblastic activity.

Gamesmanship - MDP and HDP are both bone agents so don't get confused if they say HDP to purposefully confuse you.

A brief discussion of F-18 vs Tc-MDP

The take home point is F-18 PET is way way way better than Tc-MDP. The image quality and sensitivity of F18 is multiple orders of magnitude better than Tc-MDP. It also has a shorter examination time. So, why do you never see F-18? Because it costs more, and insurances won't pay etc... Politics and Finance are the reasons. It's common gamesmanship to ask you to tell the difference between the two (discussed below). Another thing they can ask is what organ gets the highest dose? The **organ receiving the highest dose is Bone with MDP, and Bladder with F-18 (overall F-18 > Tc-MDP).**

Scan on Scan on Scan
This is a common trick, popular in case books & case conferences - asking you to distinguish F-18 bone scan vs Tc-MDP bone scan vs PET-FDG with marrow stimulation.

This is how you do it:
- **Tc-MDP** will have bone and kidney uptake. It will be a blurry fuzzy piece of crap.

- **F-18** will be beautiful, super high resolution, and look like a MIP PET.

- **FDG –PET with bone stimulation** - will look similar to the F-18, but will have brain uptake. Also, this can show increased uptake in the spleen.

What Factors will affect tracer uptake?
- OsteoBLASTIC activity (why pure lytic lesions can be cold)
- Blood Flow

Where is tracer uptake NORMAL ?
- Bone (duh)
- Kidney (not seen *or very faint = Super Scan)
- Bladder
- Breasts (especially in young women)
- Soft tissues – low levels
- Epiphyses in kids

Let's Talk About Abnormal Distribution:
Increased focal uptake is very nonspecific, and basically is just showing you bone turn over. So a metastatic deposit can do that (and this is the classic indication). But, you can also see it with arthritis (classically shoulder) and healing fractures (most commonly shown with segmental ribs).

Some Sneaky Situations:
- *Skull Sutures:* It's normal to see some persistent visualization of the skull sutures, BUT when this is **marked you may be thinking about renal osteodystrophy**.

- *Breast Uptake:* Some mild diffuse breast uptake is normal (especially in younger women), BUT **focal uptake can be cancer.**

- *Renal CORTEX activity:* You are suppose to have renal activity (not seeing kidneys can make you think super scan), BUT when the **renal cortex is hotter than the adjacent lumber spine** you should **think about hemochromatosis**.

- *Diffuse Renal Uptake:* This often occurs in the setting of chemotherapy (especially if the study is looking for bone mets). This also can be seen with urinary obstruction.

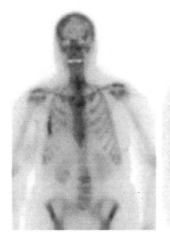 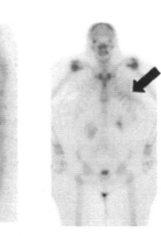 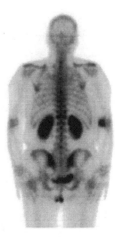

Multiple Contiguous Lesions
(Rib Fractures)

Asymmetric Breast Tissue Uptake
(Primary Breast CA)

Diffuse Renal Uptake
(Chemotherapy)

- *Liver Uptake:* This can be several things, but the main ones to think about are (1) **Too Much Al+3** contamination in the Tc, (2) Cancer – either primary **hepatoma** or mets, (3) **Amyloidosis**, (4) **Liver Necrosis**

- *Spleen Uptake:* This is a common trick to show an **auto-infarcted spleen** – common in **sickle cell patients**. These same patient's are going to have scattered hot and cold areas from multiple bone infarcts.

- *The Single Lesion:* When you see a single hot lesion, the false positive rate for attributing the finding to a met is high. Only about 15% to 20% of patients with proven mets have a single lesion (most commonly in the spine). In other words **80% of the time it's benign. A classic exception is a single sternal lesion in a patient with breast cancer.** This is due to breast CA 80% of the time.

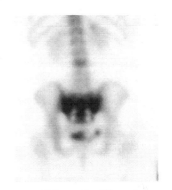

"Honda Sign"
Sacral Insufficiency Fx

- *Sacral Insufficiency fracture:* This is a hot geographic area, confined to the sacrum, often with a characteristic butterfly or **"H" shaped (Honda sign)**. Osteoporosis is the most common cause, but it can also occur in a patient who has had radiation.

- *Diffusely Decreased skeletal uptake:* This can be seen with (1) free Tc, or (2) Bisphosphonate therapy.

- *Fractures in the Elderly (including elder abuse):* In older populations, bone scans may be negative for several days. A bone scan obtained at **1 week** will exclude a fracture.

Flair Phenomenon: This is a sneaky situation shown on bone scan, where a good response to therapy will mimic a bad response. What happens is you have increased radiotracer uptake (both in number and size of lesions) seen 2 weeks to 3 months after treatment.

> *So how can you tell it's flair and not actually cancer getting worse?*
> - On plain film lesions should get more sclerotic
> - After 3 months they should improve.

Specific Cancer – Specific Trivia
- Prostate Cancer Loves Bone Mets (85% of dying patients have it)
- Prostate Cancer bone mets are uncommon with a PSA less than 10 mg/ml
- Lung Cancer bone mets tend to be in the appendicular skeleton
- Lung Cancer can have hypertrophic osteoarthropathy (10%)
- Breast Cancer bone mets are most common to the spine, but the **solitary sternal lesion is more specific**
- Neuroblastoma frequently mets to the bones (metaphysis of long bones)
- **I-123 and 131 MIBG is superior for detection of neuroblastoma bone mets**

Cold Lesions
- Radiation Therapy (usually segmental)
- Early Osteonecrosis
- Infarction *(very early or late)*
- Anaplastic Tumor (Renal, Thyroid, Neuroblastoma, Myeloma)
- Artifact from prosthesis
- Hemagioma

Bone Scan vs Skeletal Survey (Trivia)
- Bone Scan is way better (more sensitive) than skeletal survey when dealing with blastic mets
- Skeletal Survey is superior (more sensitive) for lytic mets
  - "Skeletal survey is the preferred evaluation for osseous involvement in multiple myeloma"

Hypertrophic Osteoarthopathy: This is **a "Tramline" along the periosteum of long bones**, which is associated with conditions of chronic hypoxia (CF, Cyanotic Heart Disease, Mesothelioma, Pneumoconiosis). However, when you see this – you need to think **lung cancer**. Apparently it's actually seen in 10% of patients with lung cancer.

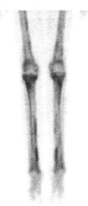

"Tramline Sign" of
Hypertrophic Osteoarthropathy

Pagets: Seen primarily in older patients (8% at 80), it's classically shown five ways: (1) Super Hot Enlarged Femur (2) Super Hot Enlarged Pelvis, (3) Super hot skull, (4) Expanded hot "entire" vertebral body (5) metabolic superscan - from widespread Pagets. As a point of gamesmanship if they show you a metabolic superscan the answer is probably hyper PTH.

Pagets Spine - Classically involves BOTH the vertebral body and posterior elements.

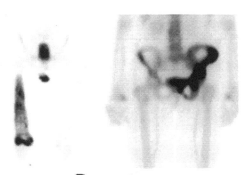

Pagets

Primary Bone Tumors: Both Osteosarcoma and Ewings will be hot. Primary utility of the bone scan is to see extent of disease. With regard to benign bone tumors the only ones worth knowing are the HOT ones and the COLD ones. Osteoid Osteoma is worth knowing a few extra things about (because they lend themselves easily to multiple choice questions).

Osteoid Osteoma: The lesion will be focal and three phase hot. A central hot nidus is often seen (**double density** or **hotter spot within hot area**). A normal bone scan excludes this entity.

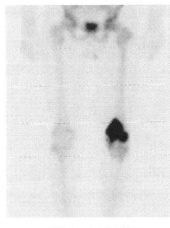
Osteosarcoma

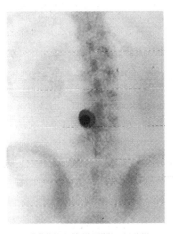
Osteoid Osteoma
-Double Density

Fibrous Dysplasia: *Be aware that in case books / case conference this is sometimes shown as a super hot mandible. Could also be shown as a leg, that looks similar to pagets.*

Benign Lesions on Bone Scan:

- **"HOT"** *(intense)*
  - Fibrous Dysplasia
  - Giant cell tumor
  - Aneurysmal bone cyst
  - Osteoblastoma
  - Osteoid osteoma
- **"COLD"**
  - Bone cyst without fracture
- VARIABLE
  - Hemangioma
  - Multiple hereditary exostosis

Heterotopic Ossification: The main reason you image this is to see if it's "mature" or not. Serial exams are used to evaluate if the process is active or not. If it's still active it has a higher rate of recurrence after it's resected. The idea is you can follow it with imaging until it's mature (cold), then you can hack it out (if someone bothers to do that).

Avascular Necrosis: AVN can occur from a variety of causes (EtOH, Steroids, Trauma, Sickle Cell, Gauchers). The trick on bone scan is the timing. **Early and late AVN is cold. Middle (repairing) will be hot.**

Super Scans

This is a common trick, where the scan shows no abnormal focal uptake, but you can't see the kidneys. The trick is that everything is hot.

This **occurs in two flavors**:

- **Diffuse Mets:** Diffuse skeletal metastatic activity (breast and prostate are the common culprits).

- **Metabolic:** From metabolic bone pathology; including *hyper parathyroid*, renal osteodystrophy, pagets, or severe thyrotoxicosis.

How can you tell them apart?

- The Skull will be asymmetrically hot on the metabolic super scan.

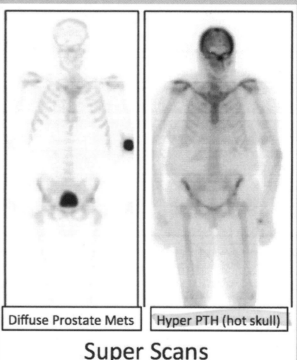

Diffuse Prostate Mets | Hyper PTH (hot skull)

Super Scans

Don't get it twisted – A common sneaky move is to show you a bone scan, with no renals. But it's because there is a horseshoe kidney in the pelvis. Could be phrased as a next step question, with the answer being look at prior CT to confirm normal anatomy.

BAD BONES!

Any bone uptake on MIBG, I-131, or Octreotide is abnormal, and concerning for skeletal mets.

Equivocal Lesion Next Step ?

If a bone scan "equivocal lesion" is found the next step is a plain film. If the plain film shows no corresponding lesion this is MORE suspicious for mets. Next step at that point would be a MRI.

The Three Phase Scan:

Bone scans can be done in a single delayed phase, or in 3 phases (flow, pool, and delayed). A lot of things can be "3 phase hot", including osteomyelitis, fracture, tumor, osteoid osteoma, charcot joint, and even reflex sympathetic dystrophy.

Cellulitis vs Osteomyelitis: The benefit of using 3 phases is to distinguish between cellulitis (which will be hot on flow and pool, but not delays), and osteomyelitis (which is 3 phase hot). In children a whole body bone scan is often performed to evaluate extent. Additionally, because of subperiosteal pus/edema you can actually have decreased vascularity to the infected area (cold on initial phases) but clearly hot on delayed phases.
In the spine, gallium (combined with bone scan) or MRI are the preferred imaging modalities.

Response: You can also use a bone scan to evaluate response to treatment. Blood flow and blood pool tend to stay abnormal for about 2 months, with delayed activity persisting for up to 2 years. This is especially true when dealing with load bearing bones. Gallium[67] and Indium[111] WBC are superior for monitoring response to therapy.

Reflex Sympathetic Dystrophy (RSD): Sometimes called "complex regional pain syndrome," it can be seen after a stroke, trauma, or acute illness. The classic description is **increased uptake on flow and blood pool**, with **periarticular uptake on delayed phase**. The uptake often involves the entire extremity. About one third of adult patients with documented RSD do not show increased perfusion and uptake *(which probably means they are faking it, and need a rheumatology consult for fibromyalgia)*. In children, sometimes you actually see decreased uptake.

Sulfur Colloid Bone Scan & WBC Imaging:

Tc can be tagged to sulfur colloid with the idea of getting a normal localization to the bone marrow. You can actually perform Tc sulfur colloid studies to map the bone marrow in patients with sickle cell (with the idea to demonstrate marrow expansion and bone infarct). However, the major utility is to use it in combination with tagged WBC or Gallium.

Both Tc Sulfur Colloid and WBCs will accumulate in normal bone marrow, in a spatially congruent way (they overlap). The principal is that infected bone marrow will become photopenic on Tc-Sulfur Colloid. Now, this takes about a week after the onset of infection, so you have to be careful in the acute setting. WBC on the other hand will obviously still accumulate in an area of infection. *Combined Tc-Sulfur Colloid and WBC study is positive for infection if there is activity on WBC image, without corresponding Tc activity on the bone marrow image.* When imaging the spine, WBC frequently fails to migrate showing a photopenic area. This is why **gallium is preferred for osteomyelitis of the spine.**

Prosthesis Evaluation: Differentiating infection from aseptic loosening is challenging and the most common reason a nuclear medicine doctor would get involved in the situation. Bone scan findings of periprosthetic activity is very nonspecific, because you can see increased tracer activity in a hip up to 1 year after placement (even longer in cementless arthroplasty). Typically, there would be diffusely increased activity on imaging with Tc-MDP in the case of infection (**more focal along the stem and lesser trochanter with loosening**) – but this isn't specific either. Combined Tc-Sulfur Colloid and WBC imaging is needed to tell the difference.

Helpful when negative - A negative bone scan excludes loosening or infection.

Neuropathic Foot: Most commonly seen in the tarsal and tarsal-metatarsal joints (60%), in diabetics. When the question is infection (which diabetics also get), it's difficult to distinguish arthritis changes vs infection with Tc-MDP. Again, combined marrow + WBC study is the way to go.

An additional pearl that could make a good "next step" question is the need for a fourth phase in diabetic feet. As these patient's tend to have reduced peripheral blood flow, the addition of a 4th phase at 24 hours may help you distinguish between bone and delayed soft tissue clearance.

Instead of In-WBC, What about Tc99 HMPAO WBC ?

When would you consider Tc99 HMPAO instead of In-WBC for infection ? Two main reasons
    (1) Kids - Tc99 will have a *lower absorbed dose & shorter imaging time*, and
    (2) Small Parts - Tc99 does better in hands and feet

Why not use Tc99 HMPAO all the time ? The downsides to Tc99 HMPAO are
    (1) It has a shorter half life *-6hrs-* which limits delayed imaging, and
    (2) It has normal GI and gallbladder activity which would obscure injection in those
       areas.

Pulmonary Nuclear Medicine

If 1940 calls and wants to rule out a PE you'll want to get the angiography room ready. In 2014, textbooks and papers still frequently lead with the following statement *"Pulmonary angiography is the definitive diagnostic modality and reference standard in the diagnosis of acute PE."* In reality, pulmonary angiography is almost never done, and CTPA is the new diagnostic test of choice. V/Q scan is usually only done if the patient is allergic to contrast or has a very low GFR. The primary reason V/Q isn't done, is that it's often intermediate probability, and the running joke is that if you don't know how to read one, just say it's intermediate and you'll probably be right.

The idea behind the test is that you give two tracers: one for ventilation and one for perfusion. If you have areas of ventilated lung that are not being perfused that may be due to PE. Normally Ventilation and Perfusion are matched, with a normal gradient (less perfusion to the apex – when standing).

Tracers:

Perfusion: For perfusion Tc-99m macroaggregated albumin (**Tc-99m MAA**) is the most common tracer used. MAA is prepared by heat denaturation of human serum albumin, with the size of the particles commercially controlled. You give it IV and the tracer should stay in the pulmonary circulation (vein-> SVC-> right heart -> pulmonary artery -> lung *STOP). The tracer should light up the entire lung. A normal perfusion study excludes PE. Areas of perfusion abnormality can be from PE or other things (more on this later). The biologic half life is around 4 hours (they eventually fall apart, becoming small enough to enter the systemic circulation to eventually be eaten by the reticuloendothelial system).

Ventilation: There are two ways to do the ventilation; you can use a radioactive gas (Xenon-133) or a radioactive aerosol (Tc-99m DTPA).

- **Xenon 133:** Also the physical half-life is 5.3 days, the **biologic half-life is 30 seconds** (you breath it out). Because it has low energy (80 keV) it **is essential to do this part of the test first** *(more on this in the physics chapter).* Additionally, because the biologic half life is so short you only can do one view (usually posterior), with a single detector (dual detector can do anterior and posterior). There are 3 phases to the study: (1) wash in (single max inspiration and breath hold), (2) equilibrium (breathing room air and xenon mix), and (3) wash out (breathing normal air)

- **Tc-99m DTPA:** This one requires patient cooperation: because they have to breath through a mouth guard with a nose clamp for several minutes. It is also essential to do this part of the test first.

5 Classic Trivia Questions about Tc99m MAA:

(1) *They show tracer in the brain*: This a classic way of showing you a **shunt** (it got into the systemic circulation somehow, maybe an ASD, VSD, or Pulmonary AVM).

(2) *How big are the particles?* A capillary is about 10 micrometers. You need your particles to stay in the lung, so they can't be smaller than that. You don't want them to be so big they block arterioles (150 micrometers). So the **answer is 10-100 micrometers**.

(3) *When do you reduce the particle amount?* A few situations. You don't want to block more than about 0.1% of the capillaries, so anyone who has fewer capillaries (**children, people with one lung**). Also you don't want to block capillaries in the brain, so anyone with a **right to left shunt**. Lastly anyone with **pulmonary hypertension (or who is pregnant)**.

(4) *Is reduced particle the same as reduced dose?* Nope. The normal dose of Tc can be added to fewer particles.

(5) *They show you multiple focal scattered hot spots:* This is the classic way of showing **"clumped MAA"**, which happens if the tech draws **blood into the syringe** prior to injection.

Classic Trivia Questions for Xenon 133:

(1) *They show you persistent pulmonary activity during washout*: This indicates **Air Trapping (COPD)**

(2) *They show you accumulation of tracer over the RUQ:* This is **fatty infiltration of the liver** (xenon is fat soluble).

Classic Trivia Questions for Tc-99m DTPA

Xenon	TC-99m DTPA
Quick Wash Out only one or two views	Slower Wash Out – **multiple projections**
Activity homogenous in the lungs	**"Clumping"** common in the mouth, central airways, and stomach (from swallowing).

Quantitative Perfusion:

You can do quantitative studies typically to evaluate prior to lung resection, or prior to transplant. You want to make sure that one lung can hold its own, if you are going to take the other one out.

Testable Trivia: Quantification is NOT possible if you use Tc-99 DTPA aerosol. You can do it with a combined Xe + Tc MAA because the Xe will not interfere with the Tc.

Gamesmanship -

Q: What if you see tracer in the thyroid or stomach on VQ Scan??
A: You should think 2 things: (1) Free Tc, or (2) Right - to - Left Shunt

Q: What do you need to call a Right - to - Left Shunt ?
A: Tracer in the Brain

Q: What if you see a unilateral perfusion defect (of the whole lung), but no ventilation defect ?
A: Get a CT or MRI. DDx is gonna be a mass, fibrosing mediastinitis, or Central PE.

Q: How do you grade this unilateral perfusion defect (of the whole lung), but no ventilation defect ?
A: It's technically high probability.

Pulmonary Infections

Using Gallium:

Gallium ^{67} Scan

The body handles Ga^{+3} the same way it would Fe^{+3} - which as you may remember from step 1 gets bound *(via lactoferrin)* and concentrated in areas of inflammation, infection, and rapid cell division. Therefore it's a very non-specific way to look for infection or tumor. Back in the stone ages this was the gold-standard for cancer staging (now we use FDG-PET). I should point out that Gallium can also bind to neutrophil membranes even after the cells are dead, which gives it some advantages over Indium WBC - especially in the setting of chronic infection.

Gallium is produced in a cyclotron via the bombardment of Zn^{68}, at which point it's complexed with citric acid to make Gallium Citrate. The half life is around 3 days (78hours). It decays via electron capture, emitting gamma rays at 4 photopeaks:

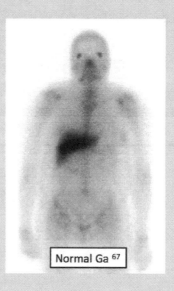

Normal Ga ^{67}

93 keV - 40%
184 keV - 20%
300 keV - 17%
393 keV - 5%

Images are not typically done sooner than 24 hours - because background is too high. *The critical organ is the colon.* Remember "critical organ" = the first organ to be subjected to radiation in excess of the maximum allowable amount.

Normal localization: Liver (*which is the highest uptake*), bone marrow (*"Poor Mans's bone scan"*), spleen, salivary glands, lacrimal glands, breasts (especially if lactating, or pregnancy). Kidneys and bladder can be seen in the first 24 (faintly up to 72 hours). Faint uptake in the lungs can be seen in < 24 hours. After 24 hours you will see some bowel. In children the growth plates and thymus.

"Poor Man's Bone Scan" - Uptake is in both cortex (like regular bone scan) and marrow. Degenerative change, fractures, growth plates, all are hot - just like bone scan.

Uptake is nonspecific and can be seen with a variety of things including infection, but also CHF, atelectasis, and ARDS.

Sarcoidosis:

The utility of Gallium in Sarcoidosis patients is to help look for active disease. Increased uptake in the lungs is 90% sensitive for active disease (scans are negative in inactive disease). Additionally, Gallium can be used to help guide biopsy and lavage – if looking to prove the diagnosis. The degree of uptake is graded relative to surrounding tissue (greater than lung is positive, less than soft tissue is negative).

Classic Signs:

- *Lambda Sign* – The nuke equivalent to the "1-2-3 Sign" on Chest x-ray. You have increased uptake in the bilateral hila, and right paratracheal lymph node.

- *Panda Sign* – Prominent uptake in the nasopharyngeal region, parotid salivary gland, and lacrimal glands. This can also been seen in Sjogrens and Treated Lymphoma.

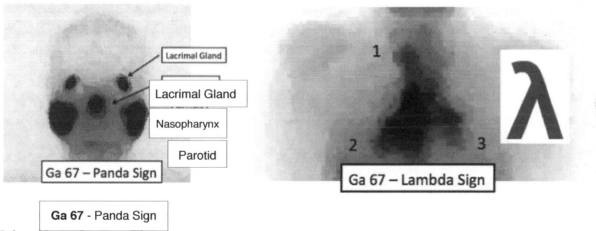

Ga 67 - Panda Sign

Other Noninfectious Things

- Gallium can be used to show early drug reaction from chemotherapy (Bleomycin) or other drugs (Amiodarone).
- Gallium is elevated in IPF (idiopathic pulmonary fibrosis) and can be used to monitor response to therapy.

Immunosuppressed Patients

- **PCP** – Gallium Hot, -- Characteristic Gallium Pattern is Diffuse Bilateral Pulmonary Uptake

- **Kaposi Sarcoma** – Gallium Negative, Thallium Positive

- **Bacterial Pneumonia** - Intense lobar configuration without parotid or nodal uptake

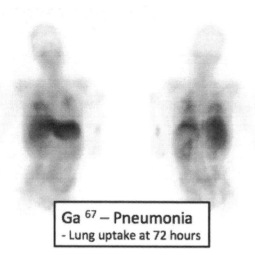

Ga ^{67} – Pneumonia
- Lung uptake at 72 hours

Misc Infections That Gallium Can Pick Up:

- *Abdominal and Pelvic Infections* – In-111 WBC is superior to Gallium (Gallium has some normal GI uptake).

- *Malignant Otitis Media* – Will be both Gallium and Bone Scan (Temporal Bone) Hot.

- *Spinal Osteomyelitis* - Gallium is superior to Indium WBC for spinal infections.

Thyroid Imaging / Treatment

The thyroid likes to drink Iodine (it's sort of its job). Imaging takes advantage of this with Iodine analogs. The distinction between "trapping" and "organification" is a common question.

- *"Trapping"* – Analog is transported into gland. ^{123}I, ^{131}I, and ^{99m}Tc all do this.

- *"Organification"* – Analog is oxidized by thyroid peroxidase and bound to tyrosyl moiety. ^{123}I and ^{131}I do this. **^{99m}Tc does NOT do this**. Instead ^{99m}Tc slowly washes out of the gland.

Tracer options / pros and cons.

I-131: The major advantage here is that it's cheap as dirt. The disadvantage is that it has a long half life (8 days), and that it's a high energy (364 keV) beta emitter. The high energy makes a crappy image with a ½ inch crystal. It's ideal for therapy, not for routine imaging. It's contraindicated in kids and pregnant women.

Trivia: Thyroid formation takes place in fetus at 8-12 weeks.

I-123: This guy has a shorter half life (13 hours) and ideal energy (159 keV). It decays via electron capture and all around makes a prettier image. The problem is that it costs more.

Tc-99m: Remember that this guy is trapped but not organified. Background levels are higher because only 1-5% of the tracer is taken up by the thyroid gland. A common scenario to choose Tc over Iodine, is when they've had a recent thyroid blocker on board (iodinated contrast is the sneaky one).

> ### *Random Trivia on Breast Feeding* (You know they love this shit):
>
> - *Tc-99m: You can resume breast feeding in 12-24 hours*
> - *I-123: You can resume breast feeding in 2-3 days*
> - *I-131: You should not breast feed – pump and dump.*

Iodine Uptake Test:

You give either 5 milli Ci of 131 or 10-20 milli Ci of 123. This is conventionally reported at 4-6 hours, and 24 hours. Normals are 6-18% (4-6 hours), and 10-30% at 24hours. A correction for background is done on measurements prior to 24 hours (using the neck counts – thigh counts).

Factors affecting the test
- Renal Function (increases stable iodine pool, reduces numbers)
- Dietary Iodine – variable and controversial
- Medications – thyroid blockers, Nitrates, IV Contrast, **Amiodarone**

Increased Uptake	Decreased Uptake
Graves	Primary or secondary causes of Hypothyroidism
Early Hashimoto	Renal Failure
Rebound after Abrupt withdrawal of antithyroid medication	Medications *(thyroid blockers, Nitrates, IV Contrast, Amiodarone)*
Dietary Iodine Deficiency	Dietary Iodine Overload

Graves Disease: About 75% of the time, if you have hyperthyroidism the cause is going to be graves. Graves is an autoimmune disease where an antibody to the thyrotropin receptor stimulates the thyroid to produce hormone. TSH will be very low, where T3 and T4 will be high. The classic clinical scenario is a middle aged women with a protracted course, pre-tibial edema, and exophthalmos. Scintigraphy is going to give you a homogeneously increased gland, with uptakes increased at both 4 hours and 24 hours. Sometimes the 24 hour uptake is lower than the 4 hours (or even at a normal range) - this is from rapid thyroid hormone production.

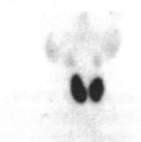

Graves
-Diffuse Homogenous Uptake

Visualization of the pyramidal lobe: The pyramidal lobe is seen in about 10% of normal thyroids. In patient's with Graves disease it is seen as much as 45% of the time. Therefore, it's suggestive when you see it.

Multi-nodular Toxic Goiter (Plummer Disease): The classic scenario is an elderly women with weight loss, anxiety, insomnia, and tachycardia. The gland is typically heterogeneous, with uptake that is only moderately elevated. The nodules will be hot on the background of a cold gland.

Toxic Multi-nodular Goiter vs Non-Toxic Multi-nodular goiter: The toxic goiter will have hot nodules on a background of cold thyroid. The Non-toxic one will have warm/hot nodules on a normal background of the thyroid.

Graves	Toxic Multi-Nodular Goiter
Uptake High :70s	Uptake Medium High: 40s
Homogenous	Heterogeneous

Hashimotos – The **most common cause of goitrous hypothyroidism** (in the US). It is an autoimmune disease that causes hyper first then hypothyroidism second (as the gland burns out later). It's usually hypo – when it's seen. It has an **increased risk of primary thyroid lymphoma**. Step 1 trivia; associated with autoantibodies to thyroid peroxidase (TPO) and antithyroglobulin. The appearance of the hypothyroid gland is typically an inhomogeneous gland with focal cold areas. The hyperthyroid (acute) gland looks very much like Graves with diffusely increased tracer.

Subacute Thyroiditis: If you have a viral prodrome followed by hyperthyroidism, and then thyroid uptake scan shows a **DECREASED %RAIU you have de Quervains (Granulomatous thyroiditis)**. During this acute phase, the disease can mimic Graves with a low TSH, high T3 and high T4. The difference is the uptake scan. After the gland burns out, it may stay hypothyroid or recover. If they ask you about this, it's most likely going to try and fool you into saying Graves based on the labs, but have a low % RAIU.

Hot Nodule vs Cold Nodule: Most thyroid nodules are actually cold, and therefore most are benign (colloid, cysts, etc..). In fact, cold nodules in a multi-nodular goiter are even less likely to be cancer compared to a single cold nodule. Having said that, cold nodules are much more likely to be cancer when compared to a functional (warm) nodule.

Discordant Nodule: This is a nodule that is HOT on Tc^{99} but COLD on I^{123}. Because some cancers can maintain their ability to trap, but lose the ability to organify a hot nodule on Tc, it shouldn't be considered benign until you show that it's also hot on I^{123}.

Radioiodine Therapy

I^{131} can be used to treat both malignant and non-malignant thyroid disease.

Cancer

Actual subtypes and pathology of thyroid cancer have been discussed at length in the endocrine chapter. However, just a few points that are relevant to discuss here. Papillary is the most common subtype (papillary is popular), and it does well with surgery + 131. Medullary thyroid CA (the one the MENs get), does NOT drink the I-131 and therefore doesn't respond well to radiotherapy. Prior treatment can also make you more resistant to treatment, and re-treatment dosing is typically 50% more than the original dose.

Things that make you treatment resistant:
- Medullary Subtype CA (will not drink the tracer)
- History or prior I-131 ("easy gland has been killed off")
- History of Methimazole treatment (even if years ago)

Medullary Subtype CA

Neuroendocrine in origin, so can occasionally (around 10%) have uptake on MIBG or Octreotide. They will be cold on thyroid scan and don't drink the treatment I-131.

Associated with MEN 2a and 2b

So, normally the patient gets diagnosed and then they go for surgery. After surgery they will come to nuclear medicine. You expect that they will have some residual thyroid (it's really hard to get it all out). Prior to actually treating them you will give them a tiny dose of 131 to see how much thyroid they have left. If the uptake is less than 5% this is ideal. Uptake more than 5% will result in a painful ablation (may need steroids on top of the NSAIDs) and may need to go back to the OR. Next, you will treat them. You want their TSH really ramped up. The higher the TSH the thirstier the cancer /residual thyroid tissue. An ideal TSH is like 50 (30 would be a minimum).

How do you get the TSH up?
- There are two ways;
  - (1) is to stop the thyroid hormone (post op they are obviously hypothyroid),
  - (2) is to give recombinant TSH "Thyrogen."

How do you decide on dosing?
- Dosing is dependent on the stage of the disease; 100 for thyroid only, 150 for thyroid + nodes, 200 for distal. They are told about the precautions etc... Then you give them the dose. Before you let them go home, you test them to see if they need to go to the hospital.

So when do patients need to be admitted to the hospital?
- NRC limit is 7mR/h measured at 1 meter from the patient's chest (some agreement states use 5mR/h). The number to remember is 33 mCi of residual activity (or 30mCi in some strict agreement states).

Possible Side Effects of Treatment:
- Can cause **pulmonary fibrosis if given to patient with lung mets**. This is really only the case of macro-nodular disease (as opposed to micronodular disease). That isn't necessarily a contraindication
- Sjogrens have a greater risk of **salivary gland damage**
- Salivary gland damage is dose related – so cancer treatment patients have a greater risk

What routes does the body use to eliminate I^{131}?
- Urine is the main way it is eliminated but sweat, tears, saliva, and breast milk are other routes.

If they don't need admitted to the hospital, what precautions should they take?
- There is a whole bunch of crap they are asked to do. Drink lots of water (increase renal excretions). Suck on hard candy (keep radiotracer from jacking your salivary glands). Patients are encouraged to stay away from people (distance principal). Sleep alone for 3 days (no sex, no kissing). Good bathroom hygiene (flush twice, and sit down if you are a guy). Use disposable utensils and plates. Clothes and linens should be washed separately. Most of these things are done for 3 days.

Is it ok to breast feed? Is it ok to try and get pregnant?
- No breast feeding. If you take I^{131}, your breast feeding days are over (at least this time around).
- No getting pregnant for at least 6-12 months after therapy

Other Trivia:
- If you participated in the therapy, you need your thyroid checked 24 hours later.
- If the patient got admitted to the hospital the RSO needs to inspect the room after discharge before the janitor can clean it or the next patient can move in.
- Thyroglobulin is a lab test to monitor for recurrence. Anything over zero – after thyroidectomy, is technically abnormal, although the trend is more important (going up is bad)
- **Severe uncontrolled thyrotoxicosis and pregnancy are absolute contraindications.**

Classic Scenario - *Patient is on dialysis and needs I^{131} Rx*

Give I^{131} immediately following dialysis to maximize the time the I^{131} is on board. Decrease dose as there is limited (essentially no) excretion until next dialysis. Dialysate can go down sewer. Dialysis tubing needs to stay in storage.

Hyperthyroidism:

I^{131} can also be used to treat hyperthyroidism. Dosing depends on the etiology; 15mCi for graves (more vascular), 30mCi for multi nodular *(harder to treat the capsule)*. Again the TSH must be high for the therapy to be effective. By 3-4 months, there should be clinical evidence of resolution of signs and symptoms of hyperthyroidism, if I-131 therapy was successful. As an aside, there is no such thing as an "emergent hyperthyroid treatment." You can always use meds to cool it down. The standard medication is Methimazole. However, if there is an allergy to Methimazole, the patient is having WBC issues (side effect is neutropenia) or the patient is pregnant -use propylthiouracil (PTU). **PTU is recommended during pregnancy.**

What about Thyroid Eye Disease? It's controversial, but some people believe that thyroid eye disease will worsen after I-131 treatment. If you are prompted, I would just have optho look at their eyes, bad outcome is likely severity related.

*You might not want to treat a bug eyed dude (depends on who you ask).

Wolff-Chaikoff Effect: Since we are talking about hyperthyroid treatment, there is no better time than to discuss the W.C. effect. Essentially, this is a reduction in thyroid hormone levels caused by ingestion of a large amount of iodine. The Wolff–Chaikoff effect lasts several days (around 10 days), after which it is followed by an "escape phenomenon." The W.C. effect can be used as a treatment principle against hyperthyroidism (especially thyroid storm) by infusion of a large amount of iodine to suppress the thyroid gland. The physiology of the W.C. effect also explains why hypothyroidism is sometimes produced in patients taking several iodine-containing drugs, including amiodarone.

Parathyroid Imaging

What Causes Hyperparathyroidism ?

- **Most common cause is a hyperfunctional adenoma** (85%).
- Second most common cause is multiple gland hyperplasia (12%).
- Third most common cause is cancer (3%).

Nuclear medicine can offer two techniques to localize these lesions; dual phase, and dual tracer.

Dual *Phase* Technique

In dual phase technique, a single tracer (Tc^{99}-Sestamibi) is administered, and both early (10 mins) and delayed (3 hours) imaging is performed. The idea is that sestamibi likes things with lots of **blood flow, and lots of mitochondria**. Parathyroid pathology tends to have both of these things, so the tracer will be more avid early, and stick around longer (after the tracer washes out of normal tissue). SPECT can give you more precise localization.

Testable Trivia: Sestamibi parathyroid imaging depends on mitochondrial density and blood flow"

False Positives:

Caused by things other than parathyroid pathology that like to drink sesamibi.
- Thyroid Nodules
- Head and Neck Cancers
- Lymphadenopathy
- Brown Fat

Sestamibi   I 123
Thallium   Pertechnatate

Dual *Tracer* Technique

In dual tracer technique two different agents are used and then subtraction is done. This first agent is chosen because it goes to both thyroid and parathyroid (options are either Tc^{99}-Sestamibi or 201- Thallium Chloride). The second agent is chosen because it only goes to the thyroid (options are either I-123 or Pertechnetate). When subtraction is done, anything left hot could be a parathyroid adenoma.

Problems:
- Motion: subtraction imaging can't tolerate much motion
- Stuff Messing with the Thyroid Tracers: recent iodinated contrast, etc…

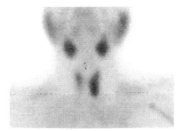  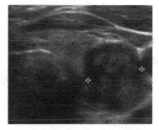

Tc - Sestamibi   I-123   Subtraction   Ultrasound Correlation

Parathyroid Adenoma – Shown on Dual Tracer Method

CNS Imaging

The goal of brain imaging in nuclear medicine is to evaluate function (more than anatomy). Typically you are dealing with SPECT brain, FDG Brain, and Cisternograms / shunt studies.

SPECT

The idea behind brain SPECT is that you can look at brain blood flow, which should mimic metabolism. You have two main tracers Tc HMPAO (hexamethylpropyleneamine oxime) and Tc ECD (ethyl cysteinate dimer). HMPAO and ECD can be used in both dementia imaging and for seizure focus localization. The two tracers have similarities and differences, and the contrast between them lends well to multiple choice tests.

HMPAO	ECD
Neutral and Lipophilic	Neutral and Lipophilic
Accumulate in the cortex proportional to blood flow (Gray Matter > White Matter)	Accumulate in the cortex proportional to blood flow (Gray Matter > White Matter)
Washout is fast	**Washout is slow (more rapid clearance from blood pool)**
Uptake favors the frontal lobe, thalamus, and cerebellum	Uptake favors the parietal and occipital lobes * *Makes comparison between HMPAO and ECD difficult*

Key points:
- Both agents pass blood brain barrier and stick to gray matter proportional to CBF
- HMPAO washes out faster
- ECD washout is slower, has better background clearance, and does not demonstrate intracerebral redistribution.

Tc DTPA - This is another agent that can be used for flow.

Key Points:
- DTPA does NOT cross the blood brain barrier and therefore cannot be used for brain parenchymal imaging. *You can NOT do SPECT
- Has the advantage over HMPAO and ECD in that it can be repeated without delay

Dementia imaging patterns: *will be discussed in the FDG brain section below.*

Seizure Focus:

The goal of nuclear imaging regarding seizures is to attempt to localize a seizure focus (sometimes they do ok if they cut it out). The idea is that **a seizure focus will be hot** (hypermetabolic and hyperperfusion) **during the seizure "ictal."** Then **cold between seizures "interictal."** You need to inject tracer (HMPAO or ECD) within 30 seconds of the seizure to get a good study. PET can be used, but is less practical.

Thallium ^{201}

Thallium is produced in a cyclotron, decays via electron capture, and has a half life of around 3 days (73 hours). The major emissions are via the characteristic x-rays of its daughter products mercury 201 - at 69 keV and 81 keV. The tracer is normally given as a chloride and will therefore rapidly be removed from the blood

Thallium **behaves like potassium**, crossing the cell membrane by active transport (Na+/ K pump). Tumors and inflammatory conditions will increase the uptake of this tracer. The higher the grade tumor, the more uptake you get. As Thallium requires active transport, it can be thought of as a viability marker - you need a living cell to transport it.

Normal Distribution: Thyroid, salivary glands, lungs, heart, skeletal muscle, liver, spleen, bowel, kidneys, and bladder. Any muscle twitching will turn hot.

If you are going to use it with Gallium, you must use the Thallium first as the Gallium will scatter all over the Thallium peaks.

High Yield Trivia / Uses:
- Toxoplasma Infection is Thallium Negative, Lymphoma is Thallium Positive
- Kaposi Sarcoma is Thallium Positive (Gallium Negative)
- Tumor is Thallium Positive, Necrosis is Thallium Negative

Tumor vs Necrosis:

The tracers used for SPECT tumor studies are different than those used for dementia or seizures. The tumor tracers are ^{201}TI (more common) and ^{99m}Tc Sestamibi (less common). ^{201}TI is a potassium analog, that enters the cell via the Na/K pump. Inflammatory conditions will increase the uptake of this tracer, but not as much as tumors. The higher the tumor grade, the more intense the uptake. Thallium can be thought of as a marker of viability, as it will localize in living tumor cells, and not necrosis. The control is the scalp (abnormalities will have greater uptake than the scalp). You can use Thallium in combination with perfusion tracers (HMPAO).

Tumor vs Necrosis	
Thallium Hot, HMPAO Cold	Tumor
Thallium Cold, HMPAO Cold	Necrosis

CNS Lymphoma vs Toxoplasmosis:

As discussed in the neuro chapter CNS lymphoma vs CNS Toxoplasmosis can be a diagnostic dilemma. **Thallium has a role in helping to distinguish the two (Toxo Cold, Lymphoma Hot).** *Please refer to the neuro chapter for additional discussion.*

Typically CNS lymphoma, toxoplasmosis, bacterial abscess, cryptococcus infection, and tuberculosis are all positive on Ga-67 scintigraphy.

Only CNS lymphoma will be positive on TI-201.

Brain Death

You are looking for the presence (or absence) of intracerebral perfusion to confirm brain death. So that you don't keep Grandma around as a piece of broccoli, you need to have a tourniquet on the scalp – otherwise you might think scalp perfusion is brain perfusion and say she's still alive. **You have to identify tracer in the common carotid – otherwise the study must be repeated. In the setting of brain death, tracer should stop at the skull base. The hot nose sign**, is seen secondary to perfusion through the external carotid to the maxillary branches. As a point of trivia – the hot nose sign cannot be used to call brain death, it is a "Secondary Sign."

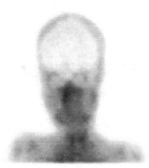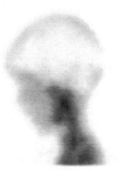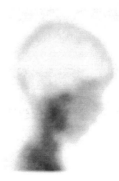

Brain Death – Hot Nose Sign

Stroke

There is no reason, ever, under any circumstances known to man, women, or beast to ever, ever use SPECT to diagnose stroke. Having said that, you can look at stroke with SPECT and will therefore likely be asked questions about it.

The big take home points are this:
- *Acute Stroke is Cold*
- *Sub Acute Stroke can be warm – from luxury perfusion* (blood flow is more than dead cells need).
- *Chronic Stroke is Cold*

Ischemia (TIAs)

You can evaluate for cerebrovascular reserve by first giving acetazolamide (Diamox) – which is a vasodilator, followed by a perfusion tracer. Normally you should get a 3-4x increase in perfusion. However, **in areas which have already maxed out their auto regulatory vasodilation (those at risk for ischemia) you will see them as relatively hypointense**. These areas of worsening tracer uptake may benefit from some revascularization therapy.

FDG-PET

PET can assess perfusion ($^{15}O\text{-}H_2O$) but typically it uses ^{18}FDG to assess metabolism (which is analogous to perfusion). Renal clearance of ^{18}FDG is excellent, giving good target to background pictures. Resolution of PET is superior to SPECT.

It's important to remember that external factors can affect the results; bright lights stimulating the occipital lobes, high glucose (>200) causes more competition for the tracer and therefore less uptake, etc…

The most common indication for FDG Brain PET is dementia imaging. Because blood flow mimics metabolism HMPAO and ECD can also be used for dementia imaging and the patterns of pathology are the same.

Dementia is discussed in detail in the neuroradiology chapter. Please refer to the masterpiece that is the neuro chapter for additional details.

FDG PET - Brain

Alzheimers	Low posterior temporoparietal cortical activity	-Identical to Parkinson Dementia -Posterior Cingulate gyrus is the first area abnormal
Multi Infarct	Scattered areas of decreased activity	
Dementia with Lewy Bodies	Low in lateral occipital cortex	Preservation of the mid posterior cingulate gyrus **(Cigulate Island Sign)**
Picks / Frontotemporal	Low frontal lobe	
Huntingtons	Low activity in caudate nucleus and putamen	

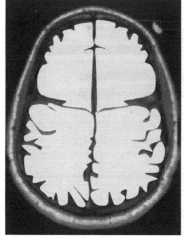

Normal

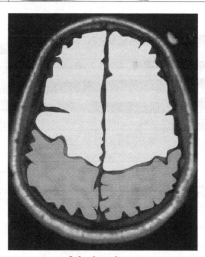

Alzheimers
-Low posterior temporoparietal

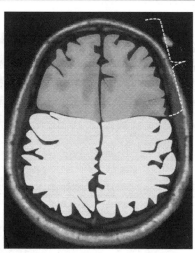

Frontotemporal
-Low Frontal Lobe

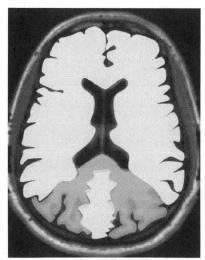

Lew Body Dementia
-Low Lateral Occipital with sparing of the cingulate gyrus

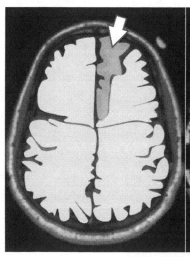

Multi-Infarct
-Scattered Areas of Low Uptake

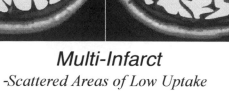

Miscellaneous Conditions For Which Pet Brain has Utility.

Crossed Cerebellar Diaschisis (CCD)

Depressed blood flow and metabolism affecting the cerebellar hemisphere after a contralateral supratentorial insult (infarct, tumor resection, radiation).

Creates an Aunt Minnie Appearance:

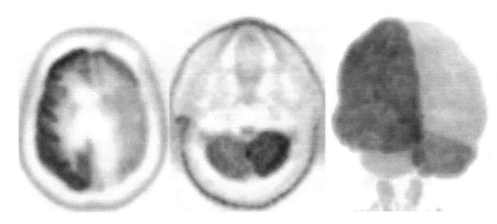

Crossed Cerebellar Diaschisis

CSF Imaging

The principle involved in imaging the CSF consists of intrathecal administration that will safely follow CSF and remains in the CSF compartment until it is absorbed through the conventional pathways. The **most common tracer used is ^{111}In – labeled DTPA.** So, you have to do an LP on the dude (it's intrathecal).

Normal Examination
- Time Zero - You do the LP
- 2-4 hours it ascends and reaches the basal cisterns
- 4 hours - 24 hours it flows around the sylvian and interhemispheric cistern
- At 24 hours it should clear from the basilar cisterns and be over the cerebral convexities

Abnormal Examination (general principles)
- Tracer in the lateral ventricles
- Failure to clear from the cisterns and localize over the convexities by 24 hours

Communicating Hydrocephalus: Normal pressure hydrocephalus is wet, wacky, and wobbly (incontinent, confused, and ataxic) clinically, and the "ventricular enlargement out of proportion to atrophy" on CT.

On scintigraphy you are looking for:
- *Early entry (4-6 hours) of tracer into the lateral ventricles*
- *Persistence of tracer in the lateral ventricle > 24 hours*
- *Delay in Assent to the parasagittal region > 24 hours*

NPH – Persistent Tracer in the Ventricles > 24hours

Since radiotracer shouldn't normally enter the ventricles, a radionuclide cisternogram cannot be used to distinguish communicating from noncommunicating hydrocephalus. Historically (1930s) you could tell by injecting the material directly into the lateral ventricles.

This vs That: *NPH vs Non obstructive (communicating) hydrocephalus.* NPH will have a normal opening pressure on LP.

CSF Leak: You can use CSF tracers to localize a leak. The most common sites of CSF leak (fistulas) are between the cribriform plate and ethmoid sinuses, from the sella turcica into the sphenoid sinus and from the ridge of the sphenoid to the ear. The study is like a bleeding scan, in that the leak must be active during the test for you to pick it up.

How is it done? You image around the time the CSF is at the basilar cisterns (1-3 hours) and also image pledgets (jammed up the nose prior to the exam). You compare tracer in serum to the pledgets (ratio greater than 1.5 is positive).

Shunt Patency: There are a bunch of ways to do this. Most commonly Tc labeled DTPA is used (^{111}In – labeled DTPA could also be used). Usually, the tracer is injected straight into the tubing.

- Normal Test will show tracer in the peritoneum – shows distal end is patent.
- You can manually occlude the distal limb to force tracer into the ventricles – shows proximal end is patent.
- If the tracer fails to reflux into the ventricles, or it does but then doesn't clear you can think proximal obstruction
- If there is delayed tracer flow into the peritoneum (> 10 minutes = delayed), this can mean partial distal obstruction.

GI Imaging

Gastric Emptying : Believe it or not, this study is actually considered the "gold standard" to evaluate gastric motor function. The primary indication is typically gastroparesis (usually in a diabetic). The exam should be performed fasting (at least 4 hours). Some texts say that it should be done in the first 10 days of the menstrual cycle to prevent hormones from interfering (I'm sure this recommendation is evidence based). Most commonly Tc labeled sulfur colloid is used, on a standardized liquid meal, solid meal (egg whites), or both. Solids are more sensitive, but you can have emptying problems from liquids only and normal emptying from solids. The most likely test question is to understand the difference in curves between solids and liquids. The main point is that solids have a "lag phase" in which the stomach helps grind up the food into smaller parts (liquids don't have this). Lag Time can be increased in diabetic patients.

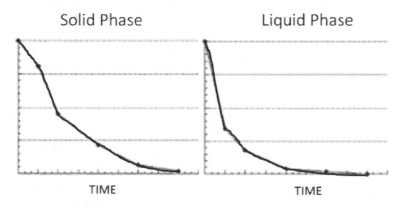

Another possible question is that **"attenuation correction"** plays a role in calculation of emptying times, as movement from the back of the stomach to the front can increase counts due to attenuation.

Esophageal Transit: Used (rarely) in the evaluation of esophageal motility disorders. The supposed advantage is the ability to give quantitative information. The patient is made to fast overnight, then fed Tc-99 sulfur colloid. Dynamic imaging is performed and transit time and / or residual esophageal activity is measured.

GI Bleeding: The goal of a GI bleeding scan is to localize the bleed (not to say there is one). Bleeding scan is sensitive to GI bleed rates as low as at 0.1ml/min (Mesenteric angiography, requires 1-1.5 ml/min bleeding).

Key Point:
- *GI bleed scan detection = 0.1 ml/min*
- *Angiogram detection = 1.0 ml/min*

First Some Technical Stuff (Very Boring and High Yield)

Before the Tc-99 can be tagged to a RBC (*beta chain of the hemoglobin*) it must first be reduced. This is accomplished with stannous ion (tin). This is referred to as "tinning."

There are 3 methods:

RBC Tagging

In Vivo

1. Tin (stannous ion) is injected into the patient
2. Then Tc-99m pertechnetate is injected
3. Tin binds to the hemoglobin then reduces the Tc (which then binds)

Although the process is super simple, you only get about 60-80% of it bound. So you have a lot of free Tc and a dirty image (poor target to background). Sometimes it fails miserably (via drug interaction – **heparinized tubing, or recent IV contrast**). The images are too crappy for cardiac wall motion studies, but can work for GI bleeding.

In Vivo – In Vitro (Modified Method)

1. Tin (stannous ion) is injected into the patient
2. After 15-30 mins you pull 3-5 cc of blood out of an IV line into a syringe with both Tc-99m pertechnetate and an anticoagulant
3. It's then re-injected 10 mins later

This one does a little better, binding close to 85%. Drug interactions (like heparin) are the most common cause of failure.

In Vitro

Blood is withdrawn and added to a kit with both Tin (stannous ion) and Tc. It's then re-injected. This method works the best (98% binding), but is the most expensive.

Image Acquisition: GI bleeding scan is acquired with DYNAMIC imaging (as opposed to 5min static, transmission, spect, or dual tracer protocol). This allows the detection of intermittent bleeds and better localization of the origin of the bleed.

Reading the Study: You are looking for the appearance of tracer (outside the vascular distribution) that **moves like bowel** (can be antegrade or retrograde). You can get faked out by a lot of stuff; renal or bladder excretion (possibly with hydro), transplant kidney (classic trick – but again it won't move), varices or angiodsyplasia (these shouldn't move), a penis with blood in it (this will look like a penis), hemangioma (this will be over the liver or spleen – and not move), and the last trick – Free Tc in the stomach. It you see gastric uptake* next look at the salivary glands and thyroid to confirm it's free Tc, and not an actual bleed.

Alternative (Stone Age) Way of Doing A Bleeding Scan; Back when dinosaurs roamed the earth, they used to do bleeding scans with **Tc Sulfur Colloid**. This had a variety of disadvantages including; fast clearance (had to do scan in 30mins), multiple blind spots (the stomach, splenic flexure, and hepatic flexures - as sulfur colloid goes to the liver and spleen normally). The only possible advantages are that it requires less prep and has good target to background.

Meckel Scan: The Meckel Diverticulum is a remnant of the omphalomesenteric duct located near the distal ileum. These things can have ectopic gastric mucosa and present with painless bleeding in the pediatric population. **Pertechnetate** is used because it is **taken up by gastric mucosal cells**. So you are looking for tracer uptake in the pelvis (usually RLQ) around the same time as the stomach.

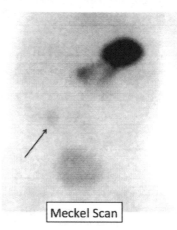

Meckel Scan

Only about 10-30% of meckels diverticulum will have gastric mucosa (these are the ones more likely to bleed).

Here are the Tricks:

- You need to **do the study when the patient is NOT bleeding** (if they are bleeding – then do a bleeding scan).

- *Pre-Treatment*: You can use a bunch of different stuff to make the exam better:
    - Pentagastrin – enhances uptake of pertechnetate by gastric mucosa (also stimulated GI activity)
    - H2 Blockers (Cimetidine and Ranitidine) block secretion of the pertechnetate out of the gastric cells making it stick around longer.
    - Glucagon – slows gastric motility.

- *False Positive*: Can occur from bowel irritation (recent scope, laxative use)

- *False Negative*: **Recent In vivo labeling or RBCs**, Recent Barium Study (attenuated)

HIDA Scan:

Function and integrity of the biliary system can be evaluated for by using Tc-99m labeled tracers that mimic bilirubin's uptake, transport, and excretion. All the tracers are basically analogs of this iminodiacetic acid stuff.

Trivia: You need higher doses of tracer if the patient has hyperbilirubinemia

Prep for the test is diet control. You need to have not eaten within four hours (so your gallbladder is ready to fill), and have eaten within 24 hours (so your gallbladder isn't so full, it can't let any tracers in). If you haven't eaten for over 24 hours, then CCK can be given.

Normally, the liver will have prompt tracer uptake (within 5 minutes), then you will have excretion into the ducts, then the bowel - pretty much the same time you see the gallbladder. If the gallbladder is sick (obstructed), it will still not have filled within 60 min. This is the basic idea.

Acute Cholecystitis: Almost always (95%) patients with acute cholecystitis have an obstructed cystic duct. If you can't get tracer in the gallbladder within 4 hours, this suggests obstruction.

Rim Sign – A curved area of increased activity along the gallbladder fossa (hot rim, or pericholecystic hepatic activity sign) suggests a **more angry gallbladder** – sometimes gangrenous.

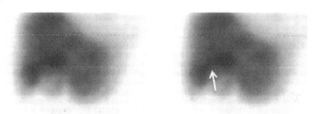

Hot Rim Sign – Hyperemia in Fossa

Mechanism of the Rim Sign: The mechanism is the *result of inflammation causing regional hepatic hyperemia, with more radiopharmaceutical being delivered to this area of hepatic parenchyma;*

Cystic Duct Sign – This sign is seen with **acute cholecystitis**. The sign describes a nub of activity in the cystic duct, with the remaining duct obstructed.

Chronic Cholecystitis: This can be shown two ways; (1) delayed filling of the GB (not seen at 1 hour, but seen at 4 hours), or (2) with a low EF (< 30%) with CCK stimulation. A reduced EF can also be seen in acute acalculous cholecystitis

Testable Trivia
- The Dose of CCK: 0.02 **microgram**/kg over 60 mins
- The Dose of Morphine 0.02-0.04 **mg**/kg over 30-60 mins

Biliary Obstruction: A lack of visualization of the biliary tree "Liver Scan Sign" can be seen with acute obstruction of the CBD.

Things that can go wrong:
- No Bowel Activity , Persistent Blood Pool = Hepatocyte Dysfunction (Hepatitis)
- No Bowel Activity, Blood Pool Goes Away Normally = Common Duct Obstruction
- No Gallbladder Activity x 4 hours (or 1 hour + morphine) = Acute Cholecystitis
- Abnormal GB emptying (EF < 30%) = Chronic Cholecystitis

Prompt Uptake - With Delayed Excretion (Medication)

Classically **Dilantin (Chlorpromazine)** and **birth control pills** can cause prompt tracer uptake and delayed clearance. This can mimic biliary obstruction

---

Biliary Atresia vs Neonatal Hepatitis

If you see a hepatobiliary scan (HIDA) in a kid, for sure this is the indication. Apparently, these two things are hard to tell apart clinically. If you see **tracer in the bowel it's hepatitis**, but just remember that it might be slow so you need super **delays (24 hours if necessary)**. If you don't see it in the bowel, you might still need to repeat the study if you didn't **charge up those hepatocytes with some phenobarb** (up regulates the cytochrome system). In other words, a lot of places pre-medicate with phenobarbital to increase the utility of the test. So, if you operate early (kasai procedure) they do a lot better, so it's important not to screw this up.

Bile Leak

You can use HIDA tracer after trauma or surgery to look for bile leak. The trick is that you need delayed images, and look in the right paracolic gutter / pelvis. You can get tracer in the gallbladder fossa, mimicking a gallbladder.

Reappearing Liver Sign - Labeled bile may track superiorly into the perihepatic space and coat the surface of the liver. This can give the appearance of **paradoxically increasing activity in the liver** after an initial decrease in activity from liver emptying into the bowel.

Sulfur Colloid Liver Scan

Not frequently done because of the modern invention of CT. Sulfur Colloid tagged with Tc is quickly eaten by the livers reticuloendothelial system. It can be used to see "hot" and "cold" areas in the liver. **Classically the multiple choice question is Focal Nodular Hyperplasia Hot on sulfur colloid (although in reality it's only hot 30-40% of the time).**

Sulfur Colloid Liver Scan	
Hepatic Adenoma	COLD
FNH	40% HOT, 30% COLD, 30% Neutral
Cavernous Hemangioma	COLD *(RBC Scan HOT)*
HCC	COLD, *(Gallium HOT)*
Cholangiocarcinoma	COLD
Mets	COLD
Abscess	COLD *(Gallium HOT)*
Focal Fat	COLD *(Xe HOT)*

Particle size is worth discussing briefly. Particles for this scan need to be 0.1 – 1.0 micrometers. This is the right size for the liver to eat them. If they are too big the spleen will eat them, and if they are too small the bone marrow will eat them. Also, realize that if they were too big they would get stuck in the lungs like a VQ on the first pass through.

Colloid Shift – In a normal sulfur colloid scan, 85% of the colloid is taken up by the liver (10% spleen, 5% bone marrow). In the setting of diffuse hepatic dysfunction, portal hypertension, hypersplenism, or bone marrow activation you can see change in uptake – shift to the spleen and bone marrow. The most specific causes of colloid shift are cirrhosis, diffuse liver mets, diabetes, and blunt trauma to the spleen.

Diffuse Pulmonary Activity – This is not normal localization of sulfur colloid. This is non-specific and can be seen with a ton of things (most commonly diffuse liver disease), but the first thing you should think (on multiple choice) is excess aluminum in the colloid. It can also be seen in primary pulmonary issues (reflecting phagocytosis by pulmonary macrophages).

Excess Al also seen in Tc MDP bone scan ī diffuse uptake →

Renal Activity on Sulfur Colloid = The most common cause is **CHF** (*maybe due to decreased renal blood flow and filtration pressure*). Alternatively, in the setting of **renal transplant – this can indicate rejection** (*due to colloid entrapment within the fibrin thrombi of the microvasculature*). Other more rare causes include coxsackie B viral infection, disseminated intravascular coagulopathy, and thrombotic thrombocytopenic purpura.

Hemangioma Scan

This can be done using Tc labeled RBCs. Delayed blood pool is typically done (30 mins – 3 hours). If it's small (< 2cm) you'll need SPECT to localize it. Otherwise planar imaging will show a hot focus. You want to see **marked HOT on delays, with no real hot spot on immediate flow or immediate pool**. Angiosarcoma could be HOT on delays but would also be hot on flow. A partially fibrosed hemangioma may be a false negative.

Spleen Scan

You can use heat damaged Tc labeled RBCs to localize to the spleen. A possible indication might be hunting ectopic spleen.

GU Imaging

Imaging of GU system in nuclear medicine can evaluate function (primary role), or it can evaluate structure.

Function (dynamic):

Normal kidney function is 80% secretion and 20% filtration. Tracer choice is based on which of these parameters you want to look at.

Tc-DTPA: Almost all filtration and therefore a great agent for determining GFR. A piece of trivia is that since a small (5%) portion of DTPA is protein bound (and not filtered) you are slightly underestimating GFR. Critical organ is the bladder.

GFR

Tc-MAG 3: This agent is almost exclusively **secreted** and therefore estimates effective renal plasma flow (ERPF). It is cleared by the proximal tubules. Critical organ is the bladder.

ERPF

Tc GH (glucoheptonate): This agent can be used for structural imaging (discussed later in this section), or functional imaging as it is filtered. Critical organ is the bladder.

Tc DTPA	Tc MAG 3	Tc GH
Filtered (**GFR**)	Secreted (**ERPF**)	Filtered
Good For Native Kidneys with **Normal Renal Function**	Concentrated better by kidneys with **poor renal function**	Good for dynamic and cortical imaging.
Critical Organ Bladder	Critical Organ Bladder	Critical Organ Bladder

There are essentially 5 indications for dynamic (functional) scanning: (1) Differential Function (2) suspected obstruction, (3) suspected renal artery stenosis, (4) Suspected Complication from Rental Transplant, (5) Suspected Urine Leak.

Some basics:

Images are obtained posteriorly (**anterior if patient has a transplant or horseshoe**). Typically dynamic exams have 3 phases; blood flow phase, cortical phase, and clearance phase.

Differential Function

This is a basic exam with the standard flow, cortical, and clearance phases.

Flow: Begins within 20 seconds of injection. Flow will first be seen in the aorta. Then as it reaches the renal arteries, the kidneys should enhance symmetrically and about equal to the aorta (at that time).

Flow	
Decreased (symmetric)	Technical Error – poor bolus
Decreased (asymmetric)	Renal Artery Thrombosis. Renal Vein Thrombosis. Chronic High Grade Obstruction. Acute Rejection. Acute Pyelonephritis.
Increased (asymmetric)	Renal Artery Aneurysm

An important piece of trivia is that **ATN, Interstitial Nephritis, and Cyclosporin toxicity will all have normal perfusion/flow.**

Cortical (parenchymal): This is the most important portion of the exam (with regard to differential function). An area of interest in drawn around the kidneys and a background area of interest is also drawn (to correct for the background). This can be screwed up by drawing your background against the liver or spleen (which is not true background since they will take up some tracer). You want to measure this at a time when the kidney is really drinking that contrast, but not so late that it is putting it in the collection system. Most places use around 1 min. A steep slope is good.

Clearance (excretory): Radiotracer will begin to enter the renal pelvis, collecting system, and bladder. In a normal patient, you will be down to half peak counts at around 7-10 mins. If you wanted to quantify retention of tracer you could look at a 20/3 or 20/peak ratio.

20/3 or 20/peak ratio: This is a method of quantifying retention of radiotracer by comparing the peak count at 20 minutes with the peak count at 3 mins (normal < 0.8) or the peak count (normal 0.3).

Suspected Obstruction ("The Lasix Renogram")

The exam is performed the same as a standard dynamic exam (blood flow, cortical, and clearance), with a 30 minute wait after clearance. If there is still activity in the collecting system, a challenge is performed with Lasix. The idea is that a true obstruction will NOT respond to the Lasix, whereas a dilated system will empty when overloaded by Lasix. The study can be done with MAG-3 or DTPA. Mag-3 does better with patients with poor renal function, and thus is used more commonly.

The exam is interpreted as follows:

- No obstruction = tracer clears from collecting system without need for Lasix
- No obstruction = Washout of 50% of the tracer within 10 minutes of Lasix administration
- Indeterminate = Washout of 50% of the tracer within 10-20 minutes of Lasix administration
  - The most common cause for this indeterminate result is a very dilated pelvis and subsequent "reservoir effect."
- Obstructed= Washout taking longer than 20 mins after Lasix administration

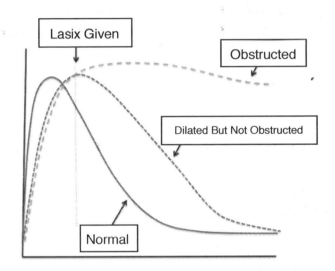

Source of False Positive for Obstruction:
- Poor response to Lasix – secondary to **bad renal function**, or **dehydration** at baseline
- "Reservoir Effect" – **very dilated renal pelvis,** delaying transit time
- Back Pressure Effects – **Full or Neurogenic Bladder** can generate back pressure and not let the kidneys empty (can be resolved with a foley catheter).

Suspected Renal Artery Stenosis ("Captopril Renogram")

The study can be performed in one of two ways (both using MAG 3 as the typical tracer). The first is a standard dynamic study, followed by ACE inhibitor. The second as a baseline study with ½ dose, followed by a full dose of ACE inhibitor. **A "normal study" will occur if there is no difference between the baseline and the captopril studies.**

The appearance of RAS will vary depending on the tracer given:
- **DTPA** – Remember this is a GFR tracer. A sick kidney will have **decreased uptake and flow**, because of loss of perfusion pressure.

- **MAG 3** – Remember this is a Secreted tracer. A sick kidney will have **marked tracer retention**, with a curve similar to obstruction.

If it's bilateral up or bilateral down, it's not RAS. If the baseline study has asymmetrically poor function, that isn't positive for RAS, you need to see it worsen (> 10%).

Trivia related to ACE inhibitor administration; they need to stop their ACE inhibitor prior to the renal study (3-5 days if captopril). They should be NPO for 6 hours prior to the test (for PO ACE inhibitors).

Suspected Complication from Renal Transplant

ATN vs Rejection: The most common indication for nuclear medicine in the setting of renal transplant is to differentiate rejection from ATN. ATN is usually in the first week after transplant, and is more common in cadaveric donors. There will be **preserved renal perfusion** with delayed excretion in the renal parenchyma (elevated 20/3 ratio, delayed time to peak). ATN usually gets better. There is an exception to this rule, but it will confuse the issue with respect to multiple choice, so I'm not going to mention it. Cyclosporin toxicity can also look like ATN (normal perfusion, with retained tracer) but will NOT be seen in the immediate post op period. Rejection will have poor perfusion, and delayed excretion. A chronically rejected kidney won't really take up the tracer.

In a Normal DMSA or ATN (with mag3 tracer), the nephrographic appearance is the same. Tracer in the cortex, and that's it.

ATN	Immediate Post OP (3-4 days post op)	Perfusion Normal	Excretion Delayed
Cyclosporin Toxicity	**Long Standing**	Perfusion Normal	Excretion Delayed
Acute Rejection	Immediate Post OP	**Poor Perfusion**	Excretion Delayed

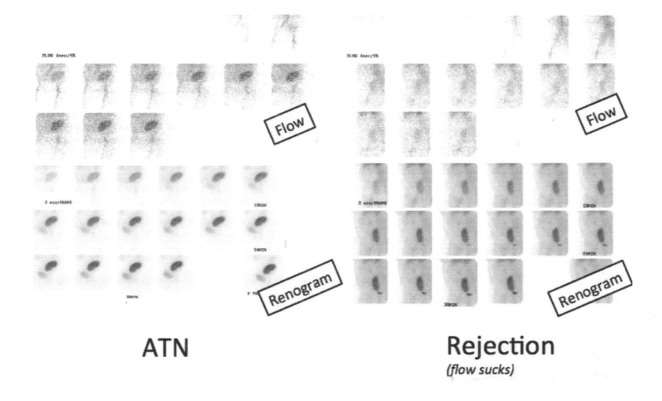

ATN

Rejection
(flow sucks)

Fluid Collections: Fluid collections seen after a transplant include urinomas, hematomas, and lymphoceles. All 3 can cause photopenic areas on blood pool imaging.

- **Urinoma**: Usually found in the first 2 weeks post op. Delayed imaging will show tracer between the bladder and transplanted kidney. A hematoma is not going to have tracer in it.

- **Lymphocele:** Usually found 4-8 weeks after surgery. The cause is a disruption of normal lymphatic channels during perivascular dissection. Most are incidental and don't need intervention. If they get huge, they can cause mass effect. This will look like a **photopenic area on the scan.**

Vascular Complications: Both arterial and venous thrombosis will result in no flow or function. If you suspect renal artery stenosis (most common at the anastomosis), you can do a captopril study, with results similar to RAS if there is a stricture.

Structure

If you want to look at the renal cortex, you will want to use an agent that binds to the renal cortex (via a sulfhydryl group). You have two main options with regard to tracer.

• Tc-DMSA: This is the more commonly used tracer. It binds to the renal cortex and is cleared very slowly. **Critical organ is the kidney** *(notice other renal tracers have the bladder as their critical organ)*.

• *Tc GH (glucoheptonate):* This is less commonly used and although it binds to the cortex, it is also filtered and therefore can be used to assess renal flow, the collecting system, and the bladder. Critical organ is the bladder.

DMSA is the preferred cortical imaging agent in pediatrics, because it has a lower dose to the gonads (even though its renal dose is higher than TcGH).

Indications for the exam:

• *Acute Pyelonephritis: Can appear as (a) focal ill defined area of decreased uptake, (b) multifocal areas of decreased uptake, (c) diffuse decreased uptake – in an otherwise normal kidney.*

  ○ *Scarring and Masses can also appear as focal areas of decreased uptake – although scarring usually has volume loss.*

• *Column of Bertin vs Mass:* Simply put, the mass will be cold. The Column of Bertin (normal tissue) will be take up tracer.

The trick on DMSA is just like reading CXR or Chest CT – you need to know if it is acute or chronic. The clinical history changes your DDx.

• *Defects on DMSA with acute renal problems = pyelo.*
• *Defects on DMSA with chronic renal problems = scar (or mass).*

Testicular

This hasn't been done in the United States since 1968, therefore it is very likely to be on the test. The study is basically a blood flow study. The primary clinical question is testicular torsion vs other causes of pain (epididymitis). The tracer used is sodium pertechnetate ($Na^{99m}TcO_4$). Oh, don't forget to tape the penis out of the way - tape it up, not down like is required for the male residents on mammography rotations.

- **Normal** – Symmetric low level flow to the testicles.

- **Acute (early) Torsion** – Focal absence of flow to the affected side ("nubbin sign").

- **Delayed (late) Torsion** – Sometimes called a missed torsion. The appearance is a halo of increased activity, with central photopenia.

- **Testicular Abscess** – Identical to delayed torsion - halo of increased activity, with central photopenia.

- **Acute Epididymitis**- Increased flow and blood pool to the affected side.

FDG PET (for cancer)

As mentioned before 18-FDG is cyclotron produced, and decays via positive beta emission to 18-O. The positron gets emitted, travels a short distance, then collides with an electron producing two 511 keV photons which go off in opposite directions. The scanner is a ring and when the two photons land 180 degrees apart at the same time the computer does math (which computers are good at) to localize the origin.

A CT component is fused over the PET portion. This is done for two reasons:
  (1) Anatomy – so you can see what the hell you are looking at.
  (2) **Attenuation Correction** – Dense stuff will slow down the photons, and the CT allows for correction of that. It also leads to errors, the classic one being a metallic pacemaker look bright hot on the corrected image (the computer overcorrected). This is a classic question. The answer is look at the source images (uncorrected).

Some other technical trivia is that FDG enters the cell via a GLUT 1 transporter and is then phosphorylated by hexokinase to FDG-6-Phosphate. This locks it in the cell. Normal bio distribution is brain, heart, liver, spleen, GI, blood pool, salivary glands, and testes. The collecting system and bladder (target organ) will also be full of it, because that's where it's getting excreted.

Variable areas of uptake: Muscles (classic forearm muscle uptake in the nervous chair squeezing patient). Breast and ovaries in females at certain stages of the menstrual cycle. Thymus in younger patients. Lastly, brown fat around the neck, thorax, and adrenals (especially in a cold room).

Ways to minimize brown fat uptake: Keep the room warm. Medications like benzodiazepines or beta blockers.

Tumors that are PET COLD	Not Cancer but PET HOT
BAC (Adeno In Situ) - Lung Cancer	Infection
Carcinoid	Inflammation
RCC	Ovaries in Follicular Phase
Peritoneal Bowel/Liver Implants	Muscles
Anything Mucinous	Brown Fat
Prostate	Thymus

Effects of Insulin and Blood Glucose

- **High Blood Glucose (> 150-200):** The more glucose the patient has, the more competition is created for the FDG and you will have artificially low SUVs.

- **Insulin:** So why not just give the patient some insulin??? It will drive it all into the muscles. This is a classic trick. PET with diffuse muscle uptake = Insulin Administration

Effects of being fat
- Fat people will have HIGHER SUV values, because the fat takes up less glucose

When do you image? Following therapy an interval of 2-3 weeks for chemotherapy, and 8-12 weeks for radiation is the way to go. This avoids "stunning" – false negatives, and inflammatory induced false positive.

Who do you image? The main utility is extent of disease, and distal metastatic spread. Local invasion is tricky with a lot of things. Usually straight up CT or MRI is better for local invasion and characterization.

What if you see the right ventricle ? The RV is not typically seen on PET unless it's enlarged. If you see the RV think about RVH.

Special Situations – Trivia

- Focal Thyroid Uptake - Requires Further Workup – might be cancer, might be nothing

- Diffuse Thyroid Uptake – Most often Autoimmune (Hashimoto) Thyroiditis

- RCC are COLD, Oncocytomas are HOT

- COLD Ground Glass Nodule = Cancer, HOT Glass Nodule = Infection

- The Reason HCC is often cold (60%) is that it has variable glucose-6- phosphatase and can't trap the FDG

- Testicular cancers skip right to the retroperitoneum. The trivia is the seminomatous CA is FDG hot, whereas non-seminomatous tends to be FDG Not.. not hot.

Non – PET Cancer Imaging

In¹¹¹- Octreoscan

Indium¹¹¹

Indium is produced in a cyclotron and decays with a 67 hour half life via electron capture. It **produces two photopeaks** at 173 keV and 247 keV. Just like Gallium, In¹¹¹ in a liquid will carry a +3 valence and behaves like Fe_{+3}, with the capability of forming strong bonds with transferrin.

The most common application is to bind it to WBC, although it can also be hooked to octreotide, or DTPA for CNS imaging (cisternography). Basically, you can hook indium to almost anything if you hook it first to a strong chelator like DTPA. As a point of trivia, you need to isolate the WBCs prior to labeling because the transferrin in the blood binds with greater affinity and will out-compete them.

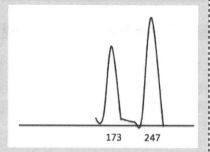

¹¹¹In Pentetreotide is the most commonly used agent for somatostatin receptor imaging. The classic use is for carcinoid tumors, gastrinomas, paragangliomas, merkel cell tumors, lymphoma, small cell lung cancer, medullary thyroid cancer, and meningiomas.

I want to stress the random fact that Meningiomas take up Octreotide (and Tc MDP).

As a point of trivia, there are 5 octreotide receptors of which ¹¹¹In Pentetreotide can bind to two of them. The scan works because 80% of neuroendocrine tumors express these two receptors.

Normal uptake is in the thyroid, liver, gallbladder, spleen, kidneys, bladder, and GI tract. Imaging is done in early and delayed phase. The advantage of the early phase (4 hours) is that the bowel activity is absent. The delayed is done to clarify that the abdominal tracer is of GI origin.

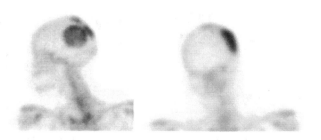

Meningioma - Hot on Octreotide and Tc MDP

MIBG

MIBG is an analog of noradrenalin and is therefore taken up by adrenergic tissue. MIBG is first line for tumors like pheochromocytoma, paraganglioma, and neuroblastoma. You can have MIBG with either I-123 or I-131. I-123 is better because it has better imaging quality. I-131 is cheaper, and the long half life allows for delayed imaging.

Blocking the Thyroid Gland: The thyroid gland should be blocked, to prevent unintended radiation to the gland from unbound I-123 or I-131. This is accomplished with Lugols Iodine or Perchlorate.

Biodistribution – Normal in liver, spleen, colon, salivary glands. The adrenals may be faintly visible. Note the kidneys are NOT seen.

Trivia: **MIBG is superior to MDP bone scan for neuroblastoma bone mets. *If you see a skeleton on MIBG the answer is diffuse bone mets.***

Trivia: MIBG is better for Pheo than In-111 Octreotide. MIBG is better than CT or MRI for the extra-adenral Pheos.

Medication Interaction with MIBG - High Yield Trivia

Certain medications interfere with the workings of MIBG and must be held. Medications include calcium-channel blockers, labetalol (other beta-blockers have no effect), reserpine, tricyclic antidepressants and sympathomimetics.

This vs That - MIBG Scans

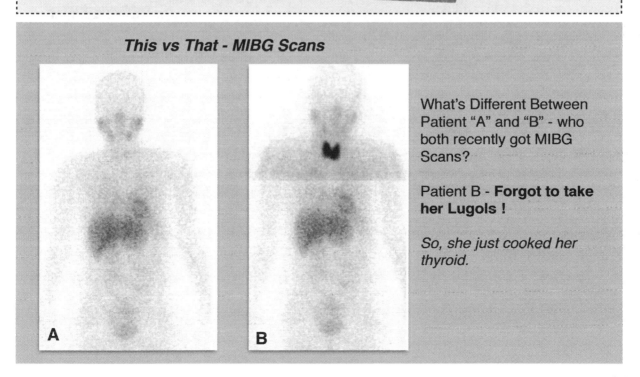

What's Different Between Patient "A" and "B" - who both recently got MIBG Scans?

Patient B - **Forgot to take her Lugols !**

So, she just cooked her thyroid.

A

B

Gallium

Gallium can be used for tumors. Remember, it's very nonspecific with regard to infection, inflammation, or tumor. Classically, Gallium was used for lymphoma imaging.

Prostascint

[111]In can be labeled to the antibody capromab Pendetide (Prostascint). Capromab is a monoclonal antibody which recognizes PSA antigen. Pendetide is the chelating agent. In my opinion, the exam is shit and doesn't work well.

When do you do the test? If you have a rising PSA and negative bone scan. The purpose of the study is to look for mets outside the prostate bed (soft tissue mets). If they do not have distal mets, they can be offered salvage therapy (radiation to the surgical bed). It's important to not obsess over the surgical bed, the real question is distal mets. Having said that the prostate bed is best seen on the lateral between the bladder and penis.

Testable Trivia: Prostascint will localize to soft tissue mets, **NOT bone mets**.

Sentinel Node Detection

A sentinel node is the node which receives afferent drainage directly from a primary lymph node. Surgeons want to know where these are at; especially with melanoma and breast cancer. The agent used for lymphoscintigraphy is **10-50nm Tc99m sulfur colloid**.

Melanoma: Sentinel node mapping is done when you have a lesion between 1mm-4mm deep. Less than 1mm you are typically safe. More than 4 mm you are totally screwed and it makes no difference. Intradermal injection in 4 spots around the lesion / excision scar and imaging is done.

Breast Cancer: Cancer drains to the internal mammary chain nodes about 3% of the time. Knowing this, and which axillary node to go for first can help avoid aggressive lymph node dissection. Injections can be done superficial or deep (into the pectoral muscle).

Size Matters

Does particle size matter for sentinel node detection? Yes and No. Albumin is typically filtered, to a size of around 0.2 microns. The size is actually not essential for the test to be diagnostic (you could use the un-filtered liver spleen scan sulfur colloid in a pinch). The primary reason for this size is speed of exam. If you used larger particles you would be waiting all day for them to get to the lymph nodes.

Test	Particle Size
Lymphoscintigraphy	< 0.2 microns (< 200 nm)
VQ	10-100 microns
Liver Spleen	"Unfiltered" – so all sizes big and small

Breast Specific Gamma Imaging

Tc99 Sestamibi will concentrate in a breast cancer 6 times more than normal background breast tissue. It does pretty good, with the sensitivity supposedly near 90%. The technique is to give 20-30 mCi of Tc99 Sestamibi in the contralateral arm then image 20 mins later. A foot injection is often done if you are going to image both breasts. A dedicated gamma camera that can mimic a mammogram and provide compression.

Does Breast Density Affect Uptake / Distribution ?

Nope. The distribution is homogeneous regardless of density. Having said that, hormonal fluctuation can increase the background uptake.

When will background activity be lowest?

Around mid-cycle in premenopausal women.

What are some causes of false positive studies ?

Fibroadenoma, fibrocystic change, or inflammation can give a false positive

What are some causes of false negative studies?

Lesions that are small (< 1cm), or deep. Lesions located in the medial breast, and/or those overlapping with heart activity.

What about lymph nodes?

If you see lymph nodes on a "mibi" scan this is NOT normal, and they are concerning for mets.

Cardiac Imaging

Myocardial Perfusion / SPECT:

Tc Sestamibi and Tc Tertrofosmin are the most common tracers. They work by crossing the cell membrane and localizing in mitochondria (passive diffusion). They don't redistribute (like Thallium), giving better flexibility.

Sestamibi vs Tetrofosmin – Tetrofosmin is cleared from the liver more rapidly and decreases the chance of a hepatic uptake artifact.

Thallium – This is historical, with regard to cardiac imaging. It mimics potassium and crosses the cell membrane first by distribution related to blood flow – second by delayed redistribution (washout). Washout is delayed in areas with poor perfusion

Imaging Timing:

Tc studies (sestamibi and tetrofosmin) are done 30-90 mins after injection – allowing for clearance from background

Thallium	Sestamibi and Tetrofosmin
Old	Newer
Crosses cell via Na/K pump	Crosses cell via passive diffusion (localizes in mitochondria)
Redistributes	Does NOT redistribute
Imaging must be done immediately after injection	Imaging typically done 30-90 mins after injection to allow for background to clear

Lung/ Heart Ratio: Only done with Thallium. If there is more uptake in the lungs, this correlates with multi-vessel disease or high grade LAD or LCX lesions.

General Principal: You will see less perfusion distal to an area of vascular obstruction (compared to normal myocardium). To improve sensitivity the heart is stressed. Under stress you need about 50% stenosis to see a defect (it needs to be like 90% without stress).

Preparation: Patient shouldn't eat for 4 hours prior to imaging (decreases GI blood flow). Patients should (ideally) stop beta-blockers, calcium channel blockers, and long acting nitrates for 24 hours prior to the exam – as these meds mess with the sensitivity of the stress portion. There are reasons to keep people on these meds (they might be getting risk stratification on medical therapy) – but I'd say for the purpose of multiple choice just know that those medication classes mess with stress imaging sensitivity.

Protocols: There are multiple ways to skin this particular cat. People will do two day exams; rest then stress. People will do one day exams stress then rest. The advantage to doing stress first is that you can stop if it's normal. Typically the dosing is low for the rest and high for the stress.

Chemical Stress: If you can't exercise, the modern trend is to give you Regadenoson – which is a specific adenosine receptor agonist. It's specific to a certain receptor having less bronchospasm than conventional adenosine or dipyridamole. If they get bronchospasm anyway you need to give them albuterol.

Findings:

Fixed Defect (seen on stress and rest)	Scar (prior infarct)
Reversible Defect (seen on stress, better on rest)	Ischemia
Fixed Defect with Reversible Defect around it	Infarct with peri-infarct ischemia
Transient Ischemic Dilation (LV cavity is larger on stress)	From diffuse subendocardial hypoperfusion producing an apparent cavity dilation. Correlated with high risk disease (left main or 3 vessel).
Fixed Cavity Dilation	Dilated cardiomyopathy -
Right Ventricular Activity on Rest	If has intensity similar to LV then think right ventricular hypertrophy
Lots of splanchnic (liver and bowel) activity	Means you aren't exercising hard enough – not shifting enough blood out of the gut.

Other Trivia:

Stunned vs Hibernating Myocardium:

Stunned: This is the result of ischemia and reperfusion injury. It is an acute situation. The **perfusion will be normal**, but contractility will be crap. It will get better after a few weeks.

Hibernating: This is a more chronic process, and the result of severe CAD causing chronic hypoperfusion. You will have areas of **decreased perfusion and decreased contractility** even when resting (just like scar). Don't get it twisted, **this is not an infarct. This tissue will take up FDG more intensely than normal myocardium, and will also demonstrate redistribution of thallium**.

> **Rapid Review**
>
> **Ischemia** = Will take up less tracer (relative to other areas) on stress, and the same amount of tracer (relative to other areas) on rest. It's not normal heart so it won't contract well.
>
> **Scar** = Won't take up tracer on rest or stress (it's dead). It's scar not muscle, so it won't contract normally either.
>
> **Stunned** = The perfusion will be normal on both stress and rest, but the contractility is not normal.
>
> **Hibernating** = Won't take up tracer on rest or stress (it's not dead, just asleep - like a bad soap opera plot). The difference between hibernating muscle and scar is that the hibernating muscle will take up FDG and redistribute thallium. The defect at rest will resolve / "redistribute" on delayed thallium imaging. Remember thallium works with the Na/K pump - so cells need to be alive to pump it in. A truly dead cell won't have a function Na/K pump and therefore won't be able to redistribute / resolve the defect.

MUGA: This is an equilibrium radionucleotide angiogram with cardiac pool images taken after the tracer has equilibrated to the intravascular space. This studies requires gating (the "G" in MUGA). The study is done using Tc 99 labeled RBCs, and the objective is to calculate an EF. Photopenic halo around the cardiac blood pool is a classic look for pericardial effusion. Regional wall motion abnormality on a resting MUGA is usually infarct (could be stunned or hibernating as well).

Most likely questions regarding MUGA: ED −ES
                                                                    ED −Background

- **False Low EF:** Screwed up LAO view can cause overlap of LV with LA or RV or even great vessels – causing a false low EF.

- **False High EF:** Wrong background ROI (over the spleen), will cause over subtraction of background and elevate the EF.

Misc Trivia:

Rubidium 82: This is a potassium analog (mechanism is Na/K pump). This is similar to TI-201, and can be used as a similar agent. You can use it for PET myocardial perfusion, although it's not used in most places because of cost limitations. Also, because of the very short half life (75 seconds) it tends to give a dirtier image compared to PET of NH_3.

I say made with a generator , you say Tc99 and Rubidium. *Rubidium is the only PET agent made like this, so that instantly makes it a testable fact.

—

Short Axis Anatomy Review - *I always found this confusing:*

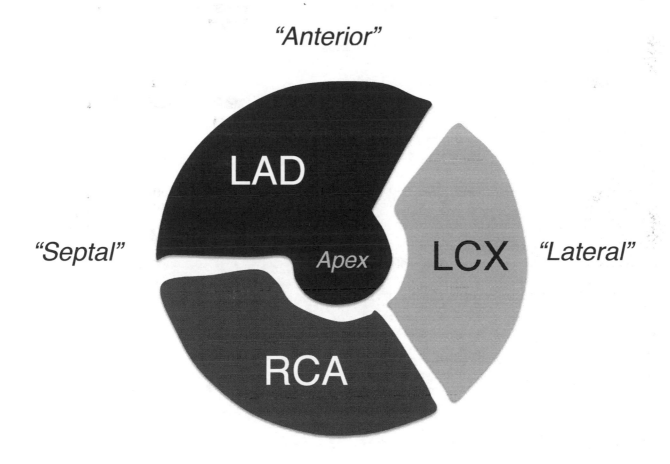

Artifacts		
Breast Tissue "Soft Tissue Attenuation"	Decreased activity in anterior wall (may also affect septal and lateral – depending on body habitus)	Check for ECG changes and wall motion. If normal, then call it artifact. If not sure can repeat in prone position.
Left Hemidiaphragm "Soft Tissue Attenuation"	Decreased activity in inferior wall	Check for ECG changes and wall motion. If normal, then call it artifact.
Subdiaphragmatic Radiotracer Activity	Increased activity in inferior wall, can mask true defect. Can also mess with "normalization" of the ventricle and make the rest of the LV look low.	Liver Excretes Tc, so you see it in the liver and bowel. Little bit of exercise can be used to reduce GI blood flow.
Patient Motion (usually respiration)	Causes all kinds of problems	You can repeat because tracer is fixed for around 2 hours
Misregistration	Causes all kinds of problems	
Left Bundle Branch Block	Reversible or Fixed Septal Defects , sparing the apex	Seen more in exercise or dobutamine stress compared to vasodilators
Normal Apical Thinning	Normal variant	Look for matching stress and rest perfusion patterns with preserved wall function to show you this is normal (and not infarct)

Medication Trivia:

	Mechanism	Trivia
Dipyridamole	Inhibits the breakdown of adenosine - which builds up. Adenosine is a potent vasodilator.	No caffeine
Adenosine	Vasodilator	No caffeine; Side effects are worse than with dipyridamole. Rare side effect is AV block - which will get better when adenosine short half life runs out.
Regadenoson	Selective A_{2A} - causes less side effects	No caffeine
Dobutamine	Beta 1 agonist - acts like exercise by increasing heart rate and myocardial contraction.	Patient Can NOT be on a beta blocker. Best used in patient's who cannot have Adenosine or Dipyridamole. Better in patients with COPD or Asthma, or who have taken caffeine in the last 12 hours.
Aminophylline	Antidote for Adenosine	Half life is shorter than Dipyridamole - so must continue to monitor.

Nuclear Therapy

Treatment for Bone Pain:

There are currently three approved agents for bone pain associated with metastatic disease from breast and prostate cancer: (1) Sr^{89}-Chloride, (2) Sm^{153} EDTMP, and (3) Ra^{223}-dichloride.

Why does cancer cause bone pain / bone problems?

Metastatic disease leads to a tumor derived factor that increases osteolytic activity. You end up with increased fracture risk, osteopenia, and hypercalcemia of malignancy.

Can the patient get external radiation treatment with the therapy?

Yes. External radiation is not a contraindication and can be used with the therapy.

Absolute contraindications (for Sr and Sm) include: Pregnancy, Breastfeeding, and renal Failure (<30GFR). *Patient's with extensive bony mets (superscan) maybe shouldn't be treated either * controversial - and therefore not likely tested.*

Sr^{89} (Metastron): It works by complexing with the hydroxyapatite in areas where bone turnover is the highest. It's the oldest, and worst of the three agents. It is a pure beta emitter. It has a high myelotoxicitiy, relative to newer agents and therefore isn't really used.

Sm^{153} (Quadramet): This is probably the second best of the three agents *"Samarium is a good Samaritan."* It works by complexing with the hydroxyapatite in areas where bone turnover is the highest. It is a beta decayer. The primary method of excretion is renal. Unlike Sr89 about 28% of the decay is via gamma rays (103 kev) which can be used for imaging. Does have some transient bone marrow suppression (mainly thrombocytopenia and leukopenia), but recovers faster than Sr.

Sr^{89} (Metastron):	Sm^{153} (Quadramet)
15-30% drops in platelet and WBC from pre-injection	40-50% drops in platelet and WBC from pre-injection
8-12 weeks needed for full recovery	6-8 weeks needed for full recovery

Ra²²³ (Xofigo): This is the most recent of the three agents, and probably the best. The idea is that Ra²²³ behaves in a similar way to calcium. It is absorbed into the bone matrix at the sites of active bone mineralization. Its primary mechanism is the emission of 4 alpha particles, causing some serious double stranded DNA breaks.

Why is it the best?

(1) It's an alpha emitter with a range shorter than Sr and Sm. This means less hematologic toxicity.

(2) At least one trial actually showed a survival benefit in prostate CA.

(3) It has a long half life (11.4 days) allowing for easy shipping.

What are the side effects?

Non-hematologic toxicities are generally more common than hematologic ones; diarrhea, fatigue, nausea, vomiting, and bone pain make the list.

Trivia: The general population is safe, as the gamma effects are low. Soiled clothing and bodily fluids should be handled with gloves, and clothes should be laundered separately. A 6 month period of contraception is recommended although none of this is evidence based (as per usual).

Sr⁸⁹	Sm¹⁵³	Ra²²³
Pure Beta Emitter	Beta Emitter, with some imagable gamma rays	Alpha Emitter
Most Bone Marrow Toxicity (longest recovery).	Less Bone Marrow Toxicity	Least Bone Marrow Toxicity
Renal excretion	Renal excretion	GI excretion
		Improves Survival (prostate mets)

Yttrium-90

This can be used as a radioembolization method, for unresectable liver tumors. This is a pure Beta emitter that spares most of the adjacent normal liver parenchyma as the maximum tissue penetration is about 10mm.

Prior to treatment with Y-90 the standard is to do a 99mTc MAA hepatic arterial injection. The primary purpose of this injection is to look for a lung shunt fraction. This fraction needs to be < 10% under ideal circumstances. You can still use Y-90 for 10-20% shunts but you need to decrease the dose. Above 20% the risk of radiation pneumonitis is too large.

Particle Size: The optimal particle size is between 20-40 um, as this allows particles to trap in the tumor nodules, but large enough to get stuck without totally obstructing. If you create a true embolization the process actually doesn't work as well because you need blood flow as a free radical generation source.

Radiation Dose: The dose is typically 100-1000 Gy delivered. The current thinking is that lesions require at least 70 Gy for monotherapy success.

Imaging: There are 175 Kev and 185 keV emissions you can use to image.

Trivia: The average half life is 2.67 days.

Radioimmune Therapy (RIT):

Monoclonal antibodies can be used with Indium[111] ibritumomab tiuxetan (Zevalin) for refractory non-Hodgkin lymphoma treatment, or as a first line treatment.

The idea is that you can give the antibody labeled with Indium[111] for diagnostic evaluation of the tumor burden and then if the bio distribution is ok you can give the antibody labeled with Y-90 for treatment.

Trivia: The antibody binds to the CD-20 receptors on B-cells.

What is considered altered distribution?

(1) Uptake in the lungs that is more intense than the heart on day one, or more intense than the liver on day 2 and 3.

(2) Uptake in the kidneys more than the liver on day 3.

(3) Uptake in the bowel that is fixed, and/or more than the liver

(4) Uptake in the bone marrow > 25%

Trivia: Don't give to patients with platelets less than 100K

Most Common Side Effect? Thrombocytopenia and neutropenia (about 90% of cases).

Can you send them home post treatment? Dose to caretakers or persons near the patient is low, and they can be released to the general population after treatment. Although some things like sleeping apart, no kissing, etc… for about a week are still usually handed out.

Protocol: You need to first give rituximab to block the CD20 receptors on the circulating B cells and those in the spleen to optimize bio-distribution. Then you can give the In^{111} labeled antibody to assess for altered bio-distribution. If you suspect altered distribution you should get delayed full body imaging at 90-120 hours. If altered you shouldn't treat. If ok, then blast'em.

Some High Yield Summary Charts

Tracer	Analog	Energy	Physical Half Life
Tc – 99m		"Low" – 140	6 hours
Iodine -123	Iodine	"Low" – 159	13 hours
Xenon - 133		"Low" – 81	125 hours *(biologic t1/2 30 seconds)*
Thallium - 201	Potassium	"Low" – 135 (2%), 167 (8%), *use 71 ^{201}Hg daughter x-rays*	73 hours
Indium -111		"Medium" – 173 (89%), 247 (94%)	67 hours
Gallium - 67	Iron	Multiple; 93 (40%), 184 (20%), 300 (20%), 393 (5%)	78 hours
Iodine -131	Iodine	"High" - 365	8 days
Fluorine -18	Sugar	"High" - 511	110 mins

Treatment Radionuclides Half Life	
Strontium 89	50.5 DAYS (14 days in bone)
Samarium 153	46 Hours
Yttrium 90	64 Hours

Cardiac Radionuclides Half Life	
Rubidium 82	75 seconds
Nitrogen 13	10 mins

Blanks for Scribbles / Notes

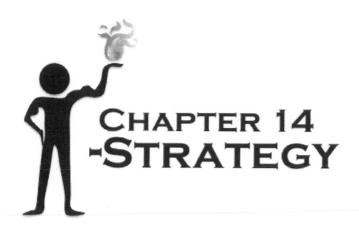

CHAPTER 14 -STRATEGY

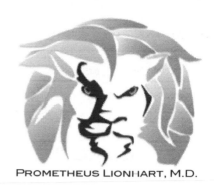

PROMETHEUS LIONHART, M.D.

There are 3 kinds of questions on multiple choice tests

1. **The ones you know** – you want to get 100% of these right
2. **The ones you don't know** – you want to get 25% of these right (same as a monkey guessing)
3. **The ones you can figure out with some deep thought** – you want to get 60-70% of these right.

If you can do that you will pass the test, especially if you've read my books.

<u>My recommendations:</u>
- For the ones you know, just get them right.
- For the ones you don't know – just say to yourself *"this is one I don't know, Prometheus says just try and narrow it down and guess."*
- For the ones you think you can figure out, mark them, and go through the entire exam. If you follow my suggestion on the first two types of questions you will have ample time left over for head scratching. Other reasons to go ahead and do the whole exam before trying to figure them out is (a) you don't want to rush on the questions you can get right, and (b) sometimes you will see a case that reminds you of what the answer is. In fact it's not impossible that the stem of another question flat out tells you the answer to a previous question.

Let your plans be dark, and impenetrable as night, and when you move, fall like a thunderbolt.
-Sun Tzu

Studying for a C-

For many of you this is the first time you truly do not need an A on the exam. I can remember in undergrad and medical school feeling like I needed to get every question right on the exam to maintain my total and complete dominance.

I felt like if I missed a single question that I wouldn't honor the class, I wouldn't match radiology, and I'd end up in rural West Virginia checking diabetic feet for ulcers in my family medicine clinic. The very thought of a career in family medicine was so horrible that I'd begin to panic.

Panic doesn't help!

Truly this exam is not like that. You can miss questions. You will miss questions. You can miss a lot of questions. You just need to miss less than about 10% of the room. No matter what they tell you, no matter what you read <u>all standardized exams are curved</u>. If they passed 100% - the exam would be called a joke. If they failed 50% the program directors would riot (after first punishing the residents with extra call). The exam will maintain a failure rate around 10-15%. What that means is that you only need to beat 10-15% of the room. You don't need 99th percentile. There is no reward for that. You need 16th percentile. 16th percentile is a C-, that is the goal.

The reason I'm perseverating on this is that you need to avoid panic. If you mark 20-30% of the questions as "not sure" - or Promethean category 2 or 3 - you might begin to freak out. Especially if the inner gunner medical student in you thinks you won't get honors. Chill Out! It's ok to miss questions. Look around the room and know that you studied harder and are smarter than 15% of the room.

Do not flee the exam in tears !

Fate rarely calls upon us at a moment of our choosing.

-Optimus Prime

Exploiting the "Genius Neuron"

Have you ever heard someone in case conference take a case and lead with "It's NOT this," when clearly "this" is what the case was? It happens all the time. Often the first thing out of people's mouths is actually the write answer, but many times you hear people say "it's not" first. Ever wondered why?

There is this idea of a "Genius Neuron." You have one neuron that is superior to the rest. This guy fires faster and is more reliable than his peers and because of this he is hated by them. He is the guy in the front row waving his hand shouting "I know the answer!" You know that guy, that guy is a notorious asshole. So, in your mind he shouts out the answer first, and then the rest of the neurons gang up on him and try and talk him out of it. So the end product is "It's NOT this."

For the purpose of taking cases in conference, this is why you should always lead with "this comes to mind," instead of "it's not." Now, the practical piece of advice I want to give you is to **trust your genius neuron**. Serious, there is a lot of material on this test. But if you read this book, there will be enough knowledge to pass the test existing somewhere between your ears. You just have to trust that genius neuron.

How?? - Do it like this:

(1) Read the entire question. Look at all the pictures.

(2) Read ALL the answer choices. Never stop at A thinking that is the answer.

(3) Look again at ALL the pictures – now that you see the choices.

(4) Choose the first answer your mind tells you is correct – the one your genius neuron thinks it correct.

(5) After you have finished the test, and you are re-reviewing your answers NEVER change the genius neuron's answer except for two criteria. (A) You read the question wrong. (B) You are 100% sure that it is another choice, and you can give a reason why. Never change based on your gut feelings. Those secondary gut feelings are the stupid neurons trying to gang up on the smart one. Just like in the real world the stupid people significantly outnumber the smart ones.

I know this sounds silly, but I really believe in this. This is a real thing. I encourage you to try it with some practice questions.

You either believe in yourself or you don't

      -Captain James T. Kirk.

Dealing with the Linked Question

It is a modern trend for multiple choice tests to have "linked" questions. You may remember that USMLE Step 3 had them, and it is rumored that the CORE Exam has them as well.

These are the questions that prompt you with "this is your final answer, you can't change your answer." When you see this STOP!

If you are 100% sure you are right, then go on. If you had it narrowed down to two choices, think about which one would be easier to write a follow up question about. This might seem obvious, but in the heat of the battle you might get too aggressive. Slow down and think twice on these.

The second point I want to make about these questions is finding some Zen if you miss it. There are a lot of questions on this test, it's ok to miss some. You will still pass (probably). People like you have always studied for the A+, not the C-. So when you miss a question it makes you freak out because you think you blew it. You don't need an A+ this time. You don't need a B. You just need to pass so they don't get any more money from you. Believe me they have taken enough from you already. I just want you to understand that you will miss questions and it's ok. If the second part reveals that you dropped one, don't let it phase you. Just do your best. The most important fight is always your next one.

It isn't the mountains ahead to climb that wears you out; it's the pebble your shoe

-Muhammad Ali

It's Possible to Know Too Much

If you were to begin studying and begin taking multiple choice practice questions and you plotted your progress as you gained more knowledge you would notice something funny. At first you would begin to get more and more questions right… and then you would start to miss them.

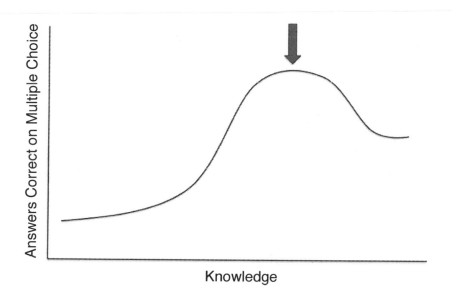

Well how can that be? I will tell you that once you know enough all choices on the exam become correction. Which of the following can occur?… well actually they can all occur - i've read case reports of blah blah blah. That is what happens.

The trick is to not over think things. Once you've achieved a certain level of knowledge, if they give you a gift — take it. It's usually not a trick (usually). Don't look for obscure situations when things are true. Yes… it's possible for you to know more than the person writing the questions. Yes… I said it and it's fucking true. These people don't know everything. You can out knowledge them if you study enough - and that is when you get yourself into trouble.

Take home point - once you've reached the peak (arrow on chart) - be careful over thinking questions past that point.

"Always remember: Your focus determines your reality"

    -Jedi Master Qui-Gon Jinn

6 Promethean Laws For Multiple Choice

#1 - If you have a gut feeling - go for it ! (trust the genius neuron)

#2 - Don't over think to the extent that you veer from a reflexive answer - especially if choices seem equally plausible (you can know too much).

#3 - Read ALL the choices carefully

#4 - If it seems too obvious to be true (trickery), re-read it and then go with it (even if it seems to easy). Let it happen - it's usually not a trick… usually.

#5 - Add up what you know you know, and compare with what you think you know. Weight your answers by what you KNOW you KNOW.

#6 - Most Importantly - <u>Don't Panic</u>

Maybe I can't win, maybe the only thing I can do is just take everything he's got. But to beat me, he's gonna have to kill me, and to kill me, he's gonna have to have the heart to stand in front of me, and to do that, he's has to be willing to die himself

- *Rocky Balboa*

SECTION 1: PEDS

*Why are you showing me a **lateral soft tissue neck x-ray?*** This could be shown for two main reasons:

(1) the thumb sign of epiglottis, or
(2) the super wide pre vertebral soft tissues for retropharyngeal abscess.

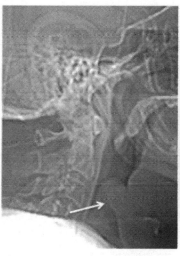 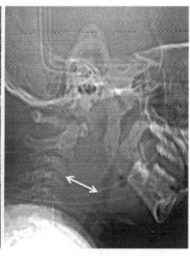

Epiglottitis – Thumb Sign   Retropharyngeal Abscess

*Why are you showing me an **ultrasound of the neck?*** In peds this can only be a few things.

- **Fibromatosis Colli** is probably the most common thing shown (mass like fibrosis of the sternocleidomastoid muscle).

- Jugular vein thrombosis - think **Lemierre syndrome** (chest will have septic emboli). Fusobacterium necrophorum, is responsible for a majority of cases.

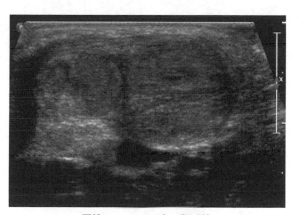

Fibromatosis Colli
(two heads of the sternocleidomastoid)

- Cysts
  - If midline think **Thyroglossal cyst**.
  - If lateral think **branchial cleft cyst.**

NG Tube Tricks: The presence of an NG tube (especially if not placed correctly) should alert you to some form of trickery.

- *The NG tube stops in the upper thoracic esophagus:* Think esophageal atresia (probably in the setting of VACTERL).

- *The NG tube curling into the chest* – it's either (1) in the lung, or (2) it's in a congenital diaphragmatic hernia. If I had to pick between the two (and it wasn't obvious), I'd say left side hernia, right side lung – just because those are the more common sides.

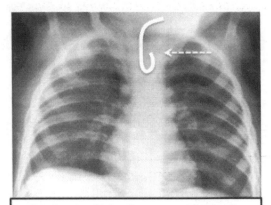

NG tube curls in the upper thoracic esophagus. First think **Esophageal Atresia.** Then think VACTERL

The Classic Congenital Lobar Emphysema Trick: They can show you a series of CXRs. The first one has an opacity in the lung (the affected lung is fluid filled). The next x-ray will show the opacity resolved. The following x-ray will show it getting more lucent, and more lucent. Until it's actually pushing the heart over. This is the classic way to show it in case conference, or case books

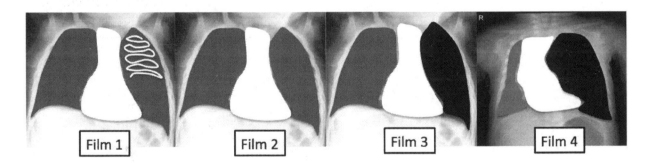

The Mandible: There are only a few things that a mandible will be shown for with regards to Peds. Think Caffeys first - especially if the picture looks blurry and old (there hasn't been a case of this in 50 years). If it's osteonecrosis think about O.I. on bisphosphonates. If it's a dwarf case, think wide angled mandible with Pycnodysostosis. A "floating tooth" could be EG.

The School Aged CXR: *Things to look for:*

- **Big Heart** - Probably showing you a sickle cell case. Look for bone infarcts in shoulders.
- **Lucent Lung** - Think foreign Body (air trapping). Remember you put the affected side down (if it remains lucent- that confirms it).

The Abdominal Plain Film - on a newborn - *Problem Solving Bubbles:*

Pattern	Path	Next Step
Single Bubble:	In a newborn this is Gastric (antral or pyloric atresia). In an older child think gastric volvulus	
Double Bubble	Duodenal Atresia	
Triple Bubble	Jejunal Atresia	
Single Bubble + Distal Gas + "Bilious Vomiting	Concern for Mid Gut Volvulus	Next Step = Upper GI
Multiple Dilated Loops	Concern for lower obstruction	Next Step = Contrast Enema

Heterotaxia: This can be inferred or asked several ways.

Heterotaxia Syndromes	
Right Sided	**Left Sided**
Two Fissures in Left Lung	One Fissure in Right Lung
Asplenia	Polysplenia
Increased Cardiac Malformations	Less Cardiac Malformations
Reversed Aorta/IVC	Azygous Continuation of the IVC

This vs That: *Neonatal pneumonia and RDS* can look similar (both with granular opacities). RDS should have low lung volumes (regular pneumonia will have increases). RDS is gonna be premature (if they give you that history). Lastly, pneumonia will often have a pleural effusion – which RDS will not.

This vs That: *Cystic Fibrosis vs Primary Ciliary Dyskinesia*

CF	PCD
Abnormal Mucus – Cilia can't clear it	Normal Mucus – Cilia don't work
Bronchiectasis (upper lobes)	Bronchiectasis (lower lobes)
Normal sperm, obliterated vas deferens	Normal vas deferens, sperm cannot swim normally

This vs That: *Vascular Impressions:*

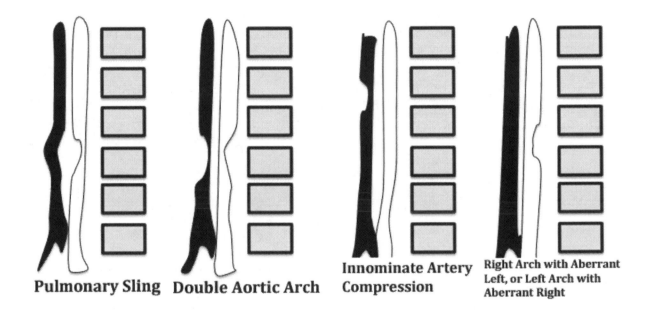

Pulmonary Sling **Double Aortic Arch** **Innominate Artery Compression** **Right Arch with Aberrant Left, or Left Arch with Aberrant Right**

This vs That: *Intralobar vs Extralobar Sequestration*

Intralobar	Extralobar
No pleural covering	Has it's own pleural covering
More Common	Less Common
Presents later with recurrent infection	Presents early with other bad congenital things (heart, etc...)

This vs That - Location:

- Intralobar Sequestration = Left Lower Lobe
- Congenital Lobar Emphysema (CLE) = Left Upper Lobe
- CCAM = No Lobar Preference

This vs That: Duodenal Atresia vs Jejunal Atresia:

Duodenal Atresia	Jejunal Atresia
Double Bubble	Triple Bubble
Failure to Canalize (often isolated atresia)	Vascular Insult * More likely associated with other atresias
Associated with Downs	

Baby Liver - This vs That:

Age 0-3		
Hemangioendothelioma	Endothelial Growth Factor Elevated	High flow heart failure, big heart on CXR.
Hepatoblastoma	AFP Elevated	Associated with Wilms, Associated with Prematurity Can cause precocious puberty
Mesenchymal Hamartoma	AFP Negative	It's really cystic

Peds Cystic Renal Mass

Unilateral →

Bilateral →

Multi Cystic Dysplastic Kidney
- *Neonate, No Renal Function*

AR-PCKD
– Enlarged, Bright, Microcystic

Multilocular Cystic Nephroma
- *Young Boy, "Herniates into Renal Pelvis"*

Cystic Wilms

This vs That:

Neuroblastoma	Wilms
Age: usually less than 2 (can occur in utero)	Age: Usually around are 4 (never before 2 months)
Calcifies 90%	Calcifies Rarely (<10%)
Encases Vessels (doesn't invade)	Invades Vessels (doesn't encase)
Poorly Marginated	Well Circumscribed
Mets to Bones	Doesn't usually met to bones (unless clear cell wilms variant).

This vs That:

Neuroblastoma	Adrenal Hemorrhage
Anechoic and Avascular	Echogenic and Vascular
Low of T2	Hight on T2
Will grow on followup	Should shrink on followup

When I Say This..... You Say That.....

- When I say "Subglottic Hemangioma," You Say PHACES Syndrome
- When I say "PHACES Syndrome," You say Cutaneous Hemangioma
- When I say "Ropy Appearance," You say Meconium Aspiration
- When I say "Post Term Delivery," You Say Meconium Aspiration
- When I say "Fluid in the Fissures," You say Transient Tachypnea
- When I say "History of c-section", You say Transient Tachypnea
- When I say "Maternal sedation", You say Transient Tachypnea
- When I say "Granular Opacities + Premature", You say RDS
- When I say "Granular Opacities + Term + High Lung Volume," You say Pneumonia
- When I say "Granular Opacities + Term + Low Lung Volume," You say B-Hemolytic Strep
- When I say "Band Like Opacities", You say Chronic Lung Disease (BPD)
- When I say "Linear Lucencies" , You say Pulmonary Interstitial Emphysema
- When I say "Pulmonary Hypoplasia," You say diaphragmatic hernia
- When I say "Lung Cysts and Nodules," You Say LCH or Papillomatosis
- When I say "Lower lobe bronchiectasis," You Say Primary Ciliary Dyskinesia
- When I say "Upper lobe bronchiectasis," You Say CF
- When I say "Posterior mediastinal mass (under 2)," You Say Neuroblastoma
- When I say "No air in the stomach", You say Esophageal Atresia
- When I say "Excessive air in the stomach", You say "H" Type TE fistula
- When I say "Anterior Esophageal Impression," You say pulmonary sling
- When I say "Pulmonary Sling," You say tracheal stenosis.
- When I say "Single Bubble," You say Gastric (antral or pyloric) atresia
- When I say "Double Bubble," You say duodenal atresia
- When I say "Duodenal Atresia", You say Downs
- When I say "Single Bubble with Distal Gas," You say maybe Mid Gut Volvulus
- When I say "Non-bilious vomiting", You say Hypertrophic Pyloric Stenosis
- When I say "Paradoxial aciduria" You say Hypertrophic Pyloric Stenosis
- When I say "Bilious vomiting - in an infant", You say Mid Gut Volvulus
- When I say "Corkscrew Duodenum" You say Mid Gut Volvulus
- When I say "Reversed SMA and SMV" You say Malrotation
- When I say "Absent Gallbladder" You say biliary atresia
- When I say "Triangle Cord Sign" You say biliary atresia
- When I say "Asplenia" , You say "cyanotic heart disease"

- When I say "Infarcted Spleen," You say Sickle Cell
- When I say "Gall Stones," You say Sickle Cell
- When I say "Short Microcolon," You say Colonic Atresia
- When I say "Long Microcolon," You say Meconium ileus or distal ileal atresia
- When I say "Saw tooth colon," You say Hirschsprung
- When I say "Calcified mass in the mid abdomen of a newborn", you say Meconium Peritonitis
- When I say "Meconium ileus equivalent," you say Distal Intestinal Obstruction Syndrome (CF).
- When I say "Abrupt caliber change of the aorta below the celiac axis" , You say Hepatic Hemangioendothelioma.
- When I say "Cystic mass in the liver of a newborn," you say Mesenchymal Hamartoma
- When I say "Elevated AFP, with mass in the liver of a newborn," you say Hepatoblastoma
- When I say "Common Bile Duct measures more than 10mm", You say Choledochal Cyst
- When I say "Lipomatous pseudohypertrophy of the pancreas," You say CF
- When I say "Unilateral Renal Agenesis" You say unicornuate uterus
- When I say "Neonatal Renal Vein Thrombosis," You say maternal diabetes
- When I say "Neonatal Renal Artery Thrombosis," You say Misplaced Umbilical Artery Catheter
- When I say "Hydro on Fetal MRI," You say Posterior Urethral Valve
- When I say "Urachus," You say bladder Adenocarcinoma
- When I say "Nephroblastomatosis with Necrosis," you say Wilms
- When I say "Solid Renal Tumor of Infancy," you say Mesoblastic Nephroma
- When I say "Solid Renal Tumor of Childhood," you say Wilms
- When I say "Midline pelvic mass, in a female," you say Hydrometrocolpos
- When I say "Right sided varicocele," you say abdominal pathology
- When I say "Blue Dot Sign," you say Torsion of the Testicular Appendages
- When I say "Hand or Foot Pain / Swelling in an Infant", You say - sickle cell with hand foot syndrome.
- When I say Extratesticular scrotal mass, you say embryonal rhabdomyosarcoma
- When I say "Narrowing of the interpedicular distance," you say Achondroplasia
- When I say "Platyspondyly (flat vertebral bodies)," you say Thanatophoric
- When I say "Absent Tonsils after 6 months" You say "Immune Deficiency"
- When I say "Enlarged Tonsils well after childhood (like 12-15)" You say "Cancer"… probably lymphatic
- When I say "Mystery Liver Abscess in Kid, "You say "Chronic Granulomatous Disease"

High Yield Trivia:

- Pulmonary Interstitial Emphysema (PIE) - put the bad side down
- Bronchial Foreign Body - put the lucency side down (if it stays that way, it's positive)
- Papillomatosis has a small (2%) risk of squamous cell CA
- Pulmonary sling is the only variant that goes between the esophagus and the trachea. This is associated with trachea stenosis.
- Thymic Rebound – Seen after stress (chemotherapy) – Can be PET-Avid
- Lymphoma – Most common mediastinal mass in child (over 10)
- Anterior Mediastinal Mass with Calcification – Either treated lymphoma, or Thymic Lesion (lymphoma doesn't calcify unless treated).
- Neuroblastoma is the most common posterior mediastinal mass in child under 2 (primary thoracic does better than abd).
- Hypertrophic Pyloric Stenosis - NOT at birth, NOT after 3 months (3 weeks to 3 months is easiest for me to remember)
- Criteria for HPS - 4mm and 14mm (4mm single wall, 14mm length).
- Annular Pancreas presents as duodenal obstruction in children and pancreatitis in adults.
- Most common cause of bowel obstruction in child over 4 = Appendicitis
- Intussusception - 3months to 3 years is ok, earlier or younger think lead point
- Gastroschisis is ALWAYS on the right side
- Omphalocele has associated anomalies (gastroschisis does not).
- Physiologic Gut Hernia normal at 6-8 weeks
- AFP is elevated with Hepatoblastoma
- Endothelial growth factor is elevated with Hemangioendothelioma
- Most Common cause of pancreatitis in a kid = Trauma (seatbelt)
- Weigert Meyer Rule - Duplicated ureter on top inserts inferior and medial
- Most common tumor of the fetus or infant - Sacrococcygeal Teratoma
- Most common cause of idiopathic scrotal edema - HSP
- Most common cause of acute scrotal pain age 7-14 - Torsion of Testicular Appendages
- Bell Clapper Deformity is the etiology for testicular torsion.
- SCFE is a Salter Harris Type 1
- Physiologic Periostitis of the Newborn doesn't occur in a newborn - seen around 3 months
- Acetabular Angle should be < 30, and Alpha angle should be more than 60.

SECTION 2: GI

Problem Solving Through MRI

Different programs have variable volume with MRI. Some of you will be excellent at it. Some of you will suck at it. An important skill to have is to understand how to problem solve with different sequences. The best way to do this is to have a list of T1 bright things, T2 bright things, dark things, and things that restrict diffusion.

T1 Bright	T2 Bright	T1 and T2 DARK	Restricts Diffusion
Fat	Fat	Flow Void	Stroke
Melanin (Melanoma)	Water	Fibrosis / Scar	Hypercellular Tumor
Blood (Subacute)	Blood (Extracellular Methemoglobin)	Metal	Epidermoid
Protein Rick Fluid	Most Tumors	Air	Abscess (Bacterial)
Calcification (Hyalinized)			Acute Demyelination
Slow Moving Blood			CJD
Laminar Necrosis			T2 Shine Through

Be able to move through sequences and problem solve.

Think about a Lipoma for example. This will be T1 bright, T2 bright, and fat sat out. Another example might be something with layers in it. What can layer? Fat could layer, water could layer, blood could layer, pus could layer. Fat would be bright/ bright. Water would be dark on T1. Pus would be dark on T2. Blood could do different things depending on it's age. Fat would sat out. Pus may restrict diffusion (like a subdural empyema). You get the idea. Run through some scenarios in your mind. The key point is to know your differentials for this.

Classic Gamesmanship: They could show you a dilated esophagus on CT or barium. Then they show you ground glass in the lung bases (and sub-pleural sparing if you are lucky). This answer is scleroderma with NSIP.

Benign Liver Masses					
	Ultrasound	CT	MR	Trivia	
Hemangioma	Hyperechoic	Peripheral Nodular Discontinuous Enhancement	T2 Bright	Rare in Cirrhotics	
FNH	Spoke Wheel	Homogenous Arterial Enhancement	"Stealth Lesion - Iso on T1 and T2"	Central Scar	Bright on Delayed Eovist (Gd-EOB-DTPA)
Hepatic Adenoma	Variable	Variable	Fat Containing on In/Out Phase	OCP use, Glycogen Storage Disease	Can explode and bleed
Hepatic Angiomyolipoma	Hyperechoic	Gross Fat	T1/T2 Bright	Unlike renal AML, 50% don't have fat	Tuberous Sclerosis

Location Location:

- **H Pylori** Gastritis – Usually in **Antrum**
- **Zollinger-Ellison** – Ulcerations in the stomach (**jejunal ulcer** is the buzzword). Duodenal bulb is actually the most common location for ulcers in ZE.
- **Crohns** – Uncommon in the stomach, but when it is, it likes the **antrum**
- **Menetrier's** – Usually in the **Fundus** (*classically spares the antrum*)
- **Lympoma** – "**Crosses the Pylorus**" – classically described as doing so, although in reality adenocarcinoma docs it more.

Infections:
- **Giardia** - Duodenum
- **Strongyloides** - Duodenum
- **TB** - Terminal Ileum
- **Yersinia** - Terminal Ileum

This vs That:
- Herpes Esophagitis = Multiple Small Ulcers
- CMV and AIDS = Solitary Large Ulcer

This vs That - *Esophageal Cancer:*
- Squamous Cell = Black Guy who drinks and smokes - mid esophagus
- Adenocarcinoma = White Guy with reflux (history of PPIs), - lower esophagus

This vs That - *Uphill vs Downhill Varices*

Uphill Varices	Downhill Varices
Caused by Portal Hypertension	Caused by SVC obstruction (catheter related, or tumor related)
Confined to Bottom Half of Esophagus	Confined to Top Half of Esophagus

This vs That - *Traction vs Pulsion Diverticulum*

Traction	Pulsion
Triangular	Round
Will Empty	Will **NOT** Empty (contain no muscle in their walls)

This vs That - *Esophageal Hernias*
- Sliding - GE Junction Above the Diaphragm
- Rolling - GE Junction Below the Diaphragm

This vs That - *Carney's Triad vs Carney's Complex*

Carney's Triad	Carney's Complex
Extra-Andrenal Pheochromocytoma,	Cardiac Myxoma * (C for Complex)
GIST	Skin Stuff
Pulmonary Chordoma (hamartoma)	Endocrine Stuff

This vs That - *Benign vs Malignant Ulcers (on Barium)*

Malignant	Benign
Width > Depth	Depth > Width
Located within Lumen	Project behind the expected lumen
Nodular, Irregular Edges	Sharp Contour
Folds adjacent to ulcer	Folds radiate to ulcer
Aunt Minnie: Carmen Meniscus Sign	Aunt Minnie: Hampton's Line

This vs That - *Inguinal Hernia*

Direct	Indirect
Less common	More Common
Medial to inferior Epigastric	Lateral to inferior epigastric
Defect in Hesselbach triangle	Failure of processus vaginalis to close
NOT covered by internal spermatic fascia	Covered by internal spermatic fascia

This vs That - *Crohns and UC*

Crohns	UC
Slightly less common in the USA	Slightly more common in the USA
Discontinuous "Skips"	Continuous
Terminal Ileum – *String Sign*	Rectum
Ileocecal Valve "Stenosed"	Ileocecal Valve "Open"
Mesenteric Fat Increased *"creeping fat"*	Perirectal fat Increased
Lymph nodes are usually enlarged	Lymph nodes are NOT usually enlarged
Makes Fistula	Doesn't Usually Make Fistula

This vs That - *Volvulus*

Sigmoid	Cecal
Old Person (Constipated)	Younger Person (mass, prior surgery, or 3rd Trimester Pregnancy)
Points to the RUQ	Points to the LUQ

This vs That -*Liver Nodules*

Regenerative	Dysplastic	HCC
Contains Iron	Contains Fat, Glycoprotein	
T1 Dark, T2 Dark	T1 Bright, T2 Dark	T2 Bright
Does NOT Enhance	Usually Does NOT Enhance	Does Enhance

This vs That -*Central Scars*

FNH	FL HCC
T2 Bright	T2 Dark (usually)
Enhances on Delays	Does NOT enhance
Mass is Sulfur Colloid Avid (sometimes)	Mass is Gallium Avid

This vs That -*Hepatic Adenoma vs FNH*

Hepatic Adenoma	FNH
Usually > 8cm	Usually < 8cm
No Bile Ducts	Normal Bile Ducts
No Kupffer Cells	Normal Kupffer Cells
Sulfur Colloid Cold	Sulfur Colloid Hot (sometimes)

This vs That -*HCC vs Fibrolamellar HCC*

HCC	FL HCC
Cirrhosis	No Cirrhosis
Older (50s-60s)	Young (30s)
Rarely Calcifies	Calcifies Sometimes
Elevated AFP	Normal AFP

This vs That -*Hemochromatosis - Primary vs Secondary*

Primary	Secondary
Genetic - increased absorption	Acquired - chronic illness, and multiple transfusions
Liver, **P**ancreas	Liver, **S**pleen
Heart, Thyroid, Pituitary	

When I Say This..... You Say That.....

- When I say "narrowed B Ring," You say Schatzki *(Schat"B"ki Ring)*
- When I say "esophageal concentric rings," You say Eosinophilic Esophagitis
- When I say "shaggy" or "plaque like" esophagus, You say Candidiasis
- When I say "looks like candida, but an asymptomatic old lady," you say Glycogen Acanthosis
- When I say "reticular mucosal pattern," you say Barretts
- When I say "high stricture with an associated hiatal hernia," you say Barretts
- When I say "abrupt shoulders," you say cancer
- When I say "Killian Dehiscence," you say Zenker Diverticulum
- When I say "transient, fine transverse folds across the esophagus," you say Feline Esophagus.
- When I say "bird's beak," you say Achalasia
- When I say "solitary esophageal ulcer," you say CMV or AIDS
- When I say "ulcers at the level of the arch or distal esophagus," you say Medication induced
- When I say "Breast Cancer + Bowel Hamartomas," you say Cowdens
- When I say "Desmoid Tumors + Bowel Polyps," you say Gardners
- When I say "Brain Tumors + Bowel Polyps," you say Turcots
- When I say "enlarged left supraclavicular node," you say Virchow Node (GI Cancer)
- When I say "crosses the pylorus," you say Gastric Lymphoma
- When I say "isolated gastric varices," you say splenic vein thrombus
- When I say "multiple gastric ulcers," you say Chronic Aspirin Therapy.
- When I say "multiple duodenal (or jejunal) ulcers," you say Zollinger-Ellsion
- When I say "pancreatitis after Billroth 2," you say Afferent Loop Syndrome
- When I say "Weight gain years after Roux-en-Y," you say Gastro-Gastro Fistula
- When I say "Clover Leak Sign - Duodenum," you say healed peptic ulcer.
- When I say "Sand Like Nodules in the Jejunum," you say Whipples
- When I say "Sand Like Nodules in the Jejunum + CD4 <100," you say MAI
- When I say "Ribbon-like bowel," you say Graft vs Host
- When I say "Ribbon like Jejunum," you say Long Standing Celiac
- When I say "Moulage Pattern," you say Celiac
- When I say "Fold Reversal - of jejunum and ileum," you say Celiac
- When I say "Cavitary (low density) Lymph nodes," you say Celiac

- When I say "hide bound" or "Stack or coins," you say Scleroderma
- When I say "Megaduodenum," you say Scleroderma
- When I say "Duodenal obstruction, with recent weight loss," you say SMA Syndrome
- When I say "Concd shaped cecum," you say Amebiasis
- When I say "Lead Pipe," you say Ulcerative Colitis
- When I say "String Sign," you say Crohns
- When I say "Massive circumferential thickening, without obstruction," you say Lymphoma
- When I say "Multiple small bowel target signs," you say Melanoma
- When I say "Obstructing Old Lady Hernia," you say Femoral Hernia
- When I say "sac of bowel," you say Paraduodenal hernia.
- When I say "scalloped appearance of the liver," you say Pseudomyxoma Peritonei
- When I say "HCC without cirrhosis," you say Hepatitis B
- When I say "Capsular retraction," you say Cholangiocarcinoma
- When I say "Periportal hypoechoic infiltration + AIDS," you say Kaposi's
- When I say "sparing of the caudate lobe," you say Budd Chiari
- When I say "large T2 bright nodes + Budd Chiari," you say Hyperplastic nodules
- When I say "liver high signal in phase, low signal out phase," you say fatty liver
- When I say "liver low signal in phase, and high signal out phase," you say hemochromatosis
- When I say "multifocal intrahepatic and extrahepatic stricture," you say PSC
- When I say "multifocal intrahepatic and extrahepatic strictures + papillary stenosis," you say AIDS Cholangiopathy.
- When I say "bile ducts full of stones," you say Recurrent Pyogenic Cholangitis
- When I say "Gallbladder Comet Tail Artifact," you say Adenomyomatosis
- When I say "lipomatous pseudohypertrophy of the pancreas," you say CF
- When I say "sausage shaped pancreas," you say autoimmune pancreatitis
- When I say "autoimmune pancreatitis," you say IgG4
- When I say "IgG4" you say RP Fibrosis, Sclerosing Cholangitis, Fibrosing Medianstinitis, Inflammatory Pseudotumor
- When I say "Wide duodenal sweep," you say Pancreatic Cancer
- When I say "Grandmother Pancreatic Cyst" you say Serous Cystadenoma
- When I say "Mother Pancreatic Cyst" you say Mucinous
- When I say "Daughter Pancreatic Cyst," you say Solid Pseudopapillary

High Yield Trivia

- Most Common benign mucosal lesion of the esophagus = Papilloma
- Esophageal Webs have increased risk for cancer, and Plummer-Vinson Syndrome (anemia + web)
- Dysphagia Lusoria is from compression by a right subclavian artery (most patients with aberrant rights don't have symptoms).
- Achalasia has an increased risk of squamous cell cancer (20 years later).
- Most common mesenchymal tumor of the GI tract = GIST
- Most common location for GIST = Stomach
- Krukenberg Tumor = Stomach (GI) met to the ovary
- Menetrier's : involves fundus and spares the antrum
- The stomach is the most common location for sarcoid (in the GI tract)
- Gastric Remnants have an increased risk of cancer years after Billroth
- Most common internal hernia, Left sided paraduodenal
- Most common site of peritoneal carcinomatosis = retrovesical space
- An injury to the bare area of the liver can cause a retroperitoneal bleed
- Primary Sclerosing Cholangitis associated with Ulcerative Colitis
- Extrahepatic ducts are normal with Primary Biliary Cirrhosis
- Anti-mitochondrial Antibodies - positive with primary biliary cirrhosis
- Mirizzi Syndrome - the stone in the cystic duct obstructs the CBD.
- Mirizzi has a 5x increased risk of GB cancer.
- Dorsal pancreatic agenesis - associated with diabetes and polysplenia
- Hereditary and Tropical Pancreatitis - early age of onset, increased risk of cancer
- Felty's Syndrome - Big Spleen, RA, and Neutropenia
- Splenic Artery Aneurysm - more common in women, and more likely to rupture in pregnant women.
- Insulinoma is the most common islet cell tumor
- Gastrinoma is the most common islet cell tumor with MEN
- Ulcerative Colitis has an increased risk of colon cancer (if it involves colon past the splenic flexure). UC involving the rectum only does not increase risk of CA.

Gamesmanship: Showing persistent nephrograms - either by plain film or CT is the classic trick for ATN - usually contrast induced nephropathy

Gamesmanship: If you are show a unilateral renal agenesis case, remember the associations with absent ipsilateral epididymis, absent vas deferens, and ipsilateral seminal vesicle cyst in a man. For a woman think about mullarian anomalies (unicornuate uterus).

Renal Cancer Syndromes

Subtype	Syndrome / Association
Clear Cell	Von Hippel-Lindau
Papillary	Hereditary papillary renal carcinoma
Chromophobe	Birt Hogg Dube
Medullary	Sickle Cell Trait

Renal Cysts Syndromes:

ADPKD	Cysts in Liver	Kidneys are BIG
VHL	Cysts in Pancreas	
Acquired (Uremic)		Kidneys are small

Gamesmanship: It they wanted to ask Oncocytoma they can show it 3 ways: (1) On CT Solid Mass with Central Scar, (2) On Ultrasound "spoke wheel" vascular pattern, (3) on PET CT it will be hotter than surrounding renal cortex.

Gamesmanship: RCC is typically colder than surrounding renal parenchyma on PET, whereas oncocytoma is typically hotter.

Gamesmanship: IVPs haven't been used since the 1970s. If you see one there are a few tricks. The most common is the medial deviation of the ureters (retroperitoneal fibrosis), or the lateral deviation of the ureters (Psoas Hypertrophy, or lymph nodes).

When I Say This..... You Say That.....

- When I say "bladder stones," you say neurogenic bladder
- When I say "pine cone appearance," you say neurogenic bladder
- When I say "urethra cancer," you say squamous cell CA
- When I say "urethra cancer - prostatic portion," you say transitional cell CA
- When I say "urethra cancer - in a diverticulum," you say adenocarcinoma
- When I say "vas deferens calcifications," you say diabetes
- When I say "calcifications in a fatty renal mass," you say RCC
- When I say "protrude into the renal pelvis," you say Multilocular cystic nephroma
- When I say "no functional renal tissue," you say Multicystic Dysplastic Kidney
- When I say "Multicystic Dysplastic Kidney," you say contralateral renal issues (50%)
- When I say "Emphysematous Pyelonephritis," you say diabetic
- When I say "Xanthogranulomatous Pyelonephritis," you say staghorn stone
- When I say "Papillary Necrosis," you say diabetes
- When I say "shrunken calcified kidney," you say TB
- When I say "big bright kidney with decreased renal function," you say HIV
- When I say "history of lithotripsy," you say Page Kidney
- When I say "cortical rim sign," you say subacute renal infarct
- When I say "history of renal biopsy," you say AVF
- When I say "reversed diastolic flow," you say renal vein thrombosis
- When I say "sickle cell trait," you say medullary RCC
- When I say "Young Adult, Renal Mass, + Severe HTN," you say Juxtaglomerular Cell Tumor
- When I say "squamous cell bladder CA," you say Schistosomiasis
- When I say "entire bladder calcified," you say Schistosomiasis
- When I say "urachus," you say adenocarcinoma of the bladder
- When I say "long stricture in urethra," you say Gonococcal
- When I say "short stricture in urethra," you say Straddle Injury

High Yield Trivia

- Calcifications in a renal CA - are associated with an improved survival
- RCC bone mcts are "always" lytic
- There is an increased risk of malignancy with dialysis
- Horseshoe kidneys are more susceptible to trauma
- Most common location for TCC is the bladder
- Second most common location for TCC is the upper urinary tract
- Upper Tract TCC in more commonly multifocal (12%) - as opposed to bladder (4%).
- Weigert Meyer Rule - Upper Pole inserts medial and inferior
- Ectopic Ureters are associated with incontinence in women (not men)
- Leukoplakia is pre-malignant; Malakoplakia is not pre-malignant
- Extraperitoneal bladder rupture is more common, and managed medically
- Intraperitoneal bladder rupture is less common, and managed surgically
- Indinavir stones are the only ones not seen on CT.
- Uric Acid stones are not seen on plain film.

SECTION 4: REPRODUCTIVE

This vs That - *Bicornuate vs Septate Uterus*

You distinguish the two by the apex of the fundal contour:

- *Apex of Fundal Contour > 5mm Above Tubal Ostia = Septate*
- *Apex of Fundal Contour < 5mm Above Tubal Ostia = Bicornuate*
- *Other important trivia is; Septate has established increased 1ˢᵗ trimester loss, bicornuates have alot less problems (maybe no increased risk - depends on who you ask.*

This vs That: *Gartner Duct Cyst vs Bartholin Cyst*
- The Gartner duct cyst is above the pubic symphysis (Bartholin is below it).

This vs That: *Central Gland Prostate CA vs BPH*
- Prostate CA is usually in the peripheral zone (not the central zone). When it is in the central zone it's T2 "smudgy" or charcoal.
- BPH nodules are usually in the central zone, and they have a sharp border. You can "draw a line around them with a pencil."

This vs That: *Symmetrical vs Asymmetrical - IUGR*

Symmetrical is a "baby problem." The head is NOT spared. It's seen early, including the first trimester. Causes include TORCHS, Fetal EtOH, and Chromosomal Abnormalities

Asymmetrical is a "placenta problem." The head is spared. It's normal until the 3rd trimester. Causing include Maternal Hypertension, Severe Malnutrition, and Ehler-Danlos

Gamesmanship - The combination of a ovarian mass and a thickened endometrium should make you think Granulosa Cell Tumors (estrogen making).

Gamesmanship - Seeing fluid in the endometrial canal of a post menopausal women should make you think the cervix is obstructed (either by cancer, or more commonly stenosis).

Gamesmanship: A met to the vagina in the anterior wall upper 1/3 is "always" (90%) upper genital tract. A met to the vagina in the posterior wall lower 1/3 is "always (90%) from the GI tract

Gamesmanship: Peritoneal inclusion cysts occur after abdominal surgery (from adhesions). If they mention in the question stem "history of abdominal surgery" , and it's a GYN case have that on your radar.

Gamesmanship: If "hyperemesis" is in the the question stem, think about things that give you an elevated B-hCG - like moles and multiple pregnancy (twins).

Gamesmanship: If they show you a varicocele, regardless of what side it's on (right being more suspicious than left), and it's a "next step" type deal you probably should look for the abdominal cancer.

When I Say This..... You Say That.....

- When I say "Unicornuate Uterus," you say Look at the kidneys
- When I say "T-Shaped Uterus," you say DES related or Vaginal Clear Cell CA
- When I say "Marked enlargement of the uterus," you say Adenomyosis
- When I say "Adenomyosis," you say thickening of the junctional zone (> 12mm)
- When I say "Wolffian duct remnant," you say Gartner Duct Cyst
- When I say "Theca Lutein Cysts," you say moles and multiple gestations
- When I say "Theca Lutein Cysts + Pleural Effusions," you say - Hyperstimulation Syndrome (patient on fertility meds).
- When I say "Low level internal echoes," you say Endometrioma
- When I say "T2 Shortening," you say - Endometrioma - "Shading Sign"
- When I say "Fishnet appearance," you say Hemorrhagic Cyst
- When I say "Ovarian Fibroma + Pleural Effusion," you say Meigs Syndrome
- When I say "Snow Storm Uterus," you say Complete Mole - 1st Trimester
- When I say "Serum β-hCG levels that rise in the 8 to 10 weeks following evacuation of molar pregnancy," you say Choriocarcinoma
- When I say "midline cystic structure near the back of the bladder of a man," you say Prostatic Utricle
- When I say "lateral cystic structure near the back of the bladder of a man," you say Seminal Vesicle Cyst
- When I say "isolated orchitis," you say mumps
- When I say "onion skin appearance," you say epidermoid cyst
- When I say "multiple hypoechoic masses in the testicle," you say lymphoma
- When I say "cystic elements and macro-calcifications in the testicle," you say Mixed Germ Cell Tumor
- When I say "homogenous and microcalcifications," you say seminoma

- When I say "gynecomastia + testicular tumor" you say Sertoli Leydig.
- When I say "fetal macrosomia," you say Maternal Diabetes
- When I say "one artery adjacent to the bladder," you say two vessel cord
- When I say "painless vaginal bleeding in the third trimester," you say placenta previa
- When I say "mom doing cocaine," you say placenta abruption
- When I say "thinning of the myometrium - with turbulent doppler," you say placenta creta
- When I say "mass near the cord insertion, with flow pulsating at the fetal heart rate," you say placenta chorioangioma.
- When I say "Cystic mass in the posterior neck -antenatal period," you say cystic hygroma.
- When I say "Pleural effusions, and Ascites on prenatal US," you say hydrops.
- When I say "Massively enlarged bilateral kidneys," you say ARPKD
- When I say "Twin peak sign," you say dichorionic diamniotic

High Yield Trivia

- Endometrial tissue in a rudimentary horn (even one that does NOT communicate) increases the risk of miscarriage.
- Arcuate Uterus does NOT have an increased risk of infertility (it's a normal variant)
- Fibroids with higher T2 signal respond better to UAE
- Hyaline Fibroid Degeneration is the most common subtype
- Adenomyosis - favors the posterior wall, spares the cervix
- Hereditary Non-Polyposis Colon Cancer (NHPCC) - have a 30-50x increased risk of endometrial cancer
- Tamoxifen increases the risk of endometrial cancer, and endometrial polyps
- Cervical Cancer that has parametrial involvement (2B) - is treated with chemo/radiation. Cervical Cancer without parametrial involvement (2A) - is treated with surgery
- Vaginal cancer in adults is usually squamous cell
- Vaginal Rhabdomyosarcoma occurs in children / teenagers
- Premenopausal ovaries can be hot on PET (depending on the phase of cycle). Post menopausal ovaries should Never be hot on PET.
- Transformation subtypes: Endometrioma = Clear Cell, Dermoid = Squamous
- Post Partum fever can be from ovarian vein thrombophlebitis
- Fractured penis = rupture of the corpus cavernosum and the surrounding tunica albuginea
- Prostate Cancer is most commonly in the peripheral zone, - ADC dark
- BPH nodules are in the central zone
- Hypospadias is the most common association with prostatic utricle

- Seminal Vesicle cysts are associated with renal agenesis, and ectopic ureters.
- Cryptorchidism increases the risk of cancer (in both testicles), and is not reduced by orchiopexy
- Immunosuppressed patients can get testicular lymphoma -hiding behind blood testes barrier
- Most common cause of correctable infertility in a man is a varicocele.
- Undescended testicles are more common in premature kids.
- Membranes disrupted before 10 weeks, increased risk for amniotic bands
- The earliest visualization of the embryo is the "double bleb sign"
- Hematoma greater than 2/3 the circumference of the chorion has a 2x increased risk of abortion.
- Biparietal Diameter - Recorded at the level of the thalamus from the outermost edge of the near skull to the inner table of the far skull.
- Abdominal Circumference - does not include the subcutaneous soft tissues
- Abdominal Circumference is recorded at the the level of the junction of the umbilical vein and left portal vein
- Abdominal Circumference is the parameter classically involved with asymmetric IUGR
- Femur Length does NOT include the epiphysis
- Umbilical Artery Systolic / Diastolic Ratio should NOT exceed 3 at 34 weeks - makes you think pre-eclampsia and IUGR
- A full bladder can mimic a placenta previa
- Nuchal lucency is measured between 9-12 weeks, and should be < 3mm. More than 3mm is associated with downs.
- Lemon sign will disappear after 24 weeks.
- Aquaductal Stenosis is the most common cause of non-communicating hydrocephalus in a neonate

SECTION 5: CHEST

Gamesmanship - AIDS

- Lungs Cysts = LIP *(LIP is AIDS defining in a pediatric patient)*
- Lungs Cysts + Ground Glass + Pneumothorax = PCP
- Hypervascular Nodes = Castlemans or Kaposi
- Most common airspace opacity = Strep Pneumonia
- If they show you a CT with ground glass = PCP
- "Flame Shaped" Perihilar opacity = Kaposi Sarcoma
- Persistent Opacities = Lymphoma

Infections in AIDS by CD4	
> 200	Bacterial Infections, TB
< 200	PCP, Atypical Mycobacterial
< 100	CMV, Disseminated Fungal, Mycobacterial

Gamesmanship: Mesothelioma

One way to show this is the "Frozen Hemithorax" - which is a lack of contralateral mediastinal shift in association with massive pleural effusion ; it's due to encasement of the lung (and fissures) by cancer.

Gamesmanship: Collagen Vascular Tricks

RA in the shoulders on Frontal CXR = Lower Lobe UIP Pattern
Ankylosing Spondylitis on Lateral CXR = Upper Lobe Fibrobullous Disease
Dilated Esophagus on CT = Scleroderma with NSIP lungs

Gamesmanship: Pulmonary Edema

After the placement of a chest tube - Re-expansion Edema
After using a bunch of crack or heroin - Drug induced Edema
After a head injury - Neurogenic Edema
After lung transplant - Reperfusion Edema related to ischemia/reperfusion (peak day 4)

Gamesmanship: Upper Lobes vs Lower Lobes

It's useful to have a list of what is upper lobe predominant and what is lower lobe predominant. The easiest way to ask a question would be "which of the follow is not upper lobe?" or "which of the following is upper lobe?"

Upper Lobe Predominant	Lower Lobe Predominant
Most inhaled stuff (not asbestosis). Coal Workers, and Silicosis. This includes progressive massive fibrosis.	Asbestosis
CF	Primary Ciliary Dsykinesia
RB-ILD	Most Interstitial Lung Diseases (UIP, NSIP, DIP)
Centrilobular Emphysema	Panlobular Emphysema (Alpha 1)
Ankylosing Spondylitis	Rheumatoid Lung
Sarcoid	Scleroderma (associated with NSIP)

This vs That: Pulmonary vs Mediastinal Origin

- Mediastinal Origin will make obtuse margin with lung
- Pulmonary Origin will make acute margin with lung

This vs That: Ground Glass Nodule (on PET)
- HOT GGO = Infection
- COLD GGO = Cancer (BAC)

Gamesmanship – Collapse

- Always be on the lookout for collapse. Anytime you see anything that could be collapse at least entertain the idea.
- Post intubation think collapse
- Placement of central line thin collapse
- ICU patient with no other details think collapse (mucous plugging)
- Outpatient with no history think collapse (cancer).

When I Say This..... You Say That.....

- When I say "obliteration of Raider's Triangle," you say aberrant right subclavian
- When I say "flat waist sign," you say left lower lobe collapse
- When I say "terrorist + mediastinal widening," you say Anthrax
- When I say "bulging fissure," you say Klebsiella
- When I say "dental procedure gone bad, now with jaw osteo and pneumonia," you say Actinomycosis.
- When I say "culture negative pleural effusion, 3 months later with airspace opacity," you say TB
- When I say "hot-tub," you say Hypersensitivity Pneumonitis
- When I say "halo sign," you say Fungal Pneumonia - Invasive Aspergillus
- When I say "reverse halo or atoll sign," you say COP
- When I say "finger in glove," you say ABPA
- When I say "ABPA," you say Asthma
- When I say "septic emboli + jugular vein thrombus," you say Lemierre
- When I say "Lemierre," you say Fusobacterium Necrophorum
- When I say "Paraneoplatic syndromes with SIADH," you say Small Cell Lung CA
- When I say "Paraneoplatic syndromes with PTH," you say Squamous Cell CA
- When I say "Small Cell Lung CA + Proximal Weakness," you say Lambert Eaton
- When I say "Cavity fills with air, post pneumonectomy," you say Bronchopleural Fistula
- When I say "malignant bronchial tumor," you say carcinoid
- When I say "malignant tracheal tumor," you say Adenoid Cystic
- When I say "AIDS patient with lung nodules, pleural effusion, and lymphadenopathy," you say Lymphoma
- When I say "Gallium Negative," you say Kaposi
- When I say "Thallium Negative," you say PCP
- When I say "Macroscopic fat and popcorn calcifications," you say Hamartoma
- When I say "Bizarre shaped cysts," you say LCH
- When I say "Lung Cysts in a TS patient," you say LAM
- When I say "Panlobular Emphysema - NOT Alpha 1," you say Ritalin Lung
- When I say "Honeycombing," you say UIP
- When I say "The histology was heterogeneous," you say UIP
- When I say "Ground Glass with Sub pleural Sparing," you say NSIP
- When I say "UIP Lungs + Parietal Pleural Thickening," you say Asbetosis
- When I say "Cavitation in the setting of silicosis," you say TB
- When I say "Air trapping seen 6 months after lung transplant," you say Chronic Rejection / Bronchiolitis Obliterans Syndrome
- When I say "Crazy Paving," you say PAP
- When I say "History of constipation," you say Lipoid Pneumonia - inferring mineral oil use / aspiration.
- When I say "UIP + Air trapping," you say Chronic Hypersensitivity Pneumonitis
- When I say "Dilated Esophagus + ILD," = Scleroderma (with NSIP)

- When I say "Shortness of breath when sitting up," you say Hepatopulmonary syndrome
- When I say "Episodic hypoglycemia," you say solitary fibrous tumor of the pleura
- When I say "Pulmonary HTN with Normal Wedge Pressure," you say Pulmonary Veno-occlusive disease.
- When I say "Yellow Nails" you say Edema and Chylous Pleural Effusions (Yellow Nail Syndrome).
- When I say "persistent fluid collection after pleural drain/tube placement," you say Extrapleural Hematoma.
- When I say "Displaced extrapleural fat," you say Extrapleural Hematoma.
- When I say "Massive air leak, in the setting of trauma," you say bronchial or tracheal injury
- When I say "Hot of PET – around the periphery," you say pulmonary infarct
- When I say "Multi-lobar collapse," you say sarcoid
- When I say "Classic bronchial infection," you say TB
- When I say "Panbronchiolitis," you say tree in bud (not centrilobular or random nodules)
- When I say "Bronchorrhea," you say Mucinous BAC

High Yield Trivia

- The tricuspid valve is the most anterior
- The pulmonic valve is the most superior
- There are 10 lung segments on the right, and 8 lung segments on the left
- If it goes above the clavicles, it's in the posterior mediastinum (cervicothoracic sign)
- Azygos Lobe has 4 layers of pleura
- Most common pulmonary vein variant is a separate vein draining the right middle lobe
- Most common cause of pneumonia in AIDS patient is Strep Pneumonia
- Most common opportunistic infection in AIDS = PCP.
- Aspergilloma is seen in a normal immune patient
- Invasive Aspergillus is seen in an immune compromised patient
- Fleischner Society Recommendations do NOT apply to patient's with known cancers
- Eccentric calcifications in a solitary pulmonary nodule pattern is considered the most suspicious.
- A part solid nodule with a ground glass component is the most suspicious morphology you can have
- Most common lung CA to present as solitary nodule
- Stage 3B lung CA is unresectable (contralateral nodal involvement ; ipsilateral or contralateral scalene or supraclavicular nodal involvement, tumor in different lobes).
- The most common cause of unilateral lymphangetic carcinomatosis is bronchogenic carcinoma lung cancer invading the lymphatics

- There is a 20 year latency between initial exposure and development of lung cancer or pleural mesothelioma
- Pleural effusion is the earliest and most common finding with asbestosis exposure.
- Silicosis actually raises your risk of TB by about 3 fold.
- Nitrogen Dioxide exposure is "Silo Filler's Disease," gives you a pulmonary edema pattern.
- Reticular pattern in the posterior costophrenic angle is supposedly the first finding of UIP on CXR
- Sarcoidosis is the most common recurrent primary disease after lung transplant
- Pleural plaque of asbestosis typically spares the costophrenic angles.
- Pleural effusion is the most common manifestation of mets to the pleura.
- There is an association with mature teratomas and Klinefelter Syndrome.
- Injury close to the carina is going to cause a pneumomediastinum rather than a pneumothorax
- MRI is superior for assessing superior sulcus tumors because you need to look at the brachial plexus.
- Leiomyoma is the most common benign esophageal tumor (most common in the distal third).
- Esophageal Leiomyomatosis may be associated with Alport's Syndrome
- Bronchial / Tracheal injury must be evaluated with bronchoscopy
- If you say COP also say Eosinophilic Pneumonia
- If you say BAC also say lymphoma
- Bronchial Atresia is classically in the LUL
- Pericardial cysts MUST be simple, Bronchogenic cysts don't have to be simple
- PAP follows a rule of 1/3s post treatment; 1/3 gets better, 1/3 doesn't, 1/3 progresses to fibrosis
- Dysphagia Lusoria presents later in life as atherosclerosis develops
- Carcinoid is COLD on PET
- Wegener's is now called Granulomatosis with Polyangiitis – Wegener was a Nazi. Apparently he was not just a Nazi, he was a Nazi before it was "fashionable." Plus, I heard he was a real asshole, and a bad tipper (which is unforgivable).

Section 6: Cardiac

Gamesmanship: Congenital Heart Disease

My idea is that you can only write 3 kinds of multiple choice questions regarding congenital heart disease: (1) Aunt Minnie, (2) Differential with crappy distractions, and (3) Associations/ Trivia

Situation 1: - The Aunt Minnie

There are a few congenital heart cases that are straight up Aunt Minnies. The usual characters that most 3rd year medical students memorize are fair game.

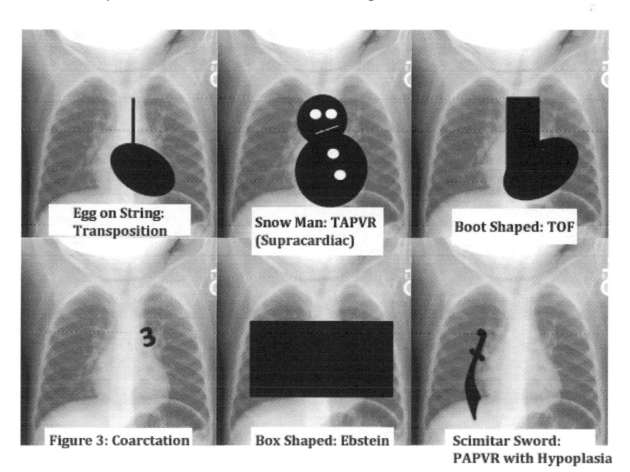

Egg on String: Transposition

Snow Man: TAPVR (Supracardiac)

Boot Shaped: TOF

Figure 3: Coarctation

Box Shaped: Ebstein

Scimitar Sword: PAPVR with Hypoplasia

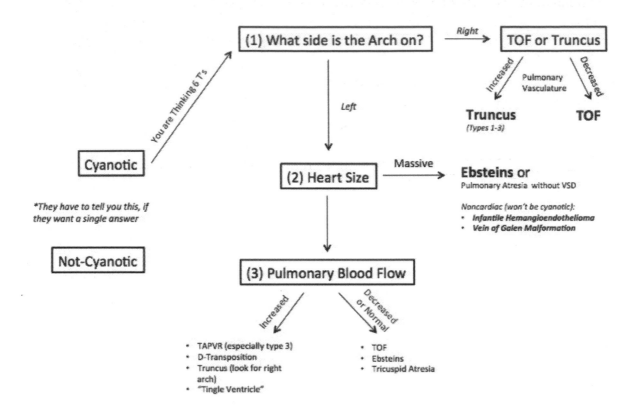

Walking through this outline. First ask yourself is it cyanotic or not? **They will have to tell you this in the stem.** Look for this in the stem every time, then cross out answers that are not cyanotic.

Cyanotic	Not Cyanotic
TOF	ASD
TAPVR	VSD
Transposition	PDA
Truncus	PAPVR
Tricuspid Atresia	Aortic Coarctation (adult type – post ductal)

Example: *Patient "X" is a newborn cyanotic, what is the most likely Dx?*

A - VSD

B- ASD

C- Demonic Possession

D - TOF

Without even looking at a picture (which they will probably show), you know the answer is D, because that is the only cyanotic one listed. If you were wondering about C - I did a google scholar search for *"Demonic Possession causing cyanosis"*, and although there were a few case reports none come down hard on cyanosis.

The next thing to ask is what side the arch is on? If you see it on the left, it's not helpful. If you see it on the right - think TOF and Truncus.

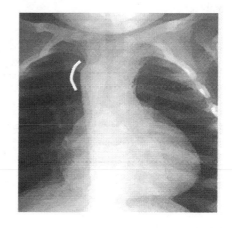

Example: *Patient "X" is a newborn cyanotic, with CXR shown. What is the most likely Dx.*

A- ASD
B- VSD
C-Tricuspid Atresia
D -TOF

So ASD, and VSD are out because the are not cyanotic. You notice the right arch - so you call it TOF.

Example: *Patient "X" is a newborn cyanotic, with CXR shown. What is the most likely Dx.*

A- ASD
B- VSD
C- Truncus
D -TOF

Now if they would give you the same picture but add the choice Truncus. Then you would have to look at the lungs. **Vasculature increased with Truncus, and normal / decreased with TOF.**

If the show you a normal left arch, the first thing I like to do is ask *is the heart is massively enlarged?*

This gives you a differential of cardiac causes, and non-cardiac causes.

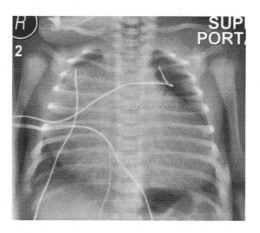

Cardiac: Ebsteins, or Pulmonary Atresia (without VSD).

Non- Cardiac: High Flow States like Vein of Galen Malformation and Hepatic Hemangioendothelioma. Obviously they have to show you a liver or brain next with these two.

Lastly the difference between increased and normal/decreased pulmonary vasculature can help eliminate distractors. I want to stress not trying to tell normal and decreased apart on crappy monitors. It's hard enough on a real viewing monitor. The distinction is not necessary for multiple choice.

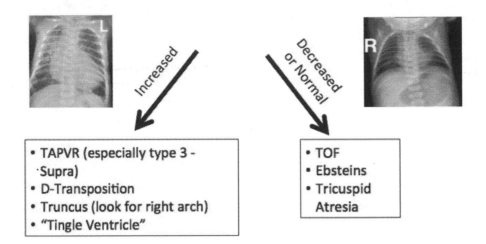

* TAPVR (especially type 3 - Supra)
* D-Transposition
* Truncus (look for right arch)
* "Tingle Ventricle"

* TOF
* Ebsteins
* Tricuspid Atresia

Example: *Patient with cyanotic heart disease, with CXR shown. What is the most likely Dx?*

A - ASD
B - VSC
C - Tricuspid Atresia
D - TAPVR

ASD and VSD are not cyanotic. Tricuspid Atresia has Decreased pulmonary vasculature (this CXR shows increased). That leaves TAPVR.

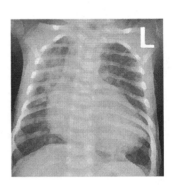

Gamesmanship - Signs of left atrial enlargement

(1) Double Density - superimposed over contour of the right heart
(2) Splaying of the carina - angle over 90 degrees
(3) Posterior displacement of the heart - seen on the lateral CXR

Gamesmanship: Which MRI sequence is best?

Pathology	Which Sequence(s) most useful?
Cardiac Myxoma	Low T1, High T2 (high myxoid content)
Acute vs Chronic MI	Look at T2 – Bright on Acute ; Dark on Chronic (fibrous scar)
Arrhythmogenic Right Ventricular Dysplasia (ARVD)	T1 Bright
Microvascular Obstruction	First Pass Perfusion (25 seconds post Gad)
Infarct	Delayed Enhancement (10-12 mins post Gad)

This vs That: Constrictive vs Restrictive Cardiomyopathy:

- Pericardium is usually thickened in constrictive

- Diastolic septal bounce is seen in constrictive (Sigmoidization of the septum).

This vs That: True vs False Ventricular Aneurysm

- *True:* **Mouth is wider** than body. Myocardium is intact. Usually anterior-lateral wall.

- *False:* **Mouth is narrow** compared to body. Myocardium is NOT intact (pericardial adhesions contain rupture). Usually posterior-lateral wall. Higher risk of rupture. .

This vs That: Valve Anatomy

Aortic Valve: *Right, Left, and Posterior Cusps*
Pulmonic Valve: *Right, Left, and Anterior Cusps*

This vs That : Stunned vs Hibernating Myocardium

- *Stunned Myocardium:* After an Acute Injury (ischemia or reperfusion injury), dysfunction of myocardium persists even after restoration of blood flow (can last days to weeks). A perfusion study will be normal, but the contractility is crap.

- *Hibernating Myocardium:* This is a more chronic process, and the result of severe CAD causing chronic hypoperfusion. You will have areas of decreased perfusion and decreased contractility even when resting. Don't get it twisted, this is not an infarct. On a FDG PET, this tissue will take up tracer more intensely than normal myocardium, and will also demonstrate redistribution of thallium. This is reversible with revascularization.

- *Scar:* This is dead myocardium. It will not squeeze normally, so you'll have abnormal wall motion. It's not a zombie. It will not come back to life with revascularization.

Stunned	Hibernating	Infract / Scar
Wall Motion Abnormal	Wall Motion Abnormal	Wall Motion Abnormal
Normal Perfusion (Thallium or Sestamibi)	Abnormal Fixed Perfusion	Abnormal Fixed Perfusion
	Will Redistribute with Delayed Thallium and will take up FDG	Will NOT Redistribute with Delayed Thallium, will NOT take up FDG
Associated with acute MI	Associated with chronic high grade CAD	Associated the chronic prior MI

This vs That: Left Atrial Myxoma vs Clot

- The myxoma will enhance

This vs That: Vegetations vs Fibroelastoma

You tell the difference by looking for valvular damage (seen with vegetations). Contrast enhancement is not very reliable because of how small these things are.

When I Say This..... You Say That.....

- When I say "ALCAPA," you say Steal Syndrome
- When I say "Supra-valvular Aortic Stenosis" you say Williams Syndrome
- When I say "Bicuspid Aortic Valve and Coarctation" you say Turners Syndrome
- When I say "Isolated right upper lobe edema," you say Mitral Regurgitation
- When I say "Peripheral pulmonary stenosis," you say Alagille Syndrome
- When I say "Box shaped heart", you say Ebsteins
- When I say "Right Arch with Mirror Branching," you say congenital heart.
- When I say "hand/thumb defects + ASD," you say Holt Oram
- When I say "ostium primum ASD (or endocardial cushion defect)," you say Downs
- When I say "Right Sided PAPVR," you say Sinus Venosus ASD
- When I say "Calcification in the left atrium wall," you say Rheumatic Heart Disease
- When I say "difficult to suppress myocardium," you say Amyloid
- When I say "blood pool suppression on delayed enhancement," you say Amyloid
- When I say "septal bounce," you say constrictive pericarditis
- When I say "ventricular interdependence," you say constrictive pericarditis
- When I say "focal thickening of the septum - but not Hypertrophic Cardiomyopathy," you say Sarcoid.
- When I say "ballooning of the left ventricular apex," you say Tako-Tsubo
- When I say "fat in the wall of a dilated right ventricle," you say Arrhythmogenic Right Ventricular Cardiomyopathy (ARVC)
- When I say "kid with dilated heart and mid wall enhancement," you say Muscular Dystrophy
- When I say "Cardiac Rhabdomyoma," you say Tuberous Sclerosis
- When I say "Bilateral Atrial Thrombus," you say Eosinophilic Cardiomyopathy
- When I say "Diffuse LV Subendocardial enhancement not restricted to a vascular distribution," you say Cardiac Amyloid.
- When I say "Glenn Procedure," you say acquired pulmonary AVMs
- When I say "Pulmonary Vein Stenosis," you say Ablation for A-Fib
- When I say "Multiple Cardiac Myxomas," you say Carney's Complex

High Yield Trivia

- The right atrium is defined by the IVC.
- The right ventricle is defined by the moderator band.
- The tricuspid papillary muscles insert on the septum (mitral ones do not).
- Lipomatous Hypertrophy of the Intra-Atrial Septum - can be PET Avid (it's brown fat)
- LAD gives off diagonals
- RCA gives off acute marginals
- LCX gives off obtuse marginals
- RCA perfuses SA and AV nodes (most of the time)
- Dominance is decided by which vessel lives off the posterior descending - it's the right 85%
- LCA from the Right Coronary Cusp - always gets repaired
- RCA from the Left Coronary Cusp - repaired if symptoms
- Most common location of myocardial bridging is in the mid portion of the LAD.
- Coronary Artery Aneurysm - most common cause in adult = Atherosclerosis
- Coronary Artery Aneurysm - most common cause in child = Kawasaki
- Rheumatic heart disease is the most common cause of mitral stenosis
- Pulmonary Arterial Hypertension is the most common cause of tricuspid atresia.
- Double most common vascular ring is the double aortic arch
- Most common congenital heart disease is a VSD
- Most common ASD is the Secundum
- Infracardiac TAPVR classically shown with pulmonary edema in a newborn
- "L" Transposition type is congenitally corrected (they are "L"ucky).
- "D" Transposition type is doomed.
- Truncus is associated with CATCH-22 (DiGeorge)
- Rib Notching from coarctations spares the 1st and 2nd Ribs
- Infarct with 50% involvement is unlikely to recover function
- Microvascular Obstruction is NOT seen in chronic infarct
- Amyloid is the most common cause of restricted cardiomyopathy
- Primary amyloid can be seen in multiple myeloma
- Most common neoplasm to involve the cardiac valves = Fibroelastoma
- Most commonly the congenital absence of the pericardium is partial and involves the pericardium over the left atrium and adjacent pulmonary artery (*the left atrial appendage is the most at risk to become strangulated*).
- Glenn shunt - SVC to pulmonary artery (vein to artery)
- Blalock-Taussig Shunt - Subclavian Artery to Pulmonary Artery (artery - artery)
- Ross Procedure - Replaces aortic valve with pulmonic, and pulmonic with a graft (done for kids).

- Aliasing is common with Cardiac MRI. You can fix it by: (1) opening your FOV, (2) oversampling the frequency encoding direction, or (3) switching phase and frequency encoding directions.
- Giant Coronary Artery Aneurysms (>8mm) don't regress, and are associated with MIs.
- Wet Beriberi (thiamine def) can cause a dilated cardiomyopathy.
- Most common primary cardiac tumor in children = Rhabdomyoma.
- 2nd most common primary cardiac tumor in children = Fibroma
- Most common complication of MI is myocardial remodeling.
- Unroofed coronary sinus is associated with Persistent left SVC.
- Most common source of cardiac mets = Lung Cancer (lymphoma #2).
- A-Fib is most commonly associated with left atrial enlargement
- Most common cause of tricuspid insufficiency is RVH (usually from pulmonary HTN / cor pulmonale).

SECTION 7: VASCULAR

Gamesmanship: Thoracic Angiogram

If you see an angiogram through the great vessels and aorta think about TOS, Takayasu, and Giant Cell. The locations are classic, and helpful. Having said that remember Takayasu is going to be a young person (probably Asian female), and Giant Cell is going to be an old person - **age trumps location.** If they show you TOS, they will show the arms up and down - dead give away.

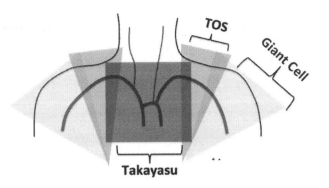

If the history is trauma, don't forget to look at the great vessels (not just the aorta).

Gamesmanship: Aortic Dissection on Angiogram

Can be shown as opacification of abdominal aortic branch vessels during aortography (catheter placed in the aortic true lumen) with the branch vessels—(celiac axis, superior mesenteric artery, and renal arteries) arising out of nowhere. They appear to be floating, with little or no antegrade opacification of the aortic true lumen. This is the so called **"floating viscera sign."**

Gamesmanship: Collateral Filling

If you inject the SMA and the celiac branches fill - infers a tight stenosis at the celiac origin. If you inject the celiac and the SMA branches fill - infers a tight stenosis at the SMA origin.

Gamesmanship: Hand Angiograms

Pathology: It's going to be either Buergers of Hypothenar Hammer Syndrome(HHS).

Ask yourself is the ulnar artery involved? If yes go with the HHS. If the ulnar nerve looks ok, but the fingers are out go with Buergers. Be careful, because the fingers can be out with HHS as well (distal emboli). Pseudo-aneurysm off the ulnar artery is a slam dunk for HHS.

Gamesmanship: Renal Artery Angiogram

Ostial Narrowing - Think Atherosclerosis - Treat with Balloon + Stent
Beading mid vessel - Think FMD - Treat with Balloon Only

Gamesmanship: Kidney Angiogram

First question should always be ? Is there an RCC or AML
Second question should be is there PAN / Speed Kidney ? A bunch of little aneurysms

Gamesmanship: Kawasaki

Two classic ways to show this: (1) CT showing a coronary artery aneurysm - the obvious one, (2)
Calcified coronary artery aneurysm shown on a CXR- this was an old oral boards favorite.

This vs That: Aortic Coarctation

- Infantile (Pre-ductal) – these guys can have pulmonary edema. More typically a long
  segment. Blood supply to the descending aorta is via the PDA.

- Adult (Ductal) – Not symptomatic until later in childhood. Often presents with differential
  arm/leg blood pressures. More typically a short segment.

This vs That: External vs Internal Carotid

Internal Carotid	External Carotid
Low Resistance	High Resistance
Low Systolic Velocity	High Systolic Velocity
Diastolic velocity does not return to baseline	Diastolic velocity approaches zero baseline
Continuous color flow is seen throughout the cardiac cycle	Color flow is intermittent during the cardiac cycle

Also you can (1) look for branches of the external carotid, or (2) use a "temporal tap" to see
ripples in the ECA spectrum.

When I Say This..... You Say That.....

- When I say "vessel in the fissure of the ligamentum venosum," you say replaced left hepatic artery.
- When I say "vessel coursing of the pelvic brim," you say Corona Mortis
- When I say "ascending aorta calcifications," you say Syphilis and Takayasu
- When I say "tulip bulb aorta," you say Marfans
- When I say "really shitty Marfan's variant," you say Loeys-Dietz
- When I say "tortuous vessels," you say Loeys-Dietz
- When I say "renal artery stenosis with HTN in a child," you say NF-1
- When I say "nasty looking saccular aneurysm, without intimal calcifications" you say Mycotic.
- When I say "tree bark intimal calcification," you say Syphilitic (Luetic) aneurysm
- When I say "painful aneurysm in smoker, sparing the posterior wall," you say Inflammatory aneurysm.
- When I say "Turkish guy with pulmonary artery aneurysm," you say Behcets
- When I say "GI bleed with early opacification of a dilated draining vein," you say Colonic Angiodysplasia
- When I say "spider web appearance of hepatic veins on angiogram," you say Budd Chiari
- When I say "non-decompressible varicocele," you say look in the belly for badness
- When I say "right sided varicocele," you say look in the below for badness
- When I say "swollen left leg," you say May Thurner
- When I say "popliteal aneurysm," you say look for the AAA (and the other leg)
- When I say "most dreaded complication of popliteal aneurysm," you say distal emboli
- When I say "Great saphenous vein on the wrong side of the calf - lateral side," you say Marginal Vein of Servelle - which is supposedly pathognomonic for Klippel-Trenaunay Syndrome
- When I say "Asian," you say Takayasu
- When I say "Involves the aorta," you say Takayasu
- When I say "Kids with vertigo and aortitis," you say Cogan Syndrome
- When I say "Nasal perforation + Cavitary Lung Lesions," you say Wegners
- When I say "diffuse pulmonary hemorrhage," you say Microscopic Polyangitis
- When I say "Smoker + Hand Angiogram," you say Buergers
- When I say "Construction worker + Hand Angiogram," you say Hypothenar Hammer
- When I say "Unilateral tardus parvus in the carotid," you say stenosis of the innominate
- When I say "Bilateral tardus parvus in the carotids," you say aortic stenosis
- When I say "Bilateral reversal of flow in carotids," you say aortic regurg
- When I say "Lack of diastolic flow on carotid US," you say Brain Death

High Yield Trivia

- Artery of Adamkiewicz comes off on the left side (70%) between T8-L1 (90%)
- Arch of Riolan - middle colic branch of the SMA with the left colic of the IMA.
- Most common hepatic vascular variant = right hepatic artery replaced off the SMA
- The proper right hepatic artery is anterior the right portal vein, whereas the replaced right hepatic artery is posterior to the main portal vein.
- Accessory right inferior hepatic vein - most common hepatic venous variant.
- Anterior tibialis is the first branch off the popliteal
- Common Femoral Artery (CFA): Begins at the level of inguinal ligament
- Superficial Femoral Artery (SFA): Begins once the CFA gives off the profunda femurs
- Popliteal Artery: Begins as the SFA exits the adductor canal
- Popliteal Artery terminates as the anterior tibial artery and the tibioperoneal trunk
- Axillary Artery: Begins at the first rib
- Brachial Artery: Begins as it crosses the teres major
- Brachial Artery: Bifurcates to the ulnar and radial artery
- Intraosseous Branch: Typically arises from the ulnar
- Superficial Arch = From the Ulna, Deep Arch = From the Radius
- The "coronary vein," is the left gastric.
- Enlarged splenorenal shunts are associated with hepatic encephalopathy.
- Aortic Dissection, and intramural hematoma are caused by HTN (70%)
- Penetrating Ulcer is from atherosclerosis.
- Strongest predictor of progression of dissection in intramural hematoma = Maximum aortic diameter > 5cm.
- Leriche Syndrome Triad: Claudication, Absent/ Decreased femoral pulses, Impotence.
- Most common associated defect with aortic coarctation = bicuspid aorta (80%)
- Neurogenic compression is the most common subtype of thoracic outlet syndrome
- Splenic artery aneurysm - More common in pregnancy, more likely to rupture in pregnancy.
- Median Arcuate Compression - worse with expiration
- Colonic Angiodysplasia is associated with aortic stenosis
- Popliteal Aneurysm; 30-50% have AAA, 10% of patient with AAA have popliteal aneurysm, 50-70% of popliteal aneurysms are bilateral.
- Medial deviation of the popliteal artery by the medial head of the gastrocnemius = Popliteal Entrapment
- Type 3 Takayasu is the most common (arch + abdominal aorta).
- Most common vasculitis in a kid = HSP (Henoch-Schonlein Purpura)

SECTION 8: IR

Gamesmanship - Self Expandable vs Balloon Expandable

Self Expandable - any where you might get external compression
Balloon Expandable - if you need more precise placement

- May Thurner Syndrome - Self Expandable
- SFA - Self Expandable
- Focal Atherosclerosis Stenosis in the Distal Aorta - Balloon Expandable
- Renal Ostium Stenosis - Balloon Expandable (needs precise placement)

This vs That -Biliary Duct Anatomy

The Right Posterior Duct drains 6&7 - runs more horizontal
The Right Anterior Duct drains 5& 8 - runs more vertical

This vs That - Dialysis

The surgically created AV Fistula has superior longevity. A fistula typically needs 3-4 months to "mature" (vein to enlarge enough for dialysis). A synthetic graft will be ready for use in 2 weeks. A synthetic graft is usually easier to declot (the clot is usually confined to the synthetic graft).

"My Leg Hurts"		
Viable	Normal Capillary Return Normal Sensation Normal Strength	Lytic Therapy
Acute Threatened	Slow Capillary Return Minimal Sensory Loss Normal Strength	Lytic Therapy
Immediately Threatened	More Sensory Loss Mild-Moderate Weakness	Lytic Therapy ONLY if patient is a poor surgical candidate
Irreversible	Profound Sensory Loss Paralysis	Surgery

Gamesmanship - TIPS

There are several sneaky things that can be shown related to TIPS.

- CO_2 run during hepatic vein wedge- Blowing the liver dome off, because the injection was too strong. Anytime you see a CO_2 run over the liver think about this.

- TIPS placed into the hepatic artery (not portal vein). Remember to confirm that you are in the right structure - pay attention to the anatomy.

- They could tell you the portal systemic gradient was normal (3-6). Remember - that TIPS treats portal hypertension. Don't do a a TIPS on someone who does NOT have portal HTN.

When I Say This..... You Say That.....

- When I say "Hairpin turn - during bronchial angiography," you say anterior medullary (spinal cord) artery
- When I say "Fever, WBC, Nausea, and Vomiting after Uterine Artery Embolization," you say Post Embolization Syndrome (obviously could also be infection)
- When I say "Most medial vessel in the leg," you say posterior tibial
- When I say "the source of 85% of upper GI bleeds," you say left gastric
- When I say "the source of bleeding from a duodenal ulcer," you say GDA
- When I say "Pulmonary AVM," you say HHT
- When I say "most feared complication of bronchial artery embolization," you say spinal cord infarct
- When I say "high risk of bleeding for liver transplant," you say transjugular approach
- When I say "most feared complication of brachial arterial access," you say compartment syndrome
- When I say "cold painful fingers during dialysis," you say "Steal syndrome"
- When I say "ulcer on medial ankle," you say venous stasis
- When I say "ulcer on dorsum of foot," you say ischemia or infected ulcer
- When I say "ulcer on plantar surface of foot," you say neutropenic ulcer

High Yield Trivia

- "Significant lesion" = A systolic pressure gradient > 10 mm Hg at rest
- Things to NOT stick a drain in: Tumors, Acute Hematoma, and those associated with acute bowel rupture and peritonitis
- Renal Artery Stenting for renal failure - tends to not work if the Cr is > 3.
- Persistent sciatic artery is prone to aneurysm
- Even if the cholecystostomy tube instantly resolves all symptoms, you need to leave the tube in for 2-6 weeks (until the tract matures), otherwise you are going to get a bile leak.
- MELD scores greater than 24 are at risk of early death with TIPS
- The target gradient post tips (for esophageal bleeding) is between 9 and 11.
- Absolute contraindication for TIPS - Heart Failure, Severe Hepatic Failure
- Most common side effect of BRTO is gross hematuria
- Sensitivity = GI Bleed Scan = 0.1mL/min , Angiography = 1.0mL/min
- For GI Bleed - after performing an embolization of the GDA (for duodenal ulcer), you need to do a run of the SMA to look at the inferior pancreaticoduodenal
- Most common cause of lower GI bleed is diverticulosis
- TACE will prolong survival better than systemic chemo
- TACE: Portal Vein Thrombosis is considered a contraindication (sometimes) because of the risk of infracting the liver.
- Go above the rib for Thora
- Left Bundle Branch Block needs a pacer before a Thoracic Angiogram
- Never inject contrast through a swan ganz catheter for a thoracic angiogram
- You treat pulmonary AVMs at 3mm
- Hemoptysis - Active extravasation is NOT typically seen with the active bleed.
- UAE - Gonadotropin-releasing medications (often prescribed for fibroids) should be stopped for 3 months prior to the case
- The general rule for transgluteal is to avoid the sciatic nerves and gluteal arteries by access through the sarcospinous ligament medially (close to the sacrum, inferior to the piriformis).
- When to pull an abscess catheter; As a general rule – when the patient is better (no fever, WBC normal), and output is < 20cc over 24 hours.
- If the thyroid biopsy is non-diagnostic, you have to wait 3 months before you re-biopsy.
- Posterior lateral approach is the move for percutaneous nephrostomy
- You can typically pull a sheath with an ACT < 150-180
- Notice that 0.039, 0.035, 0.018 wires are in INCHES
- 3 French = 1 mm
- French size is the OUTSIDE of a catheter and the INSIDE of a sheath

- Artery calcifications (common in diabetics) make compression difficult, and can lead to a false elevation of the ABI.
- Type 2 endoleaks are the most common
- Circumaortic left renal vein: the anterior one is superior, the posterior one is inferior, and the filter should be below the lowest one.
- Risk of DVT is increased with IVC filters
- Acute Budd Chiari with fulminant liver failure = Needs a TIPS
- Pseudoaneurysm of the pancreaticoduodenal artery = "Sandwich technique" - distal and proximal segments of the artery feeding off the artery must be embolized
- Median Arcuate Ligament Syndrome - First line is surgical release of the ligament
- Massive Hemoptysis = Bronchial artery - Particles bigger than 325 micrometers
- Acalculous Cholecystitis = Percutaneous Cholecystostomy
- Hepatic encephalopathy after TIPS = You can either (1) place a new covered stent constricted in the middle by a loop of suture - deployed in the pre-existing TIPS, (2) place two new stents - parallel to each other (one covered self expandable, one uncovered balloon expandable).
- Recurrent variceal bleeding after placement of a constricted stent - balloon dilation of the constricted stent
- Appendiceal Abscess - Drain placement * just remember that a drain should be used for a mature (walled off) abscess and no frank pertioneal symptoms
- Inadvertent catheterization of the colon (after trying to place a drain in an abscess) - wait 4 weeks for the tract to mature - verify by over the wire tractogram, and then remove tube.
- DVT with severe symptoms and no response to systemic anticoagulation = Catheter Directed Thrombolysis

SECTION 9: NUKES

Tracer	Analog	Energy	Physical Half Life
Tc – 99m		"Low" – 140	6 hours
Iodine -123	Iodine	"Low" – 159	13 hours
Xenon - 133		"Low" – 81	125 hours *(biologic t1/2 30 seconds)*
Thallium - 201	Potassium	"Low" – 135 (2%), 167 (8%), *use 71 ^{201}Hg daughter x-rays*	73 hours
Indium -111		"Medium" – 173 (89%), 247 (94%)	67 hours
Gallium - 67	Iron	Multiple; 93 (40%), 184 (20%), 300 (20%), 393 (5%)	78 hours
Iodine -131	Iodine	"High" - 365	8 days
Fluorine -18	Sugar	"High" - 511	110 mins

Treatment Radionuclides Half Life	
Strontium 89	50.5 DAYS (14 days in bone)
Samarium 153	46 Hours
Yttrium 90	64 Hours

Cardiac Radionuclides Half Life	
Rubidium 82	75 seconds
Nitrogen 13	10 mins

***Gamesmanship:* -** Tc-99 DTPA vs Xe-133

Distinguishing these two: The DTPA can be done in multiple projections. The DTPA tends to clump in the central airways.

This vs That - Tc WBC vs In WBC

Tc WBC	In WBC
Renal	**NO** Renal
GI	**NO** GI

This vs That - Tc WBC at 4 hours, Tc WBC at 24 hours

4 hours - lung uptake
24 hours - lung uptake has cleared, start to get bowel uptake

This vs That - Tc MDP vs F-18 Bone Scan - organ with higher dose

Tc MDP - Bone
F-18 - Bladder

This vs That - Bone Met Therapy

Sr^{89}	Sm^{153}	Ra^{223}
Pure Beta Emitter	Beta Emitter, with imagable some gamma	Alpha Emitter
Most Bone Marrow Toxicity (longest recovery).	Less Bone Marrow Toxicity	Least Bone Marrow Toxicity
Renal excretion	Renal excretion	GI excretion
		Improves Survival (prostate mets)

This vs That - Renal Tracer Mechanisms

Tc DTPA	Tc MAG 3	Tc GH
Filtered **(GFR)**	Secreted **(ERPF)**	Filtered
Good For Native Kidneys with **Normal Renal Function**	Concentrated better by kidneys with **poor renal function**	Good for dynamic and cortical imaging.
Critical Organ Bladder	Critical Organ Bladder	Critical Organ Bladder

This vs That - ATN vs Rejection vs Drug Tox

ATN	Immediate Post OP (3-4 days post op)	Perfusion Normal	Excretion Delayed
Cyclosporin Toxicity	**Long Standing**	Perfusion Normal	Excretion Delayed
Acute Rejection	Immediate Post OP	**Poor Perfusion**	Excretion Delayed

This vs That - Cancer vs Maybe Not Cancer (clinical correlation)

Tumors that are PET COLD	Not Cancer but PET HOT
BAC (Adeno In Situ) - Lung Cancer	Infection
Carcinoid	Inflammation
RCC	Ovaries in Follicular Phase
Peritoneal Bowel/Liver Implants	Muscles
Anything Mucinous	Brown Fat
Prostate	Thymus

This vs That - Why is Granny is confused?

FDG PET - Brain		
Alzheimer	Low posterior temporoparietal cortical activity	Identical to Parkinson Dementia
Multi Infarct	Scattered areas of decreased activity	
Dementia with Lewy Bodies	Low in lateral occipital cortex	Preservation of the mid posterior cingulate gyrus (**Cigulate Island Sign**)
Picks / Frontotemporal	Low frontal lobe	
Huntingtons	Low activity in caudate nucleus and putamen	

This vs That - Graves vs Toxic Multi-Nodular Goiter

Graves	Toxic Multi-Nodular Goiter
Uptake High :70s	Uptake Medium High: 40s
Homogenous	Heterogeneous

When I Say This..... You Say That.....

- When I say "hot clumps of signal in the lungs on Liver Spleen sulfur colloid," you say too much Al in the Tc.
- When I say "HOT spleen," you say WBC scan or Octreotide (sulfur colloid will be like warm spleen.
- When I say "Bone Scan with Hot Skull Sutures," you say renal osteodystrophy
- When I say "Bone Scan with Focal Breast Uptake," you say breast CA
- When I say "Bone Scan with Renal Cortex Activity," you say hemochromatosis
- When I say "Bone Scan with Liver Activity," you say either too much Al, Amyloid, Hepatoma, or Liver Necrosis
- When I say "Bone Scan with Sternal Lesion," you say breast CA.
- When I say "Bone Scan with Diffusely Decreased Bone Uptake," you say (1) Free Tc, or (2) Bisphosphonate Therapy.
- When I say "Tramline along periosteum of long bones," you say lung CA
- When I say "Super Hot Mandible in Adult," you say Fibrous Dysplasia
- When I say "Super Hot Mandible in Child," you say Caffeys
- When I say "Periarticular uptake of delayed scan," you say RSD
- When I say "Focal uptake along the lesser trochanter," you say Prosthesis loosening
- When I say "Tracer in the brain on a VQ study," you say Shunt
- When I say "Tracer over the liver on Ventilation with Xenon," you say Fatty Liver
- When I say "Gallium Negative, Thallium Positive," you say Kaposi
- When I say "High T3, High T4, low TSH, - low thyroid uptake," you say Quervains (Granulomatous thyroiditis).
- When I say "persistent tracer in the lateral ventricles > 24 hours," you say NPH
- When I say "Renal uptake on sulfur colloid," you say CHF
- When I say "Renal transplant uptake on sulfur colloid", you say Rejection
- When I say "Filtered Renal Agent," you say DTPA (or GH)
- When I say "Secreted Renal Agent," you say MAG-3
- When I say "PET with increased muscle uptake," you say insulin
- When I say "Diffuse FDG uptake in the thyroid on PET," you say Hashimoto
- When I say "I see the skeleton on MIBG," you say diffuse neuroblastoma bone mets
- When I say "Cardiac tissue taking up FDG more intense than normal myocaridum," you say hibernating myocardium
- I say "made with a generator" , you say Tc99 and Rubidium

High Yield Trivia

- Geiger Mueller - maximum dose it can handle is about 100mR/h
- Activity level greater than 100 mCi of Tc-99m is considered a major spill.
- Activity level greater than 100 mCi of Tl-201 is considered a major spill.
- Activity level greater than 10 mCi of In-111, is considered to represent a major spill.
- Activity level greater than 10 mCi of Ga-67, is considered to represent a major spill.
- An activity level greater than 1 mCi of I-131 is considered to constitute a major spill.
- Annual Dose limit of 100 mrem to the public
- Not greater than 2 mrem per hour – in an "unrestricted area"
- Total Body Dose per Year = 5 rem
- Total equivalent organ dose (skin is also an organ) per year = 50 rem
- Total equivalent extremity dose per year = 50 rem (500mSv)
- Total Dose to Embryo/fetus over entire 9 months – 0.5rem
- NRC allows no more than 0.15 micro Ci of Mo per 1 mili Ci of Tc, at the time of administration.
- Chemical purity (Al in Tc) is done with pH paper
- The allowable amount of Al is < 10 micrograms
- Radiochemical purity (looking for Free Tc) is done with thin layer chromatography
- Free Tc occurs from - lack of stannous ions or accidental air injection (which oxidizes)
- Prostate Cancer bone mets are uncommon with a PSA less than 10 mg/ml
- Flair Phenomenon occurs 2 weeks - 3 months after therapy
- Skeletal Survey is superior (more sensitive) for lytic mets
- AVN - Early and Late is COLD, Middle (repairing) is Hot.
- Particle size for VQ scan is 10-100 micrometers
- Xenon is done first during the VQ scan
- Amiodarone - classic thyroid uptake blocker
- Hashimotos increases risk for lymphoma
- Hot nodule on Tc, shouldn't be considered benign until you show that it's also hot on I^{123}. This is the concept of the discordant nodule.
- History of methimazole treatment (even years prior) makes I-131 treatment more difficult
- Methimazole side effect is neutropenia
- In pregnancy PTU is the blocker of choice
- Sestamibi in the parathyroid depends on blood flow and mitochondria
- You want to image with PET - following therapy at interval of 2-3 weeks for chemotherapy, and 8-12 weeks for radiation is the way to go. This avoids "stunning" – false negatives, and inflammatory induced false positive.
- ^{111}In Pentetreotide is the most commonly used agent for somatostatin receptor imaging. The classic use is for carcinoid tumors

- Meningiomas take up octreotide
- Prior to MIBG you should block the thyroid with Lugols Iodine or Perchlorate
- Left bundle branch block can cause a false positive defect in the ventricular septum (spares the apex)
- Pulmonary uptake of Thallium is an indication of LV dysfunction
- MIBG mechanism is that of an Analog of Norepinephrine - actively transported and stored in the neurosecretory granules
- MDP mechanism is that of a Phosphate analog - which works via Chemisorption
- Sulfur Colloid mechanism = Particles are Phagocytized by RES

SECTION 10: NEURO

Foramen	Contents
Foramen Ovale	CN V3, and Accessory Meningeal Artery
Foramen Rotundum	CN V2 ("**R2V2**"),
Superior Orbital Fissure	CN 3, CN 4, CN V1, CN6
Inferior Orbital Fissure	CN V2
Foramen Spinosum	Middle Meningeal Artery
Jugular Foramen	Jugular Vein, CN 9, CN 10, CN 11
Hypoglossal Canal	CN12
Optic Canal	CN 2, and Opthalmic Artery

This vs That: *HIV Encephalitis vs PML*

- HIV Encephalitis is symmetric (T2 bright, T1 normal)
- PML is asymmetric (T2 bright, T1 dark)

This vs That: AIDS Infections

AIDS Encephalitis	PML	CMV	Toxo	Cryptococcus
Symmetric T2 Bright	Asymmetric T2 Bright	Periventricular T2 Bright	Ring Enhancement	Dilated Perivascular Spaces
	T1 dark	Ependymal Enhancement	Thallium Cold	Basilar Meningitis

This vs That: *Toxo vs Lymphoma*

Toxo	Lymphoma
Ring Enhancing	Ring Enhancing
Hemorrhage more common after treatment	Hemorrhage less common after treatment
Thallium Cold	**Thallium HOT**
PET Cold	Pet Hot
MR Perfusion: Decreased CBV	MR Perfusion: Increased (or Decreased) CBV

This vs That: *LeForts Unique Components*

- LeFort 1: Lateral Nasal Aperture
- LeFort 2: Inferior Orbital Rim, and Orbital Floor
- LeFort 3: Zygomatic Arch, and Lateral Orbital Rim/Wall

This vs That: Temporal Bone Fractures:

Longitudinal	Transverse
Long Axis of T-Bone	Short Axis of T-Bone
More Common	Less Common
More Ossicular Dislocation	More Vascular Injury (Carotid / Jugular)
Less Facial Nerve Damage (around 20%)	More Facial Nerve Damage (>30%)
More Conductive Hearing Loss	More Sensorineural Hearing Loss

This vs That: *Porencephalic Cyst vs Open Lip Schizencephaly*

- Open Lip Schizencephaly - cleft lined by gray matter (malformation)
- Porencephalic Cyst - hole from prior ischemia

This vs That: Vocal Cord Paralysis vs Cancer

• Affected side is dilated with vocal cord paralysis
• Opposite side is dilated with cancer

This vs That: Syndromes with Tumors

NF-1	Optic Nerve Gliomas
NF-2	MSME; Multiple Schwannomas, Meningiomas, Ependymomas
VHL	Hemangioblastoma (brain and retina)
TS	Subependymal Giant Cell Astrocytoma, Cortical Tubers
Nevoid Basal Cell Syndrome (Gorlin)	Medulloblastoma
Turcot	GBM, Medulloblastoma
Cowdens	Lhermitte-Dulcos (Dysplastic cerebellar gangliocytoma)

This vs That: Meningioma vs Schwannoma

Meningioma	**Schwannoma**
Enhance Homogeneously	Enhance Less Homogeneously
Don't Usually Invade IAC	Invade IAC
Calcify more often	IAC can have "trumpeted" appearance

This vs That: Where'd all that blood come from?

Maximum Bleeding – Aneurysm Location	
ACOM	Interhemispheric Fissure
PCOM	Ipsilateral Basal Cistern
MCA Trifurcation	Sylvian Fissure
Basilar Tip	Interpeduncular Cistern, or Intraventricular
PICA	Posterior Fossa or Intraventricular

Sinus Mass Summary

Path	Demographics	Typical Location	Trivia	Imaging Characteristics
Inverting Papilloma	40-70 M>F (4:1)	Lateral nasal wall centered at the middle meatus, with occasional extension into the antrum	40% show "entrapped bone" *Cerebriform Pattern* **10% Harbor a Squamous Cell CA**	Cerebriform Pattern May have focal hyperostosis on CT
Esthesioneuroblastoma	Bimodal 20s & 60s	Dumbbell shaped with waist at the cribiform plate		**AVID homogeneous enhancement**
SNUC	Broad Range (30s-90s)	Ethmoid origin more common than maxillary	**Large,** typically > 4cm on presentation	**Fungating and Poorly defined** Heterogeneous enhancement with necrosis
Squamous Cell CA	95% > 40 years old	Maxillary Antrum is involved in 80%	**Most Common Malignancy of Sino-Nasal track**	Aggressive Antral Soft Tissue Mass, with destruction of sinus walls **Low signal on T2 (highly cellular)** Enhances less than some other sinus malignancies
JNA *(Juvenile Nasopharyngeal Angiofibroma)*	**Nearly Exclusively Male Rare < 8 or > 25**	**Origin in the Spenopalantine Foramen (SPF)**	Radiation alone cures in 80%	**Enhancing mass arising from the SPF in adolescent male** Dark Flow Voids on T1 **Avidly Enhances**
Sinonasal Lymphoma	Usually older, peak is 60s	Nasal Cavity > Sinuses	Highly variable appearance	Homogeneous mass in nasal cavity with bony destruction **Low Signal on T2 (highly cellular)**

When I Say This..... You Say That.....

- When I say "cervical kyphosis" , you say NF-1
- When I say "lateral thoracic meningocele," you say NF-1
- When I say "bilateral optic nerve gliomas," you say NF-1
- When I say "bilateral vestibular schwannoma," you say NF-2
- When I say "retinal hamartoma," you say TS
- When I say "retinal angioma," you say VHL
- When I say "brain tumor with restricted diffusion," you say lymphoma
- When I say "brain tumor crossing the midline," you say GBM (or lymphoma)
- When I say "Cyst and Nodule in Child," you say Pilocystic Astrocytoma
- When I say "Cyst and Nodule in Adult," you say Hemangioblastoma
- When I say "multiple hemangioblastoma," you say Von Hippel Lindau
- When I say "Swiss cheese tumor in ventricle," you say central neurocytoma
- When I say "CN3 Palsy," you say posterior communicating artery aneurysm
- When I say "CN6 Palsy," you say increased ICP
- When I say "Ventricles out of size to atrophy," you say NPH
- When I say "Hemorrhagic putamen," you say Methanol
- When I say "Decreased FDG uptake in the lateral occipital cortex," you say Lewy Body Dementia
- When I say "TORCH with Periventricular Calcification," you say CMV
- When I say "TORCH with hydrocephalus," you say Toxoplasmosis
- When I say "TORCH with hemorrhagic infarction," you say HSV
- When I say "Neonatal infection with frontal lobe atrophy," you say HIV
- When I say "Rapidly progressing dementia + Rapidly progressing atrophy," you say CJD
- When I say "Expanding the cortex," Oligodendroglioma
- When I say "Tumor acquired after trauma (LP)," you say Epidermoid
- When I say "The Palate Separated from the Maxilla / Floating Palate," you say LeFort 1
- When I say "The Maxilla Separated from the Face" or "Pyramidal" you say LeFort 2
- When I say "The Face Separated from the Cranium," you say LeFort 3
- When I say "Airless expanded sinus," you say mucocele
- When I say "DVA," you say cavernous malformation nearby
- When I say "Single vascular lesion in the pons," you say Capillary Telangiectasia
- When I say "Elevated NAA peak," you say Canvans
- When I say "Tigroid appearance," you say Metachromatic Leukodystrophy
- When I say "Endolymphatic Sac Tumor," you say VHL
- When I say "T1 Bright in the petrous apex," you say Cholesterol Granuloma
- When I say "Restricted diffusion in the petrous apex," you say Cholesteatoma
- When I say "Lateral rectus palsy + otomastoiditis," you say Grandenigo Syndrome
- When I say "Cochlea and semicircular canal enhancement," you say Labrinthitis
- When I say "Conductive hearing loss in an adult," you say Otosclerosis
- When I say "Noise induced vertigo," you say Superior Semicircular Canal dehiscence

- When I say "Widening of the maxillary ostium," you say Antrochonal Polyp
- When I say "Inverting papilloma," you say squamous cell CA (10%)
- When I say "Adenoid cystic," you say perineural spread
- When I say "Left sided vocal cord paralysis," you say look in the AP window
  When I say "Bilateral coloboma," you say CHARGE syndrome
- When I say "Retinal Detachment + Small Eye" you say PHPV
- When I say "Bilateral Small Eye," you say Retinopathy of Prematurity
- When I say "Calcification in the globe of a child," you say Retinoblastoma
- When I say "Fluid-Fluid levels in the orbit," you say Lymphangioma
- When I say "Orbital lesion, worse with Valsalva," you say Varix
- When I say "Pulsatile Exophthalmos," you say NF-1 and CC Fistula
- When I say "Sphenoid wing dysplasia," you say NF-1
- When I say "Simitar Sacrum," you say Currarino Triad
- When I say "bilateral symmetrically increases T2 signal in the dorsal columns," you sat B12 (or HIV)
- When I say "Owl eye appearance of spinal cord," you say spinal cord infarct
- When I say "Enhancement of the nerves root of the cauda equina," you say Guillain Barre
- When I say "Subligamentous spread of infection," you say TB

High Yield Trivia

- The order of tumor prevalence in NF2 is the same as the mnemonic MSME (schwannoma > meningioma > ependymoma).
- Maldeveloped draining veins is the etiology of Sturge Weber
- All phakomatosis (NF 1, NF -2, TS, and VHL) EXCEPT Sturge Weber are autosomal dominant - family screening is a good idea.
- Most Common Primary Brain Tumor in Adult = Astrocytoma
- "Calcifies 90% of the time" = Oligodendroglioma
- Restricted Diffusion in Ventricle = Watch out for Choroid Plexus Xanthogranuloma (not a brain tumor, a benign normal variant)
- Pituitary - T1 Bright = Pituitary Apoplexy
- Pituitary - T2 Bright = Rathke Cleft Cyst
- Pituitary – Calcified = Craniopharyngioma
- CP Angle – Invades Internal Auditory Canal = Schwannoma
- CP Angle - Invades Both Internal Auditory Canals = Schwannoma with NF2
- CP Angle – Restricts on Diffusion = Epidermoid
- Peds – Arising from Vermis = Medulloblastoma
- Peds- 4th ventricle "tooth paste" out of 4th ventricle = Ependymoma
- Adult myelination pattern: T1 at 1 year, T2 at 2 years
- Brainstem and posterior limb of the internal capsule are myelinated at birth.
- CN2 and CNV3 are not in the cavernous sinus
- Persistent trigeminal artery (vertebral to carotid) increases the risk of aneurysm
- Subfalcine herniation can lead to ACA infarct
- ADEM lesions will NOT involve the calloso-septal interface.
- Marchiafava-Bignami progresses from body -> genu -> splenium
- Post Radiation changes don't start for 2 months (there is a latent period).
- Hippocampal atrophy is first with Alzheimer Dementia
- Most common TORCH for CMV
- Toxo abscess does NOT restrict diffusion
- Small cortical tumors can be occult without IV contrast
- JPA and Ganglioglioma can enhance and are low grade
- Nasal Bone is the most common fracture
- Zygomaticomaxillary Complex Fracture (Tripod) is the most common fracture pattern and involves the zygoma, inferior orbit, and lateral orbit.
- Supplemental oxygen can mimic SAH on FLAIR
- Putamen is the most common location for hypertensive hemorrhage
- Restricted diffusion without bright signal on FLAIR should make you think hyperacute (< 6 hours) stroke.
- Enhancement of a stroke; Rule of 3s - starts at day 3, peaks at 3 weeks, gone at 3 months
- PAN is the Most Common systemic vasculitis to involve the CNS
- Scaphocephaly is the most common type of crainosynostosis

- Piriform aperture stenosis is associated with hypothalamic pituitary adrenal axis issues.
- Cholesterol Granuloma is the most common primary petrous apex lesion
- Large vestibular aqueduct syndrome has absence of the bony modiolus in 90% of cases
- Octreotide scan will be positive for esthesioneuroblastoma
- The main vascular supply to the posterior nose is the sphenopalatine artery (terminal internal maxillary artery).
- Warthins tumors take up pertechnetate
- Sjogrens gets salivary gland lymphoma
- Most common intra-occular lesion in an adult = Melanoma
- Enhancement of nerve roots for 6 weeks after spine surgery is normal. After that it's arachnoiditis
- Hemorrhage in the cord is the most important factor for outcome in a traumatic cord injury.
- Currarino Triad: Anterior Sacral Meningocele, Anorectal malformation, Sarcococcygeal osseous defect
- Type 1 Spinal AVF (dural AVF) is by far the more common.
- Herpes spares the basal ganglia (MCA infarcts do not)

SECTION 11: MSK

This vs That: Forearm Fractures:

Essex-Lopresti	Galeazzi Fracture (MUGR)	Monteggia Fracture (MUGR)
Fracture of the radial head + Anterior dislocation of the distal radial ulnar joint	Radial Shaft fracture, with anterior dislocation of the ulna at the DRUJ.	Fracture of the proximal ulna, with anterior dislocation of the radial head.

This vs That: Femoral Neck Stress Fractures

-Medial Side - Stress Fracture, Compressive Side, Dose Well
-Lateral Side - Bisphospohate, Tensile Side, Dose Terrible

Shoulder - Bankart Spectrum

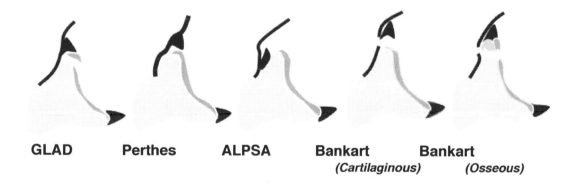

GLAD   Perthes   ALPSA   Bankart *(Cartilaginous)*   Bankart *(Osseous)*

GLAD	Perthes	ALPSA	True Bankart
Superficial partial labral injury with cartilage defect	Avulsed anterior labrum (only minimally displaced). Inferior GH complex still attached to periosteum	Similar to perthes but with "bunched up" medially displaced inferior GH complex	Torn labrum
No instability	Intact Periosteum (lifted up)	Intact Periosteum	***Periosteum Disrupted***

This vs That: Avulsion from where?

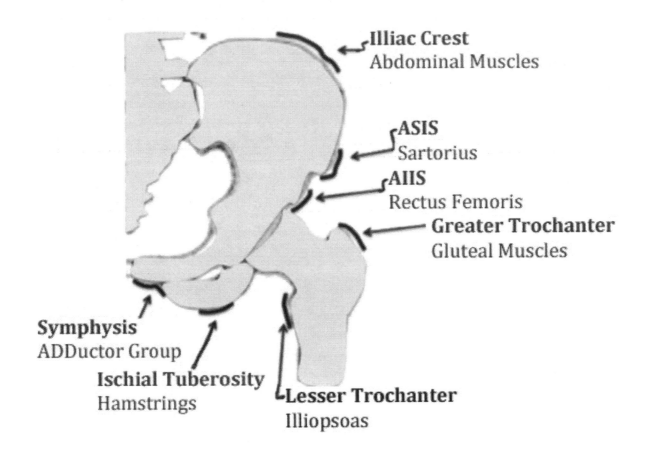

Illiac Crest
Abdominal Muscles

ASIS
Sartorius

AIIS
Rectus Femoris

Greater Trochanter
Gluteal Muscles

Symphysis
ADDuctor Group

Ischial Tuberosity
Hamstrings

Lesser Trochanter
Illiopsoas

This vs That: Impingement Types

Pincer Impingement	Cam Impingement
Middle Aged Women	Young Man
Over Coverage of the femoral head by the acetabulum	Bony protrusion on the antero-superior femoral head-neck junction
"Cross Over Sign"	*"Pistol Grip Deformity"* Describes the appearance of the femur

This vs That: **Osteochondroses**

Kohlers	Tarsal Navicular	Male 4-6. Treatment is not surgical.
Freiberg Infraction	Second Metatarsal Head	Adolescent Girls – can lead to secondary OA
Severs	Calcaneal Apophysis	Some say this is a normal "growing pain"
Panners	Capitellum	Kid 5-10 "Thrower" ; does not have loose bodies.
Perthes	Femoral Head	White kid; 4-8.
Kienbock	Carpal Lunate	Associated with negative ulnar variance. Seen in person 20-40.

Gamesmanship - Wrist Compartments

Gamesmanship Wrist Compartments	
Isolated 1st	De Quervains
1st + 2nd	Intersecting
Isolated 6th	Early RA
Multiple Flexors	RA

This vs That - Finger Tumors

Finger Tip Tumors / Masses		
Glomus	T1 Dark, T2 Bright, Enhances avidly.	T2 Bright, Enhance Avidly.
Giant Cell Tumor Tendon	T1 Dark, T2 Dark, Variable Enhancement, Bloom on Gradient	Bloom on Gradient
Fibroma	T1 Dark, T2 Dark. No Blooming	Does NOT Bloom on Gradient.

When I Say This..... You Say That.....

- When I say, "Posterior elbow dislocation," you say Capitellum fracture
- When I say "Chondroblastoma in an adult", you say "Clear Cell Chondrosarcoma"
- When I say "Malignant epiphyseal lesion", you say "Clear Cell Chondrosarcoma"
- When I say "Permeative lesion in the diaphysis of a child" , you say "Ewings"
- When I say "T2 bright lesion in the sacrum" , you say "Chordoma"
- When I say "Lytic T2 DARK lesion" , you say "Fibrosarcoma"
- When I say "Sarcomatous transformation of an infarct", you say "MFH"
- When I say, "Epiphyseal Lesion that is NOT T2 Bright" , You say Chondroblastoma
- When I say, "short 4th metacarpal," You say pseudopseudohypoparathyroidism and Turner Syndrome
- When I say, "band like acro-osteolysis," You say Hajdu-Cheney
- When I say "fat containing tumor in the retroperitoneum," you say liposarcoma
- When I say "sarcoma in the foot" you say synovial sarcoma.
- When I say "avulsion of the lesser trochanter," you say pathologic fracture
- When I say "cross over sign," you say pincher type Femoroacetabular Impingement
- When I say "Segond Fracture," you say ACL tear
- When I say "Reverse Segond Fracture," you say PCL
- When I say "Arcuate Sign," you say fibular head avulsion or PCL tear
- When I say "Deep Intercondylar Notch," you say ACL tear
- When I say "Bilateral Patellar Tendon Ruptures," you say chronic steroids
- When I say "Wide ankle mortise," you say show me the proximal fibula (Maisonneuve).
- When I say "Bilateral calcaneus fractures," you say show me the spinal compression fracture ("lover's leap")
- When I say "Dancer with lateral foot pain," you say avulsion of 5th MT
- When I say "Old lady with sudden knee pain with standing," you say SONK
- When I say "Looser's Zones," you say osteomalacia or rickets (vitamin D)
- When I say "Unilateral RA with preserved joint spaces," you say RSD
- When I say "T2 bright tumor in finger," you say Glomus
- When I say "Blooming in tumor in finger," you say Giant Cell Tumor of Tendon Sheath (PVNS)
- When I say "Atrophy of teres minor," you say Quadrilateral Space syndrome
- When I say "Subluxation of the Biceps Tendon," you say Subscapularis tear
- When I say "Too many bow ties," you say Discoid Meniscus
- When I say "Celery Stalk ACL - T2" you say Mucoid Degeneration
- When I say "Drumstick ALC - T1" you say Mucoid Degeneration
- When I say "Acute Flat foot," you say Posterior Tibial Tendon Tear
- When I say "Boomerang shaped peroneus brevis," you say tear - or split tear

- When I say "Meniscoid mass in the lateral gutter of the ankle," you say Anteriolateral Impingement Syndrome
- When I say "Scar between 3rd and 4th metatarsals," you say Morton's neuroma
- When I say "Osteomyelitis in the spine," you say IV drug user
- When I say "Osteomyelitis in the spine with Kyphosis," you say TB (Gibbus Deformity)
- When I say "Unilateral SI joint lysis," you say IV Drug User
- When I say "Psoas muscle abscess," you say TB
- When I say "Rice bodies in joint," you say TB - sloughed synovium
- When I say "Calcification along the periphery," you say myositis ossificans
- When I say "Calcifications more dense in the center," you say Osteosarcoma - reverse zoning
- When I say "Permeative lesion in the diaphysis of a child," you say Ewings
- When I say "Long lesion in a long bone," you say Fibrous Dysplasia
- When I say "Large amount of edema for the size of the lesion," you say Osteoid Osteoma
- When I say "Cystic bone lesion, that is NOT T2 bright," you say Chondroblastoma
- When I say "Lesion in the finger of a kid," you say Periosteal chondroma
- When I say "looks like NOF in the anterior tibia with anterior bowing," you say Osteofibrous Dysplasia.
- When I say " RA + Pneumoconiosis," you say Caplan Syndrome
- When I say " RA + Big Spleen + Neutropenia," you say Felty Syndrome
- When I say "Reducible deformity of joints - in hand," you say Lupus.
- When I say "destructive mass in a bone of a leukemia patient," you say Chloroma

High Yield Trivia

- Arthritis at the radioscaphoid compartment is the first sign of a SNAC or SLAC wrist
- SLAC wrist has a DISI deformity
- The pull of the Abductor pollucis longus tendon is what causes the dorsolateral dislocation in the Bennett Fracture
- Carpal tunnel syndrome has an association with dialysis
- Degree of femoral head displacement predicts risk of AVN
- Proximal pole of the scaphoid is at risk for AVN with fracture
- Most common cause of sacral insufficiency fracture is osteoporosis in old lady
- Patella dislocation is nearly always lateral
- Tibial plateau fracture is way more common laterally
- SONK favors the medial knee (area of maximum weight bearing)
- Normal SI joints excludes Ank Spon
- Looser Zones are a type of insufficiency fracture
- T score of -2.5 marks osteoporosis
- First extensor compartment = de Quervains
- First and Second compartment = intersection syndrome
- Sixth extensor compartment = early RA
- Flexor pollicis longus goes through the carpal tunnel, flexor pollicis brevis does not
- The pisiform recess and radiocarpal joint normally communicate
- The periosteum is intact with both Perthes and ALPSA lesions. In a true bankart it is disrupted.
- Absent anterior/superior labrum, along with a thickened middle glenohumeral ligament is a Buford complex.
- Medial meniscus is thicker posterior.
- Anterior talofibular ligament is the most commonly torn ankle ligament
- TB in the spine - spares the disc space (so can brucellosis).
- Scoliosis curvature points away from the osteoid osteoma
- Osteochondroma is the only benign skeletal tumor associated with radiation.
- Mixed Connective Tissue Disease requires serology (Ribonucleoprotein) for Dx
- Medullary Bone Infarct will have fat in the middle
- Bucket Handle Meniscal tears are longitudinal tears

SECTION 12: MAMMO

Gamesmanship: "The calcifications don't change configuration on CC and MLO views. This is the so called "tattoo sign" for dermal calcifications. Next step would be a tangential view to prove it.

Gamesmanship: Remember that secretory calcifications occur after menopause. Don't call them secretory in a premenopausal patient (no matter how much they look like them).

Gamesmanship: If they show you a ML view for calcifications. Think hard about milk of calcium - is it tea cupping?

Gamesmanship: If a test writer wants you to say DCIS they can prompt it 3 ways: (1) suspicious calcifications (fine linear branching or fine pleomorphic), (2) non mass like enhancement on MRI, or (3) multiple intraductal masses on galactography.

Gamesmanship: Skin thickening and trabecular thickening should get progressively better with time. It should start out worst, then better, then better. If it gets worse - this recurrent disease.

Gamesmanship: Gynecomastia looks like a cancer on ultrasound. This is why a male breast cancer workup (palpable finding) always begins with a mammogram

When I Say This..... You Say That.....

- When I say "shrinking breast," you say ILC
- When I say "thick coopers ligaments," you say edema
- When I say "thick fuzzy coopers ligaments - with normal skin," you say blur
- When I say "dashes but no dots," you say Secretory Calcifications
- When I say "cigar shaped calcifications," you say Secretory Calcifications
- When I say "popcorn calcifications," you say degenerated fibroadenoma
- When I say "breast within a breast," you say hamartoma
- When I say "fat-fluid level," you say galactocele
- When I say "rapid growing fibroadenoma," you say Phyllodes
- When I say "swollen red breast, not responding to antibiotics," you say Inflammatory breast CA
- When I say "lines radiating to a single point," you say Architectural distortion.
- When I say "Architectural distortion + Calcifications," you say IDC + DCIS
- When I say "Architectural distortion without Calcifications," you say ILC
- When I say "Stepladder Sign," you say Intracapsular rupture on US
- When I say "Linguine Sign," you say Intracapsular rupture on MRI
- When I say "Residual Calcs in the Lumpectomy Bed," you say local recurrence
- When I say "No cacls in the core," you say milk of calcium (requires polarized light to be seen).

High Yield Trivia

- No grid on mag views.
- BR -3 = < 2% chance of cancer
- BR-5 = > 95% chance of cancer
- Nipple enhancement can be normal on post contrast MRI - don't call it Pagets.
- Upper outer quadrant has the highest density of breast tissue, and therefore the most breast cancers.
- Majority of blood (60%) is via the internal mammary
- Majority of lymph (97%) is to the axilla
- The sternalis muscle can only be seen on CC view
- Most common location for ectopic breast tissue is in the axilla
- The follicular phase (day 7-14) is the best time to have a mammogram (and MRI).
- Breast Tenderness is max around day 27-30.
- Tyrer Cuzick is the most comprehensive risk model, but does not include breast density.
- If you had more than 20Gy of chest radiation as a child, you can get a screening MRI
- BRCA 2 (more than 1) is seen with male breast cancer
- BRCA 1 is more in younger patients, BRCA 2 is more is post menopausal
- BRCA 1 is more often a triple negative CA
- Use the LMO for kyphosis, pectus excavatum, and to avoid a pacemaker / line
- Use the ML to help catch milk of calcium layering
- Fine pleomorphic morphology to calcification has the highest suspicion for malignancy
- Intramammary lymph nodes arc NOT in the fibroglandular tissue
- Surgical scars should get lighter, if they get denser - think about recurrent cancer.
- You CAN have isolated intracapsular rupture.
- You CAN NOT have isolated extra (it's always with intra).
- If you see silicone in a lymph node you need to recommend MRI to evaluate for intracapsular rupture
- The number one risk factor for implant rupture is the age of the implant
- Tamoxifen causes a decrease in parenchymal uptake, then a rebound.
- T2 Bright things - these are usually benign. Don't forget colloid cancer is T2 bright.

Blank for Notes and Scribbles

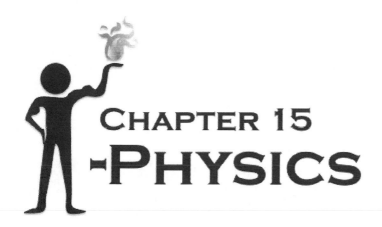

CHAPTER 15
PHYSICS

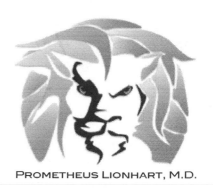

PROMETHEUS LIONHART, M.D.

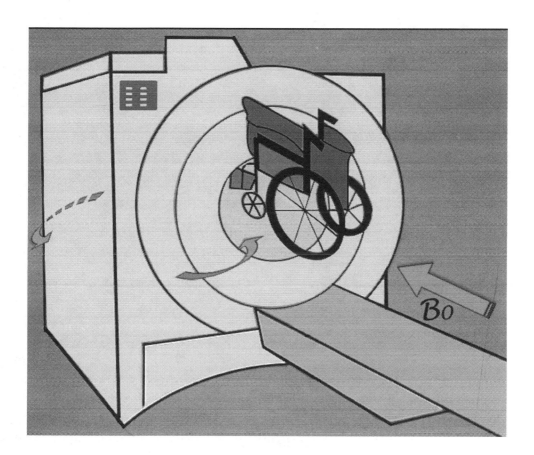

Highest Yield Tip:

It's not a math test.

Focus on problem solving, safety, and artifact reduction.

What is Electromagnetic Radiation? This is basically a wave of energy that does not require a media to travel in (it can travel in a vacuum). Its velocity is fixed at 3×10^8 m/s

Remember these from general chemistry?

Velocity = Frequency x Wavelength
Energy = Frequency x some constant "h" $E = f h$

Because the velocity is fixed, frequency and wavelength have an inverse relationship. As one goes up, the other goes down.

Depending on the frequency and wavelength – an electromagnetic wave has different qualities. For example, long wavelengths (low frequency) can carry radiant heat. Whereas, shorter wavelengths (high frequency) can carry radio, tv, and radar signals.

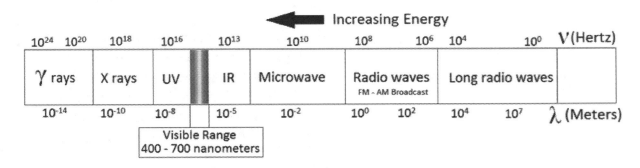

As the x-ray frequency increases the wave gets more energetic and will have the ability to remove electrons from an atom. This is called **"ionizing radiation."** Since it takes 15eV of energy to remove an electron from an atom, **a photon with energy greater than 15ev would be ionizing.**

Atomic Structure: Everyone knows electrons orbit the nucleus of protons and neutrons. Each one of these orbits has defined energy levels. **The inner most electron orbit is known as the K shell.** As the negatively charged electrons are attracted to the positively charged nucleus the K shell is the most desired location for electrons. It's not going to leave this desired spot unless energy is added to it. The electrons in higher orbits are in a "higher energy state" and require much less energy to remove. The outer most electrons require the least amount of energy to remove. Electrons can move between atomic shells, which requires the exchange of energy. Because an interior shell is a lower energy state, an electron from an outer shell will naturally "fall" closer to the nucleus to fill the vacancy.

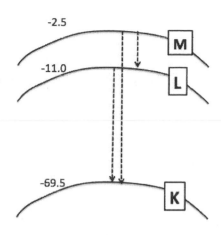

When an outer electron moves to an inner shell, energy is released. If the energy is enough an x-ray may be produced. These x-rays are called "characteristic x-rays". More on these later.

X-Ray Production: X Rays are made by *"Thermionic Emissions of Electrons."* This is done by taking a filament and running some current through it. The filament is typically made of Tungsten – because Tungsten has a very high melting temperature (it can tolerate a lot of heat). Sometimes rhenium (10%) is added to keep the Tungsten from cracking from heating and cooling. This current is considered "small" , but it still makes the Tungsten really hot (over 2000 degrees) and therefore makes the electrons in the Tungsten atoms very energetic – until they "boil off."

The filament is a cathode (negatively charged). This repels the electrons as they boil off. They fire down the vacuum chamber towards a positively charged anode (also usually made of Tungsten).

Why is the anode also made of Tungsten?

- Because it can tolerate a lot of heat.
- Because of its high Z, *X ray yield is proportional to Z squared*

Vocab:

- *Space Charge Limited* - At low peak voltage, the potential is not enough to cause all the electrons to be pulled away from the filament, leaving a residual space charge remaining

- *Saturation Voltage* - All electrons are immediately pulled away from the filament, and the tube current is maximized.

- *Emission Limited* - Above 40 kVp, the filament current is proportional to and determines the tube current

The free electrons accelerate toward this target (the anode) because of the potential difference between the cathode and anode. As they accelerate, they gain kinetic energy (keV). When the energetic electrons strike the tungsten target, they lose their kinetic energy via 3 different methods (excitation, ionization, and radiative losses i.e. Bremsstrahlung). X-rays are produced as described below.

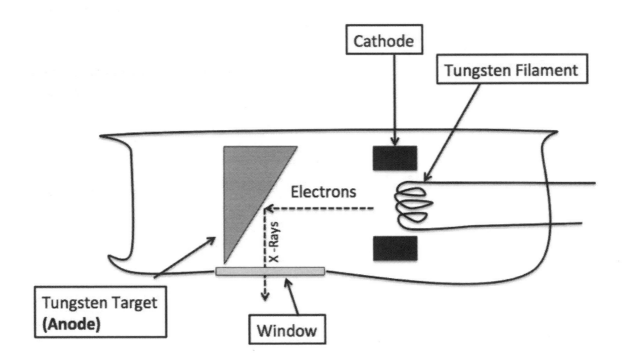

Excitation – This occurs when you have energy transfer from the incident particle to an orbital electron in the target. The transfer moves the electron to a high energy state, but not high enough to actually remove it from the shell. When it finally calms down (returns to a lower energy state) **there is emission of heat - but no x-ray production.**

Ioniziation - If the energy of the incident particle is enough to eject an electron then you have ionization.

Characteristic Radiation (characteristic x-rays): When a vacancy in an inner shell is created, an electron in an outer shell promptly jumps in to fill the vacancy. Energy released in this process is equal to the difference in binding energies between the two shells. The energy may appear as an x-ray photon. Since the binding energies have exact characteristic values, the emitted x-rays carry exact and discrete energies and are called characteristic x-rays. The characteristic x-rays are depicted as two sharp peaks over the Bremsstrahlung continuum. The peaks noted on the figure

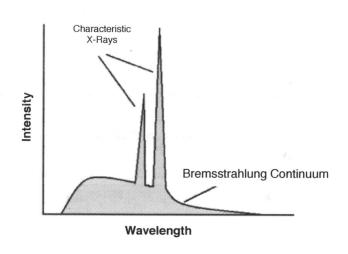

correspond to the energy difference between the inner vacated shell (secondary to the inner shell electron being ejected upon collision with an incident high energy electron) and the outer shell which is vacated to fill the inner shell.

Testable Point: The K-shell binding energy of tungsten is -69.5 keV.

Testable Trivia: "No resultant (created) photon can have more energy than the incident electron"

Testable Trivia: K shell binding energy is proportional to Z^2 – so lower Z gives lower energy x-rays

Auger Electrons: If the energy released from the filling of an inner shell vacancy by an outer shell electron is imparted to another electron (instead of being emitted as a photon), which is then also ejected, the second ejected electron is referred to as an Auger electron. No x-rays are emitted in this process. In general, *heavy elements are likely to emit x-rays and lighter elements are more likely to emit Auger electrons.*

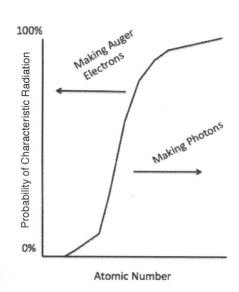

Secondary Ionization: Secondary ionization results when the electron which is ejected from the atom has enough kinetic energy to cause additional ionization events (i.e. eject additional electrons). The ejected electrons are sometimes called "delta rays."

Bremsstrahlung (radiative losses) – Energized electrons are slowed down (braking) by the positively charged nucleus. As they slow down and approach the nucleus they have basically three responses. They can (1) strike the nucleus and give off maximum energy to the x-ray, (2) come close to the nucleus and give off medium energy to the x-ray, or (3) travel distant to the nucleus and give off a little energy to the x-ray. Most (80%) x-rays are produced this way.

The amount of bremsstrahlung interactions is proportional to the energy of the incoming charged particle and the atomic number Z of the absorber.

Testable Trivia: Higher Z = More Bremsstrahlung

Testable Trivia: In nuclear medicine, low Z materials (plastic) are used to shield Beta emitters (classical example = 90 Yttrium) in order to minimize bremsstrahlung production. Lead would make this much worse.

There are a range of energies produced. The critical point (highly testable) is that the maximum energy is equal to the max kVp.

Testable Trivia: Max energy = Max kVp.

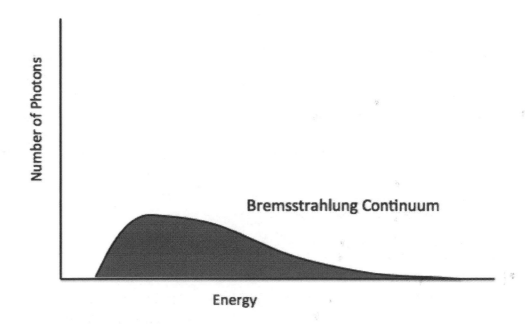

There is a hump, because the low energy x-rays are immediately attenuated.

X-Ray Generator:

Acceleration of electrons from the cathode to the anode requires a large voltage. The characteristics of said voltage will contribute to the changes in the x-ray spectrum.

Three main factors are manipulated; kVp, mA, and the duration (time)

Factor	Trivia
mA	Controls the current through the cathode.
	Controls the amount of thermionic emission.
	Determines the *Quantity*
kVp	Controls the voltage between the anode and cathode
	Controls the kinetic energy given to electrons
	Determines the *Quality* of the spectrum
	Defines the maximum energy

mA vs kVp on intensity: X-ray production increases in a linear direction with mA. Doubling mA will double intensity of the x-ray spectrum. Increasing kVp by 15% will double the intensity of the spectrum.

mAs - This is the product of mA x expose time in seconds. You can think about this as the total amount of x-rays made and the total amount of heat made.

Heat Production Math: A general idea of how much "heat" is being produced may help you wiggle through some multiple choice questions.

Tube Power = kV x mA   Heat Units = kVp x mA x Seconds

Example = 130 kv x 190 mA = 24,700 watts or 24,700 J for 1 sec exposure.

Remember a "Watt" is a Joule per Second

For regular diagnostic imaging, because your exposure times are so short you can have really high mA (like 1000). The limits of mA and kVp are based on tube heating and cooling specifics (now automatically controlled). Back in the stone ages, x-ray techs had to pick mA, kVp, and exposure time by guessing how fat someone was (sorta like one of those circus booths). They had charts on the wall to show max settings, otherwise they would melt the tube.

"Average Energy" - This is based on how much attenuation occurs at the target, as the x-ray exits the window, and as it's collimated.

Testable Trivia: In a standard Tungsten target x-ray tube with normal filtration, the average energy is going to be between 1/3 to 1/2 the maximum energy.

X-Ray Spectrum Manipulation

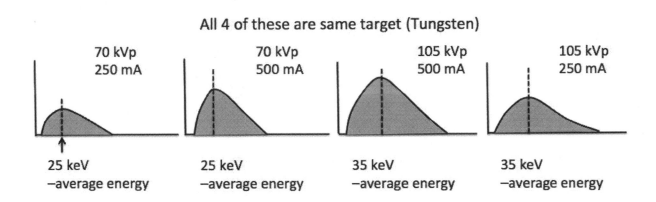

All 4 of these are same target (Tungsten)

* We are ignoring characteristic x-ray (they are all the same target)
* Notice the change in the area under the curve with increasing mA
* Notice the change in average energy with changing kVp

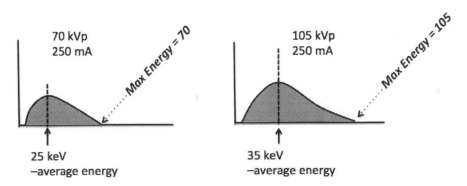

* Notice the change is Max energy with changing kVp

Now let's look at some sneaky things you can do with the characteristic peaks.

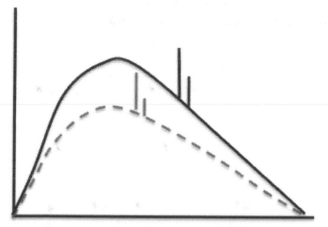

Two Superimposed Curves

Changing Targets

*Notice the characteristic peaks changed - this is how you know the target material is changed

Loss of Characteristic X-rays

*If you drop the kVp below the threshold for k shell electrons you are going to lose those characteristic peaks

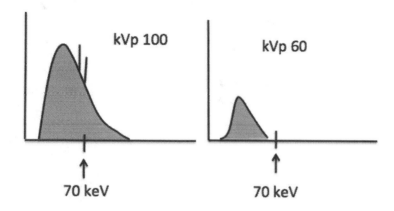

kVp 100   kVp 60

70 keV   70 keV

I believe in repetition for learning - so I'll mention this more than once. You don't need to understand this - but you do need to remember it.

— An increase in kVp by ~15% —> doubling of radiation intensity at the image detector
— With all other variables held constant, entrance skin dose will change as the square of the change in kVp (tube voltage).

↑dose
↑exposure, double mA, ↑ kVp by 15%

Contrast and Dose:

Remember I mentioned that there is a "15% Rule of Thumb" - if you want to increase the x-ray exposure you can either (1) double your mAs or (2) increase the kVp by 15%.

Why you might do one vs the other depends on the need of the study. Don't forget that the average energy of the x-ray spectrum defines the attenuation characteristics and defines the contrast between objects and tissue.

Want to visualize low contrast objects / tissue ? - Keep the kVp constant and increase the mAs.

Want to lower dose but maintain a constant exposure ? Raise the kVp by 15%, then lower the mAs by 50%. *This works because the higher kVp x-rays will penetrate more easily and delivers a lower dose.

The study is contrasted ? You are going to want the kVp set at least twice the binding energy of the contrast agent being used. This maximizes your contrast (lets you see white on black).

- Iodine - K edge is 33 keV; so you want it set at least 66 kVp
- Barium - K edge is 37 kev, so you want it set at least 74 kVp

The Pediatric (Newborn) X-Ray:

When you x-ray an infant you are going to do a couple of things differently (which makes them testable).

(1) You **do NOT use a Grid.**
(2) You **lower the kVp** - "good technique is around 65 kVp." They are small and don't require a lot of juice to penetrate. *Most adult CXRs are around 120-140 kVp.
(3) You use around the same or lower mAs - "good technique is around 2-4 mAs." Adults are typically around 4 mAs (portables are usually closer to 2.5).

Voltage Transformer:

Voltage is what gets the electrons accelerated to the anode. Moving these electrons actually requires a lot of voltage, and because AC current is used it needs to be stepped up through a transformer to the kilovolt range. The problem with alternating current is that it alternates. This essentially turns the tube on and off - no good. This was fixed by removing the voltage in the wrong direction with a circuit called a *"rectifier circuit."*

"Voltage Ripple" - Older generators just turned the current with a "rectifier circuit". This voltage varied a lot (zero to max), causing "ripples." An uneven x-ray voltage is not efficient. The most efficient tube voltage is constant at maximum value. This was fixed by engineering multiple single phase circuits or a higher frequency inverter. Modern generators are either three phase or have higher inverters - so voltage ripple just doesn't happen anymore. So, because this problem has been fixed and you will never encounter it in your entire career - it's probably high yield.

Gamesmanship: Ripple results in a more polyenergetic spectrum which increases tissue contrast. Solving the ripple problem creates a less polyenergetic beam. They may try to apply tissue contrast to this and want you to say that ripple results in more tissue contrast - which should be hard for you to do because if we wanted ripple, we'd still have it, but we don't, but that's still what the doofi (plural for doofus) will want you to say.

The Focal Spot:

The focal spot is the area of electron bombardment (and x-ray production) on the anode. Generally speaking a smaller anode has better spatial resolution. The trade off is that a smaller anode can't disperse heat as well and can melt (so you deal with more heat limitation). This is addressed in two main ways: (1) angling the anode - gives a larger surface area, (2) using a rotating anode.

Testable Trivia:
- Mammo uses a focal spot of 0.3 and 0.1mm
- General X-ray uses a focal spot of 0.6 and 1.2mm
- Portable x-ray device often use a stationary anode (doesn't rotate to dissipate heat). This limits their tube rating.

Vocab:

- *Actual Focal Spot:* This is where the x-rays land on the target anode.
- *Apparent Focal Spot:* This is where the x-rays land on the patient. This **defines the amount of blur** (not the actual spot).

- *"Line Focus Principal"* - This is the method of angling the anode to give you a smaller apparent focal spot (less blur).

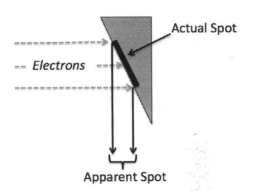

Changes in Angle:

The goal is the smallest focal spot possible (best resolution) - the trade off is heat tolerance.

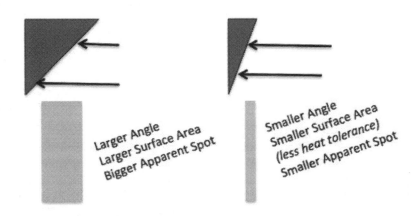

The Effect of mA / kVp on Focal Spot

The actual focal spot will enlarge with an increase in mA. The reason is, you have more electrons and they start to repel each other *"elbow each other out of the way."* This results in *"blooming"* or widening of the beam. This repulsion is most significant at low kVs. With increased kV you can get a slight decrease or *"thinning"* of the focal spot.

High mA , Low kVp = Wider Spot "blooming"
High kVp = Smaller Spot "thinning"

The Heel Effect:

Because x-rays on the anode side must pass through a greater thickness of the anode, you have a reduction in the intensity of these x-rays.

Testable Trivia: The heel effect can be decreased by increasing the anode angle or decreasing the size of the x-ray field.

Testable Trivia: This is used in mammo, where the thicker part of the breast / chest wall are aligned with the cathode *("C"athode on the "C"hest wall).*

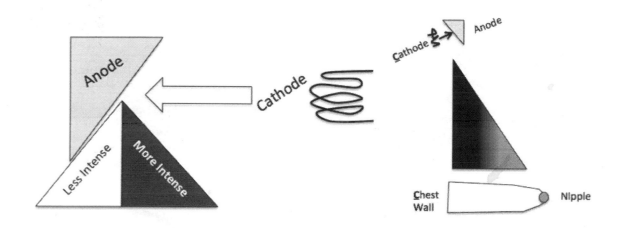

Magnitude of the Heel Effect
Depends on 3 Factors

(1) Anode Angle - *Worse with Small Angle*
(2) Source to Image Distance - *Worse with Decreased SID*
(3) Field Size - *Worse with Bigger Field*

Heel Effect on Field of View: Because the energy decreases on the anode side, this also decreases your field of view on that side (the side of the nipple). To compensate for this the entire tube is angled up to 20 degrees.

"Effective Anode Angle" - This is the sum of the anode and tube angles.

Understanding How the Anode Angle Changes the Heel Effect:

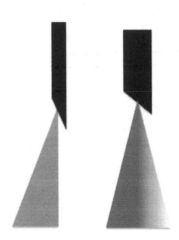

The sharper the angle, the more abrupt the change in intensity and therefore the more heel effect. I like to think about this as the "heel cut off." As, you get a sharp transition with a small angle, and a more gradual change with a larger angle.

Smaller Angle = Greater Heel Effect (heel cut off)

Another way to show the Heel Effect:

The classic way to show the heel effect is with a mammogram (cathode on the chest wall). However, there is another sneaky way to show this principal and that is with a chest x-ray.

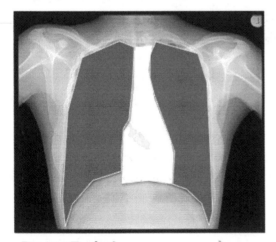

Proper Technique:
-Anode – Cathode
Oriented Vertically
With the Cathode Down

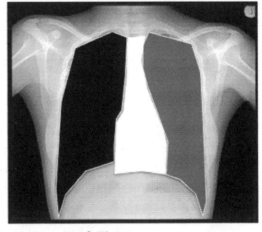

Wrong Technique:
-Anode – Cathode
Oriented Horizontal
Creates a Unilateral
Lucent Lung

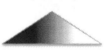

Misc Topics:

Off-Focal Radiation: This is scatter from the anode outside the focal area. This leads to an *increase in patient exposure and blurring*. This can be reduced with a small lead collimator near the tube output. Tubes constructed with metal enclosures and/or with the anode at electric ground potential will have less off-focal radiation (metal envelope attracts the scattered electrons).

X-Ray Tube Insert: X-ray tube is sealed under high vacuum. This vacuum is needed to prevent electrons from interacting with gas molecules. The x-ray port is necessary because x-rays are produced in all directions. Only the x-rays heading towards the patient are "useful." The port is typically made of the same stuff as the housing (except with mammography in where it's made of beryllium to minimize low energy x-ray absorption).

Unwanted Radiation Vocab:

- *Leakage* - X-rays that are transmitted though the housing
- *Secondary* - Characteristic radiation that is made from electron interaction with materials other than the target (glass, housing, etc.).
- *Scattered* - X rays that are deflected in direction once they leave the tube
- *Stray* - The sum total of leakage and scatter

Collimation: This is the process of restricting the size and shape of the x-ray beam emerging from the port. It's done to reduce both primary and secondary radiation. It improves image quality (less fog). The tech can gauge how much they are collimating by using a beam of light reflected by a mirror of low x-ray attenuation that mimics the x-ray beam. By order of various regulatory bodies, the light field and x-ray field must closely align.

Grid Controlled: This has nothing to do with an actual grid. Instead it refers to a way to turn the tube on and off fast by using a little cup around the filament to "suck electrons out." You are not actually shifting the big voltage across the tube, just diverting the electrons. This is how *pulse fluoro* is done.

Half Value Layer (HVL):

This is a measurement that is done to help understand beam quality. It is the amount of material required to attenuate an x-ray to 1/2 the original output. The higher the average photon energy the more penetrating it will be, and the larger its HVL.

Beam Filtration: If the beam is filtered the whimpy low energy photons will be removed first (leaving the higher ones). This will increase the average photon energy. Since **average photon energy determines penetration capacity** this will increase the HVL.

• **More filtration = Higher HVL**
• **Less filtration = Lower HVL**

Testable Trivia: With each HVL the average photon energy goes up.
3rd HVL > 2nd HVL > 1st HVL

Key points:
- HVL of an xray beam does NOT depend on mAs
- HVL does depend on beam filtration
- HVL does depend on anode material (e.g. tungsten)

Lets look at some sneaky ways this can get graphed out:

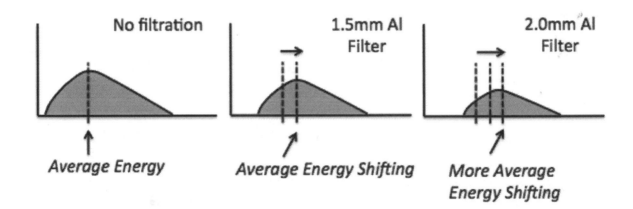

No filtration — Average Energy

1.5mm Al Filter — Average Energy Shifting

2.0mm Al Filter — More Average Energy Shifting

• Notice the average energy increases with more filtration
• Notice the area under the curve is decreasing as well (you are losing x-rays).

Testable Trivia: A mono-energetic beam would have a higher HVL than a poly-energetic beam (at the same kVp).

10th HVL ("TVL")

This is the thickness of material that can attenuate an x-ray to **90%**. This is used for shielding calculations.

"If you will it, it is no dream" - Theodor Herzl

Interactions with "matter," really means interactions with "people." Several types of interactions that can take place, but … but from a clinical standpoint only three matter: Coherent, Compton, and Photoelectric.

Coherent Scattering (Rayleigh Scattering): This occurs when a photon excites the entire atom. Eventually you get de-excitement and a photon is emitted (same energy but different direction as the original photon). If the photons produced with this kind of scatter reach the image receptor they can cause some loss in contrast.

Key Points:
*   This *(Coherent Scattering)* does NOT result in ionization (no electron is lost).
*   This does NOT result in the net transfer of energy.
*   This does NOT result in any dose to the patient.
*   This does NOT generate an X-ray
*   Seen primarily at low energies – i.e. mammography ; wasting about 15% of photon interaction below 30 keV.

Compton Scattering (the bad guy): This occurs when an x-ray hits an *outer shell* electron. The energy from this x-ray is transferred to the electron, which is then ejected. The incoming x-ray/photon (now with slightly less energy) changes direction and flies off. The amount of energy transferred has to do with the angle at which it strikes the electron (direct hit more energy, glancing blow less energy).

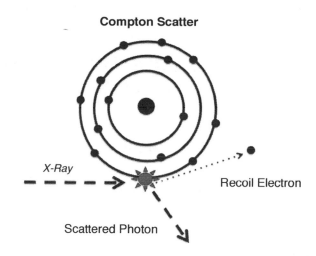

Compton Scattering produces 3 things:
   (1) Free Electron
   (2) Ionized Atom (missing an electron)
   (3) Photon of energy

Key Point:

- Probability of a Compton scatter does NOT depend of the Z of the atom – because the energy of these outer shell electrons is low.
- Probability of a Compton scatter is dependent on the density of the material – more tightly packed atoms, means more electrons to crash into
- Above 25-30 keV Compton scatter is the dominant photon interaction in soft tissue

Photoelectric Effect (the good guy): This occurs when an x-ray hits an inner shell electron. If the energy is great enough to overcome the k-shell binding energy then the inner shell electron will get ejected -this is an *all or nothing* reaction. The ejected electron is called the *"photo electron."*

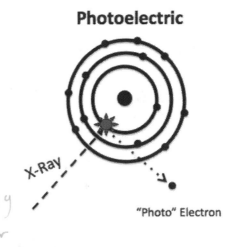

Photoelectric

"Photo" Electron

With this inner electron spot missing you get downward cascade and release of a characteristic x-ray or you get the production of an Auger electron. Because Auger electron production tends to dominate in biologic tissue (unlike Tungsten, a the target with a high Z) you still end up with biologic damage from these free electrons. P.E. is still good because this actually contributes to image contrast (Compton just makes noise).

release of energy as e⁻ cascade down → Auger

Key Points:

- Probability of P.E. directly proportional to the atomic number cubed. *(Compton does not care about Z)*
- Probability of P.E. is increased with object density
- Probability of P.E. is inversely proportional to the energy cubed

Compton (Bad Guy)	Photoelectric (Good Guy)
Outer Shell Electron	Inner Shell Electron
Variable Energy Transfer	All or None
Does not care about Z	Depends on Z^3
Depends on Density	
Dominates above 30 keV	Dominates below 30 keV

K Edge: The chance of the photoelectric effect happening sharply increases when the photon energy and electron binding energy are the same. This is taken advantage of in imaging by using iodine (33 keV) and barium (37 keV) which are right in the diagnostic range (when the kVp is set between 65 -90). The result is that iodine and barium will really soak up those x-rays, because of their K–edges, resulting in high contrast.

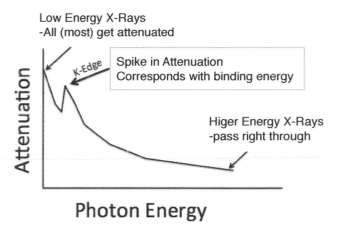

X-Ray Attenuation in Tissue:

Depends on 3 things:
- •Effective Atomic Number in Tissue
- •X Ray Beam Quality (energy)
- •Tissue Density

Linear Attenuation vs Mass Attenuation:

- **Linear:** This is the actual fraction of photons interacting per unit thickness of an absorber. In other words, it is the fraction of photons removed from the x-ray in a certain distance factoring in effects from compton scatter, PE effect, and coherent scatter. In contrast to "mass attenuation," the linear attenuation of ice, water, and water vapor is different (they have different lengths for the same amount of molecules).

  Factors to consider
    - More attenuation occurs with denser object
    - More attenuation occurs with higher Z material
    - Lower attenuation occurs with higher kVp
    - Higher attenuation occurs at K-edge

- **Mass:** This is the fraction of photons interacting – scaled per gram of tissue. This is *supposed to reflect the attenuation*. The important point is that the mass attenuation of ice, water, and water vapor is the same.

Is this your homework, Larry?

Image Noise - This is unwanted variation in image density. Noise varies from multiple factors including the thickness of film used. Quantum mottle obviously plays a role in general background graininess *(yes that's a word)*.

Testable Trivia: Noise will increase as the distance between the tube and detector increase, with the increase in noise described by the inverse square law.

Geometric Relationship - Influences Performance:

Geometric Unsharpness: This occurs because of several factors:

- Focal Spot: Small Focal Spot = Less Blur
- Source-Object Distance: Closer the source is to the image = More Blur
- Object Detector Distance: Closer the object is to the detector = Less Blur
- Magnification: **More Magnification = More Blur**

Below is a diagram showing how a change in focal spot will change the size of geometric unsharpness. As you can see, a smaller focal spot has less "unsharpness."

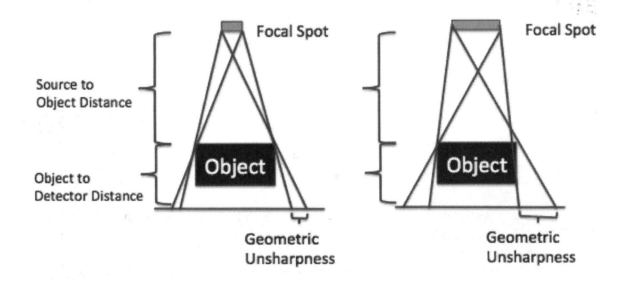

Now let's look at some different distances. If you are asked about "source to object", or "object to detector" distances I recommend you draw them out. If you can draw it, it will save some room in your brain for memorizing stuff that really maters (like the dose for temporary epilation, or how often you do the "flood test").

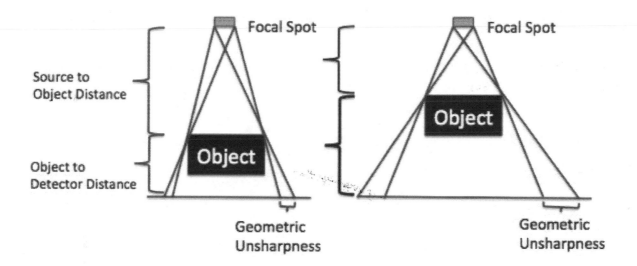

Magnification:

Let's take another look at that diagram. Notice the magnification difference between when you change the source to object distance?

Magnification is calculated by:

The tube to patient distance + patient to detector distance / tube to patient distance.

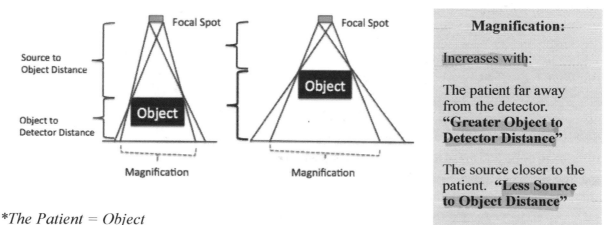

Magnification:
Increases with:
The patient far away from the detector. **"Greater Object to Detector Distance"**
The source closer to the patient. **"Less Source to Object Distance"**

*The Patient = Object

*More on Magnification in the Fluoro Chapter

Scatter:

They say scatter is a "violation" of the most basic law of radiography, because it doesn't originate in a straight line from the focal spot. Instead it is the **result of compton scatter in the body.**

Scattering depends on:
  (1) The collimated field - *less field = less scatter*
  (2) Thickness of the imaged body part
       - *thinner part = less scatter*
  (3) The energy that is chosen - *compton dominates above 26 kVp in soft tissue, and above 35 kVp in bone.*

Scatter
• Collimation
• "Thickness" of Patient
• Energy of the Beam

Reducing Scatter:

Grid - You can use a grid. Grids have different ratios. The more strips the higher the ratio and the more scatter reduction. If you are using a "linear" grid it needs to align parallel with the anode-cathode, to avoid "grid cut-off." Cross-hatched or "cellular" grids don't have this issue.

"Bucky Grids" - This is a moving grid. They wiggle back and forth rapidly - too fast to be seen. If the grid motion fails (and it stops moving) you will end up with grid lines.

"Bucky Factor" - The bucky factor describes the increased mAs required when a particular grid is used compared with a study using no grid.

Air Gap - This is basically only done with mag view on mammo. The idea is that the primary x-rays will shoot straight and go further than the scatter ones. So, if you create a little distance between the patient and the detector you can reduce the scattered photons actually being registered.

"Screwing up the Grid" - You can put the grid on upside down, off centered, or skewed. The chance of this happening is way more with a portable.

What does the Grid do to Dose ?: The **tradeoff to using a grid is that dose is increased** (because the automatic brightness control turns up the juice to compensate). There is a thing called the "bucky factor" which is basically the dose with the grid / dose without the grid. The most common bucky factor is around 2-3.

The Grid	
Pros	**Cons**
Reduces Scatter (improves contrast)	**Increased Dose**
	Increased Exposure time (possible motion artifact)

Digital vs Analog

Long ago, when dinosaurs roamed the earth, radiology was done on film screen. Now in the modern age it is digital. The comparison of film screen vs digital radiology could lend itself to multiple choice questions.

Film Screen Limitations: Screen systems are intolerant to errors in exposure (under or over leads to a loss of contrast). Noise - both on film and fluoro is an issue ,with compton scatter increasing with increasing film size. The quality of films breaks down over time. Film can't be manipulated post processing.

Possible Film Screen Advantage: **Spatial resolution of film screen is slightly better** than CR (5 line pairs per mm, vs 2.5 line pair per mm).

Digital Radiography Advantages: Digital images can easily be stored, and manipulated post processing. They don't break down chemically. **There is a higher dose efficiency (potential for less radiation) and wider dynamic range of detection.** Although the spatial resolution of film screen is slightly better, the superior contrast resolution of digital radiography more than compensates.

Digital: If you are working anywhere in the United States this is all you will use. If you are working in certain parts of Africa or have traveled back in time about 20 years you may still be using film.

Digital Pixels: Most systems use pixels with 8 bits, so this is 2^8 or 256 possible brightness values. Why did I use "2" ? - it's a binary thing - black and white.

Digital detectors can be broken down like this:

- Storage Phosphor (CR) - Type of Indirect
- Flat Panel Detectors (DR)
  - Direct
  - Indirect

Computed Radiography (CR)	Digital Radiography
Uses a photostimulable phosphor plate enclosed in a cassette. Has a two stage process for image capture and image readout (done separately)	Uses a detector that can capture and read out information. Further classified into direct and indirect methods.

Storage Phosphors (CR) : These can work with a conventional x-ray machine (just like a normal cassette). The system uses a special phosphor *(Barium Fluorohalides)* that does not emit the absorbed energy as light after interaction with an x-ray. Instead, the x-ray causes an electron in the phosphor to change to a metastable state (one that it can hold for several days).

The idea is that the storage phosphor is holding a "latent" x-ray image. The information is read by using a red point laser to scan the detector and count how much **blue-green** light is emitted as the high energy electron gets knocked out of it's metastable state.

Testable Trivia: The amount of light detected is proportional to the intensity of the incident x-ray.

The photostimulated phosphors have a wide detectable range, tolerating x-ray intensities 100 times higher and 100 times lower than the 5 micro Gy needed for an old school screen film.

The plate is reset by forceable exposure to bright white light - which erases it. If you forget to do this you will get ghosting artifacts.

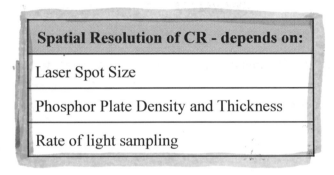

Spatial Resolution of CR - depends on:
Laser Spot Size
Phosphor Plate Density and Thickness
Rate of light sampling

Flat Panel Detectors (DR): When most people say "digital detector," this is what they are talking about. It's much faster than conventional film development or CR plate reading. These are composed of amorphous (not crystalline) selenium. The photon from the x-ray is stored as an electric charge within a square array of pixels. The information is read out by scanning the information a row at a time with all columns read in parallel.

What is the difference between direct and indirect?
- Indirect (scintillators) = X rays ⟶ Light ⟶ Charge
- Direct (photoconductors) = X rays ⟶ Charge

This vs That - Scintillators vs Phosphor
Scintillators usually have 2-3 times the efficiency in x-ray absorption of a Phosphor - at the same thickness.
Scintillators produce more visible light per x-ray
Scintillators emit a wavelength of light that is a better match for the a TFT detector

How does an indirect FPD take an x-ray and make it a picture? The x-ray activates the thallium doped Cesium Iodide (CsI), which emits light. The photodiode turns the light into an electric signal which can be read out.

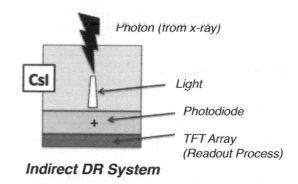

Indirect DR System

What is this "Lateral Dispersion"? This is a problem you run into with particular phosphors. Light tends to diffuse laterally after it leaves the site of conversion from an x-ray. This creates issues with spatial resolution, that get worse with increasing thickness of the crystal. Making the crystal thin has its own problems as your sensitivity for collecting x-rays is going to drop off (they just fly right through).

Is there a difference in "Lateral Dispersion" between phosphors? Yes - Gadolinium Oxysulfide has more lateral dispersion (light scatter) than CsI.

How does one solve the problem of "Lateral Dispersion"? Luckily someone much smarter than you or me already did. They invented a columnar structure that forms a "lead pipe" like matrix. With this design you can make a nice thick crystal without worry.

What is this "Thin-Film Transistor" (TFT)? These are active electronic elements that can be used in both direct and indirect systems. It's basically a layer of elements typically starting with readout electrons at the bottom and charge collector arrays on the top.

How does a direct FPD take an x-ray and make it "charge", without first making it "light"? - It uses a magical substance called amorphous selenium.

Step 1: Apply a homogeneous "bias" charge to the surface of the selenium.
Step 2: Fire the x-rays through the patient, into the selenium. The x-rays are absorbed by the selenium and electrons are released.
Step 3: Released electrons *("electron hole pair")* travel to the surface of the selenium and neutralize a portion of the applied charged. This is done in proportion to the radiation intensity. An important testable point is there is **no lateral dispersion.**
Step 4: These electrical charges are drawn in along the electric field lines to the charge storage capacitor electrodes connected to the TFT.
Step 5: The pattern of charges is scanned and converted to a digital signal stored by each TFT.

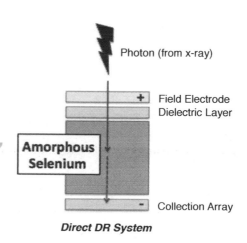

Direct DR System

Amorphous Selenium

The material is magical, likely originating from the underground dwarf mines of middle earth. Selenium is essentially a photoconductor. When it is exposed to radiation, its electrical conductivity is altered in proportion to the intensity of the radiation.

It is very susceptible to humidity and temperature. Don't try and use it outside in the Amazon jungle.

What is this "Fill Factor" ? This is the area of the detector which is sensitive to x-rays (in relation to the entire detector area). The higher the fill factor, the more efficient the detector.

Fill Factor Differences:

With DR systems, the electric field shaping essentially allows for a fill factor of nearly 100%. This is not seen with Indirect (CR) systems. Remember, differences between things make good multiple choice questions.

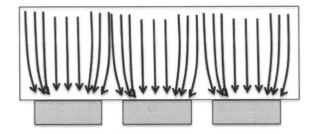 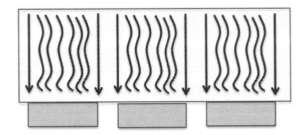

Direct – Amorphous Selenium   Indirect – Cesium Iodide

Spatial Resolution: In the digital world the term "spatial frequency" is often used, which is good because it helps me remember that the more frequently an object is sampled the better the resolution.

Some General Pearls / Points (possibly testable):
- Increased sampling frequency = Increased Resolution
- More pixels = Higher spatial resolution
- Images with high resolution need large file sizes
- Increasing x-rays will NOT improve Maximum spatial resolution
- Spatial resolution for Selenium based (direct) DR is higher than indirect detectors *newer systems are pretty close actually
- Structured scintillators are better than unstructured ones (less lateral dispersion)

What is this "Modular Transfer Function?" (MTF)

Buzzword = Contrast.
Buzzword = "Function of Spatial Resolution (Frequency)"

Objects with different sizes and different densities are recorded at different gray scale values. The easiest way to think of "MTF" is that it is a method to describe the displaying of object contrast and size. It is the ability to take the contrast values (object contrast) and turn it into intensity levels in an image (image contrast).

Another way to think about MTF is a ratio of input and output. The fraction of signal contrast that will be maintained in the captured image.

MTF changes as a function of spatial frequency (resolution) - 100% at low spatial resolution, to zero at high spatial resolution.

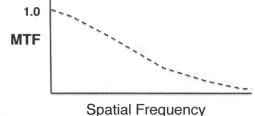

What is this "Detective Quantum Efficiency?" (DQE) This is efficiency of a detector in converting x-ray energy into an image signal. People who like math calculate this by comparing the signal to noise ratio at output with the signal to noise ratio at input as a function of spatial frequency. In a perfect world you want this to be "1.0" (all radiation energy is absorbed and converted to image). Factors that influence it are the radiation exposure, spatial frequency (resolution), modular transfer function, detector material, kVp, and mAs. The better your DQE the less radiation you need to maintain your signal. Just like MTF, DQE is better at low spatial resolution. In general the DQE of DR is around 0.45, significantly better than that of CR or plain films - which is around 0.25.

Radiation Exposure: If you have fewer repeat exams (because you can actually do post processing) then you have less radiation - obvious advantage of digital radiography. Additionally, because DR systems have superior quantum efficiency, you can lower dose compared to CR or plain films and get the same quality. **DR has less dose.**

Screen Films: It's true that **board exams tend to lag behind reality** for several years (sometimes decades), but I've put a lot of thought into this, and I refuse to include a complete section on screen films in this book. I don't even know if they will actually have questions on screen films (*how much acetic acid do you need in your fixing solution?*) , but if they do... well then just miss them.

Seriously, this has gone to far. It's over the line. This isn't Nam, there are rules.

OK fine, in the mammo chapter I'll talk a little about the film screen and lateral light diffusion , but that's it! I mean it... I'm not gonna say anything else about plain films.

Just know this: Screen films have a higher spatial resolution (sometimes) than digital systems.

Direct Conversion	Indirect Conversion
Directly converts x-rays to electrical signal	X-Ray -> Light -> Electrical Signal
Detector material is amorphous selenium	Phospor material is usually thallium doped cesium iodine
Signal does not "laterally disperse", as the applied voltage separates the electrons and holes made by x-rays	Light can scatter (worse with thicker crystal), better if columnar structure is used.
Fill Factor is high (near 100%)	Moderate fill factor (depends on size of pixel)
Higher Detector Quantum Efficiency (DQE)	Moderate Detector Quantum Efficiency (DQE)

Film Artifacts

Fogging - This is the adding of charge to the detector (a blackening of the film). This can happen if you leave the cassette in the room with scattered x-rays. You can get a big black blob on it.

Double Exposure: This happens when the cassette is used twice without changing the film or erasing the receptor. The film will look like it has two images on it.

Quantum Mottle: This is noise from a lack of photons. The film will look underexposed.

Incomplete Erasure: This looks like a double exposure.

Ghosting: This is the result of prior exposure leading to difference in x-ray sensitivity of different parts of the detector. This looks like a dark object that doesn't belong on the image.

—*The testable point is that this occurs in DR more than CR.*

We're talking about unchecked aggression here, dude.

Why is mammo different than regular x-ray? The difference in attenuation of a breast cancer and just regular breast tissue is very small. So you have to use lower energy and a nearly mono-energetic beam to enhance the attenuation differences. Also, an increase in spatial resolution is required to see micro calcifications.

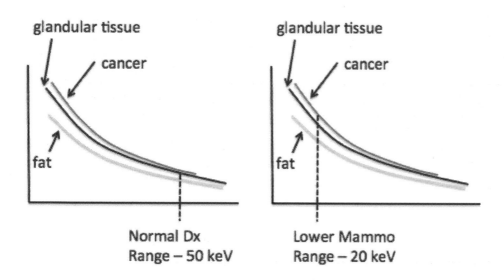

Optimal kVp: The ideal energy for mammo is between 16-23 keV. To get this energy a voltage of 25-30 kVp is used (general Dx uses between 50-120).

Target Anodes: Mammo uses a **molybdenum or rhodium anode** (general radiology uses tungsten).

The Normal Spectrum of Molybdenum:

The combination of low kVp and a low Z give Moly high characteristic x-rays, with low Bremsstrahlung.

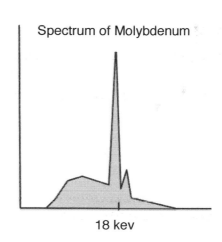

K Edge Filtration - A K edge filter is placed on the outside of the tube with the goal of creating a nearly mono-energetic beam in the target range of 16-23 keV. Moly is classically used for this, taking advantage of the 20 keV K edge and subsequent rise in photoelectric absorption. Energies lower than 15 and greater the 20 get filtered out.

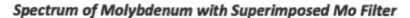

Spectrum of Molybdenum with Superimposed Mo Filter

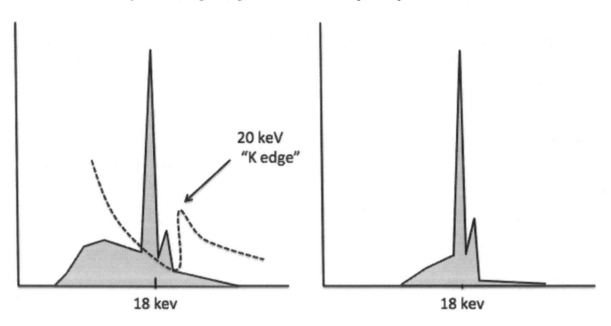

Rhodium: An alternative to Moly is Rhodium, which has a similar (slightly stronger) spectrum, and a binding energy of 20.2 keV.

High Yield:
- Filters block BOTH high and low photons, with the benefit of removing the low energy photons which only give you dose and the high energy photons which won't help with contrast.
- Rh/Rh is used for larger or denser breasts – because it's higher energy compared to Mo/Mo.
- Mo anode with Rhodium filter is also used to produce an intermediate energy spectra between a Mo/Mo and Rh/Rh combination.
- **NEVER use a Rh Target (21 kev) with a Mo Filter (20 Kev K edge)**
- Mo anode can also be combined with an aluminum filter, for a harder beam to penetrate denser breasts.
- Some digital systems will use Tungsten / Rho and Tungsten / Silver- this creates a higher energy spectrum for increased penetration and lower dose. Contrast is lost – but some post processing can bring it back.

Focal Spot Size: As mentioned before, mammo requires a better spatial resolution than you get with normal imaging. To achieve this you use a smaller focal spot:

High Yield:
- •Mammography uses a focal spot of 0.3 and 0.1mm
- •General X-ray uses focal spots of 0.6 and 1.2mm

A smaller focal spot is not going to tolerate heat as well. To address this you have to use a lower mA (otherwise you'd melt the anode). The mA is limited to 50 for 0.1mm, and 100 for 0.3mm. Another issue is that since you are using a lower mA you need a longer exposure time. Generally you still try and keep the exposure time under 2 seconds.

Heel Effect: I mentioned this before. Just remember the cathode side goes near the chest wall. Also, the loss of energy on the anode side (nipple side) is compensated for by angling the tube up to about 20 degrees.

Effective Anode Angle = Anode Angle + Tube Angle

The Beryllium Window: Most diagnostic tubes use pyrex glass – this is NOT used in mammo because it causes excessive attenuation of the energies used in mammo. Instead a beryllium exit window is used.

Compression: The breasts are placed in compression. This does several good things:

- Reduced Thickness = Less Scatter = Lower kVp can be chosen
- Lower kVp and Less Scatter = Improved Contrast
- Reduced Thickness = Less mAs needed = Less Dose
- Breast Doesn't Move = Less Motion Artifact
- Breast Smashed Closer to Bucky = Less Geometric Magnification
- Less Motion and Less Geometric Mag = Improved Spatial Resolution
- Less Tissue overlap

Anti-Scatter Grid: Since the breast is placed in compression and you are using lower kVp (both of which intrinsically reduce scatter) a smaller grid ratio is used.

Mammo uses a 4-5 grid ratio (general x-ray uses a 6-16).

Dose with the Grid – The grid removes scattered photons – which reduces some dose. However, the same technique can't be used with a grid or you will underexpose. So, the technique is turned up. Ultimately the **dose is INCREASED with a grid**.

What is a "Grid Ratio"?
Grid Ratio = H/W H= height, W= width between grids

"The Bucky Factor" – The higher the grid ratio the more you have to turn up the juice. 2x dose = 2x Bucky Factor.

Bucky Factor is 2 for Mammo and 5 for general x-ray

Magnification: Magnification is done with a smaller focal spot, a smaller paddle, and no grid (air gap technique is used instead).

Contact Mode vs Magnification Mode	
Contact Mode – The normal Mammogram	**Magnifications – 1.5x – 2x**
Breast is in direct contact with the bucky	
The Grid is on	**No Grid** – *Air Gap used to reduce scatter*
Larger Focal Spot – 0.3mm	Small Focal Spot 0.1mm
Regular Paddle	Smaller Paddle
	Increased exposure time

Testable Trivia: If you increase the air gap, you will increase the magnification.

Testable Trivia: If you increase the air gap, you will also increase the dose (because of the automatic exposure rate control ramping up the setting to compensate for less photons hitting the detector).

Film/Screen Combination:

Mammo uses a single emulsion film – matched to a single intensifying screen in the cassette. There are numerous benefits to this.

Pros and Cons of the Single Emulsion	
Pros	**Cons**
Less Parallax	**Increased Dose**
Less Crossover	
Better Spatial Resolution	

Orientation within the Cassette and Halation:

How the screen and film are oriented inside the cassette can affect spatial resolution. Bottom line is you want the film on top of the intensifying screen.

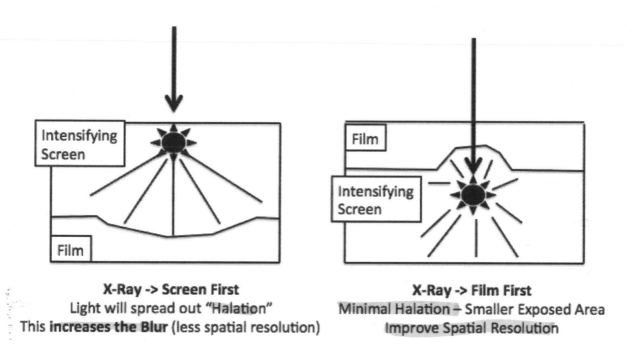

X-Ray -> Screen First
Light will spread out "Halation"
This **increases the Blur** (less spatial resolution)

X-Ray -> Film First
Minimal Halation – Smaller Exposed Area
Improve Spatial Resolution

What is this "Screen" ? The "film screen" is a sheet of film with an emulsion on one side (or two – in mammo). The screen is basically a scintillator which takes x-rays and turns them into light. The actual x-ray film responds better to light from the screen, then a x-ray. The advantage of a screen is that you can use less dose (less exposure time). The down side is that lateral light diffusion within the screen will reduce your spatial resolution.

Testable Trivia: A screen does NOT reduce scatter.

What if you increase the thickness of the screen? A thicker screen will reduce your dose, but will also worsen the lateral light diffusion and therefore also worsen your spatial resolution.

What is this optic density? The actual x-ray film does NOT respond in a linear fashion to the light from the intensifying film. The classic look has a "toe" (caused by film base and fog), and then a shoulder. Digital systems has a pure linear curve.

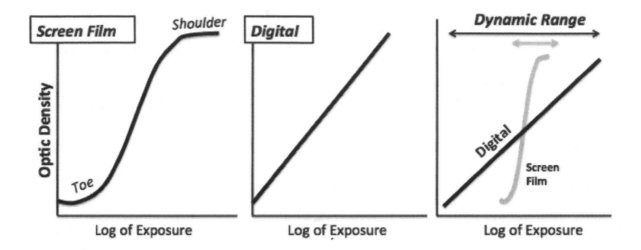

Testable Trivia: Digital systems have a wider dynamic range with a linear characteristic curve (no shoulder and toe), compared to screen films.

Just Plain Trivia: Some Geezers refer to dynamic range as "latitude"

Processing Time: It's much slower in Mammo. This extra time in the developer allows for more silver bromide crystals to develop and that can increase contrast and speed. Reduces patient dose.

Viewboxes:

- Mammo = 3000 cd/m2
- General Radiology = 1500 cd/m2
- Reading Room Light – Should not exceed 50 lux

Digital Mammography

Digital systems have the major advantage of allowing you to change the contrast and brightness after the acquisition of the image by adjusting the widow and level.

Pixel Size and Spatial Resolution: Remember that smaller pixels = better spatial resolution. Additionally, you can lose spatial resolution from spread of electronic or light signal inside the digital or computed detectors.

- In general, most digital systems have lower spatial resolution (around 5-11 lp/mm) – relative to analog (11 – 13 lp/mm).

- Another point of trivia is that the **MQSA does NOT have specific line pair requirements for digital**; instead they are linked to the manufacturers specs.

Dose: Digital machines have 15% less dose compared to analog (1.8mGy for analog, 1.6 for digital). This is because the beam quality is better. Digital also has fewer repeat exams (because you can window and level). Also, the dose is not fixed – like it is with screens; you can turn the juice up and down as needed.

Noise Limited Images: The primary factor affecting the total noise is the number of photons interacting with the detector. Although digital images can have variable contrast, the noise is fixed after the exposure is taken.

Dark Noise: This is an additional type of noise from electronic fluctuations within the detector element. The effect is proportional to the temperature of the detector – that is why coolers are needed. You see these more with underexposed regions.

Flat Field Test: Imaging of a large piece of acrylic. This is done to improve image quality, and calibrate the digital detectors.

Digital Artifacts:

Ghosting: This is caused by a residual image from the prior exposure - burned into the detector. You see this when highly attenuating objects are placed in the beam. This is why *lead is not allowed on flat panel digital systems*.

Pixels Gone Bad: This can manifest as a square or a streak.

Comparing and Contrasting Mammo to General Dx – Summary

Mammo	General Radiology
Low Energy 25-35 kVp	High Energy: 50-120 kVp
Most Common Anode is Moly	Most Common Anode is Tungsten
Low Tube Current 100mA	High Tube Current 500mA
Long Exposure Times: 1000 ms	Fast Exposure Times: 50 ms
High Receptor Air Kerma 100µGy	Low Receptor Air Kerma 5 µGy
Beryllium Window	Pyrex Glass Window
Small Focal Spot	Larger Focal Spot
Lower Grid Ratio: 5-1	Higher Grid Ratio 10-1
High Optic Density	Low Optic Density
Brighter View boxes – 3000cd/m^2	Darker View boxes – 1500cd/m^2
Longer Processing Times	Shorter Processing Times

PPV$_1$ PPV$_2$ and PPV$_3$

In an attempt to make things overly complicated the ACR and MQSA set up guidelines for data collection with sub categories for positive predictive value. Things with different types or categories make great multiple choice questions.

PPV$_1$ - This refers to cases from positive screening (anything other than a recommendation to return to screening). In other words, BR-0, BR-3, BR-4, BR-5. "Call backs" - we call them. *Benchmark for this is 4.4%*

A screening only facility only obtains data as PPV$_1$ - because they don't do call backs or biopsy.

PPV$_2$ - This refers to cases where biopsy was recommended. In other words, times you BR4 or BR5'd something. How many times you sent someone to the "room of tears" - where you tell them they need a biopsy. *Benchmark for this is 25.4%*

PPV$_3$ - This refers to the results of the biopsy. Some people call this the "*PBR*" or positive biopsy rate. Other people will call it the "*biopsy yield of malignancy.*" What will your examiner call it?... The most likely answer is the name you didn't remember it was called - so remember all of them. *Benchmark for this is 31.0%*

Synonyms: PPV$_3$ = PBR = Biopsy Yield of Malignancy

MQSA -

Appropriate Target Range for Medical Audit	
Recall Rate	5-7%
Cancers/ 1000 Screened	3-8

Specific Tasks That You Should Memorize	
Processor QC	Daily
Darkroom Cleanliness	Daily
Viewbox Conditions	Weekly
Phantom Evaluation	Weekly
Repeat Analysis	Quarterly
Compression Test	Semi-Annually
Darkroom Fog	Semi-Annually
Screen-Film Contrast	Semi-Annually

Name	Duty	Acceptable Range	Benchmark
PPV$_1$	Abnormal Screener *"Call Back"*	3-8%	4.4%
PPV$_2$	Recommended Biopsy (4 or 5)	15-40% (25-50% if palpable)	25.4%
PPV$_3$	Biopsy Done - Actual Cancer	20-45%, (30-55% if palpable)	31.0%

MQSA Rules for Male Residents on the Mammography Service:
A tie must be worn (pink is the recommend color - although not required).
General gaze should be in the downward direction (submissive posture)
You will not speak unless spoken to first
Penis must be taped either down or to the side
Urination may only be performed in the seated position

Spatial Resolution and the Line Pair Phantom:

* *RSNA says: 13 LP/mm in the Anode – Cathode Direction*
* *RSNA says: 11 LP/mm in the left-right direction*
* *Huda Says:* MQSA requires a resolution of 12 line pairs per mm for screen-film, and manufacturer specs for digital (~ 7 lp/mm).

Mean Glandular Dose:

The MQSA has some breast phantom which is suppose to be an "average breast." This thing is 4.2cm of compressed breast that is 50% adipose and 50% glandular.

The measured dose is with a grid.

Testable Trivia: Dose under **300 millirads (3mGy)**. This **required dose is ONLY for the phantom**, not a real human breast. There is no actual regulation for what a human breast can endure.

I myself dabbled in pacifism once

SECTION 5: FLUORO

Fluoro is different than regular diagnostic radiology. Radiographic images are static, and fluoroscopic imaging can be performed to view dynamic processes like swallowing or blood flow.

Regular Dx	Fluoro
mA 200-800	mA 0-5
kVp 50 -120	kVp 50-120
Very short exposure times	Longer exposure times
Focal Tube Spot 1.0 -1.2mm	Focal Spot 0.3-0.6

Things to Know:

- *Regular Dx – done with 200-800 mA, with very short exposure times*
- *Fluoro – much lower mA, with longer exposure times (this reduces the chance of overheating, so it can stay on longer)*
- Small (0.3-0.6) Focal Spot is used for Fluoro – in order to limit geometrical blurring
- Larger Focal Spot is used for the "Spot Image" – because greater tube current is needed
- A "Spot Image" is the same thing as a conventional x-ray
- A Fluoro Frame Shot has more quantum mottle than a Spot Image (less photons)
- Fluoro uses a Grid – just like regular x-ray 10:1

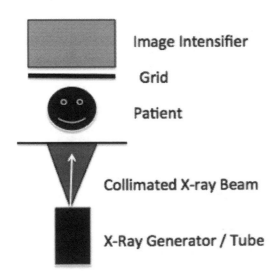

What does the Collimator do?

Multiple sets of shutter blades define the shape of the x-ray beam. By "coning down" the beam, you get less scatter and better image contrast. It also reduces dose.

What does the Image Intensifier do?

Converts the x-rays to electrons, accelerates them, and then converts that to a visible image.

414

Fluoro systems can be used in GI and GU radiology.

- *GI:* Camera below table
- *GU:* camera above table – bladder closer to image receptors; reduces focal spot blur
  - They have ~~higher operator lens do~~se

WTF is "Quantum Mottle" ?

It is the most important source of noise is radiography. It depends on the number (concentration) of x-ray photons used to produce an image (more photons = less mottle). It's apparently too complicated a concept to really understand much past this, other than to say it's caused by the statistical fluctuation (standard deviation) of the number of quanta of photons per unit size absorbed by the screen.

- ~~Increasing the speed (kvp) increases the mott~~le
- ~~Increasing the number of photons decreases the mott~~le

Image Receptor Types:

There are two kinds:

–(1) Image Intensifiers (I.I.) – the old kind
–(2) Flat Panel Detectors (F.P.D) – the new kind

Image Intensifier:

Image Intensifier

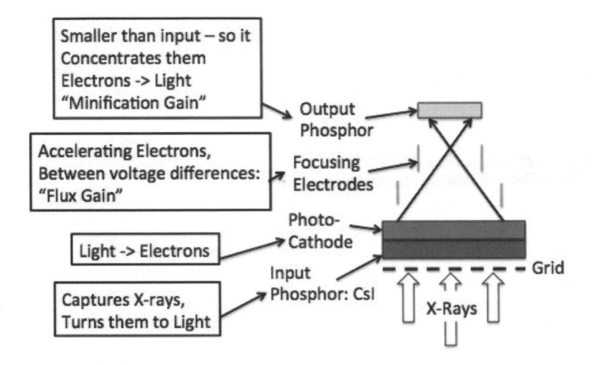

Smaller than input – so it
Concentrates them
Electrons -> Light
"Minification Gain"

Accelerating Electrons,
Between voltage differences:
"Flux Gain"

Light -> Electrons

Captures X-rays,
Turns them to Light

Output Phosphor

Focusing Electrodes

Photo-Cathode

Input Phosphor: CsI

Grid

X-Rays

The purpose of an image intensifier is to convert x-rays to light and then back to electrons. Along the course of this conversion, the electron flux and energy are amplified by the image intensifier with the end result being a greater amount of light emerging from the output phosphor. To actually view the pictures, you must couple an image intensifier through lenses to a TV camera.

"Flux Gain" This describes the increase in magnitude of light coming from the output phosphor, relative to the input. This increase in magnitude is accomplished with a high voltage between the photocathode and the output phosphor (25-35 kV). The voltage causes electrons to accelerate and yields a gain in energy.

"Minification Gain" - Electrons from the large photocathode surface are concentrated on a *small output phosphor*. This increases the number of electrons per unit area, and therefore the energy per unit area.

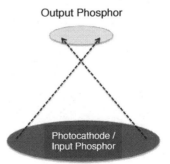

Output Phosphor

Photocathode /
Input Phosphor

Q: When you "Mag" something you are actually doing what?
A: Minifying it less

"Brightness Gain" - This is a term describing the increase in emitted light from the I.I. compared to the amount of light you would have obtained if the I.I. was never invented (and you just directly exposed the phosphorescent screen).

Testable Point: Brightness Gain is due to the combined effects of Flux Gain and Minification Gain.

- *BG = Flux Gain x Minification Gain*

"Conversion Gain" (Gx)- This is a term describing the ~~efficiency of an I.I. in changing incident x-rays into light at the output surface~~. *The older an I.I. is, the more it sucks at this.*

Dealing with an Elderly I.I.

Solution 1: ~~Use an aperture with a large hole in it.~~ The down side to this is it ~~increases the image noise.~~

Solution 2: Let the ~~Automatic Brightness Control system~~ do its job and crank up the juice (use more radiation). The down side to this is it ~~increases the dose.~~

Solution 3: Put it in a nursing home, then get another one. The general rule for this is the Image Intensifier is usually replaced when the conversion gain falls to 50%. The down side to this is that it costs money to replace things, but it's ok you can offset the cost by cutting the Resident's benefits / salary....and hire a million $/year VP or chairman to oversee the cost savings transition.

The Gains:

Flux Gain = Accelerating electrons between voltage differences.

Minification Gain = Electrons from large surface, concentrated on smaller surface

Brightness Gain = Light increase from the acceleration and concentration processes. Flux Gain x Minification Gain.

Conversion Gain: How good the I.I. is at turning the electrons back into light.

Field-of-View: Collimation is electronically controlled with positioning changes made to irradiate a small region of anatomy *when you change to a smaller input surface*. The trick is that you are actually *minifying the image less*, as a smaller input surface is projected on the same output surface.

With a smaller input and unchanged output, the minification gain is decreased. If you did not change the dose, this decrease in minification gain would translate to less light from the output phosphor.

Geometric vs Electronic Magnification

Geometric Magnification – I touched on this earlier, but I want to make a few more points. To magnify something, you generally bring it closer to the x-ray source (Mag = SID/ SOD). People usually think about the "inverse square law" for reducing radiation, but obviously it works the other way too. If you get closer to the tube you get more radiation-- **and it doesn't double, it squares**.

Electronic Magnification (Zoom) –

If you decrease the input field of view by half, then only one fourth of the input phosphor will be irradiated. If all other parameters are held constant, the brightness will also drop to one quarter. This gets the attention of the automatic exposure control which will ramp up the juice.

Testable Trivia: Both Electronic and Geometric Magnification Increase Dose. Geometric Magnification increases it more.

What is this "Automatic Brightness Control" ? This is a feedback circuit in the image intensifier / x-ray generator system thats sole purpose in life is to **maintain brightness at the output phosphor**. It does this in a variety of ways; adjusting the kVp (mA fixed), adjusting the mA (kV fixed), or both (kV and mA) to maintain the brightness at the output phosphor. The consequence to the patient is an increase in dose.

Dose Compensation For Geometric Mag:

(1) You can try and collimate.
(2) You might be able to get rid of the grid, if you kept the receptor stationary and moved the patient closer to the source. This would introduce an air gap, and naturally reduce scatter. Be careful how they word this question. That air gap is not gonna happen if you brought the tube closer, you need to move the patient closer to the tube and keep the receptor stationary.

Radiation Dose:

What regulates radiation dose? –Automatic Brightness Control System (ABC). It watches the light from the output phosphor and adjusts accordingly (increases kVp, increases mA, makes the x-ray pulse width longer, less x-ray filtration, or some combination).

What is the general radiation change with each magnification? –Increases dose by 1.4 – 2.0 times –You get less light out, the ABC turns up the juice to maintain the picture

Where is the ideal place to stand? On the same side of the patient as the imaging intensifier –It is preferable to position the C arm x-ray tube under the table

Best Position of the I.I. and X-ray Tube? X- ray tube far away, with the I.I. close.

Having the image intensifier as close to the patient as possible does 3 things:

(1) Decreases patient dose.
• The ABC tries to make pretty pictures and more incident x-rays are detected when the I.I. is close so the ABC doesn't increase mA (to increase the number of x-rays generated) to make an adequate image.

(2) Decreases scatter to the operator.
• Less x-rays are made to scatter and less scatter escapes to irradiate the operator.

(3) Increases image sharpness. Decreases focal spot blur and magnification.

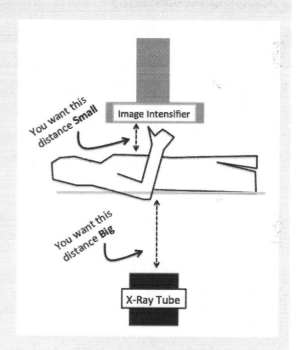

Raising the Imaging Receptor will ? Increases the dose – the machine will increase dose to compensate for the "source to image" receptor distance

Double the distance from the tube does what to dose?
• Decreases it by a factor of 4 *(inverse square law)*.

A smaller field of view, does what to dose?
• With I.I. systems – increases it
• With FPD system – also increases it (usually), but doesn't have to

Semantics:
- Radiation dose is proportional to the inverse of the distance squared (1/d^2)
- Dose reduction is proportional to the distance squared.

Does the order of mA and kVp adjust matter with regard to dose? - yes

- If mA is increased before kVp the dose gets higher
- If kVp is increased first the dose goes up less

Effect of x-ray beam filtration on dose?

- More filtration – less low energy x-rays = less dose

How does adding an "Aperture" to an I.I system affect dose?

- An aperture with a smaller hole (larger F#) to block more light from the output phosphor results in a greater radiation dose rate to the patient compared with a system with a smaller F#.
- The idea is that, the size of the hole in the aperture should balance the amount of Quantum Mottle to an acceptable dose

How does kvp selection affect dose?

- Higher kVps result in more penetrating x-rays.
- Higher kVp's result in lower patient radiation doses

How good are lead aprons? When should you wear one?

- 1mm of Pb stops about 90% of radiation (it's not 100%)
- If you are within 6 feet of a fluoroscope you should lead up

Techniques to reduce dose to patient?

- Positioning away from the source
- Using the smallest field of view by collimating (this also improves resolution)
- Avoiding magnification

Seemingly Random Trivia

Various federal regulatory bodies limit the patient entrance dose rate to a maximum value of **"87" mGy per minute** ("10" R/minute) in the normal mode of operation.

A *"high level mode"* can be used, you just have to have audible or visual alarms (in addition to the normal time alarm used in normal fluoroscopy.)

In *"high level mode"*, the maximum patient entrance dose rate must be less than ~~"174"~~ mGy per minute ("20" R/minute).

~~"5x10" digital spot films~~ = the dose of 1 minute of fluoroscopy (assuming same FOV).

Artifacts:

Pincushion Distortion: With a large field of view you can sometimes get the appearance of bent lines at the periphery (lines that should be straight). The inward bowing pattern is said to resemble a pincushion.

S Distortion: This is a similar artifact to the pincushion, also seen more in larger fields of view. The etiology with this artifact is an interference of the earth's magnetic field on the flow of electrons heading towards the I.I.

Making it better? The addition of a mythical material called "mu metal" supposedly can deflect the magnetic field (and protect against vampires).

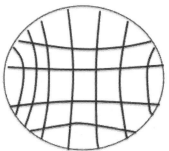

Pincushion Distortion
- Due to Large FOV

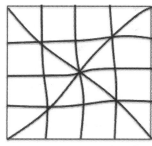

S-Distortion
- Due to Earth's magnetic field

Flair or Glare Artifact: If you have a transition from heavy attenuation to minimal attenuation - you can see bright white "Glare" at the periphery near the decreased attenuation. This is from an overproduction of x-rays in this thin area, to compensate for the nearby thick area.

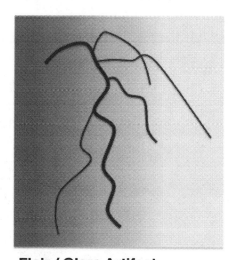

Flair / Glare Artifact
- Image becomes brighter with transition to less attenuation

Lag Artifact: You move the I.I. and the ghosted image is still superimposed from the prior field.

Vignetting Artifact: Because distances from the focusing point to the outer phosphor tend to vary, with the closest path in the center and the farthest path at the edge you can end up with a dark periphery and a light center.

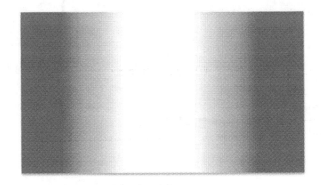

Vignetting Artifact
– Edges are darker than center

Saturation Artifact: If the dose is cranked up to try and penetrate a very dense object (classically metal) you can end up with regions around the metal appearing very bright.

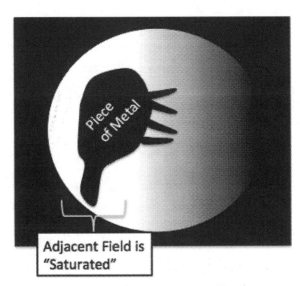

Piece of Metal

Adjacent Field is "Saturated"

Saturation Artifact

Image Receptor Types:

There are two kinds:

—(1) Image Intensifiers (I.I.) — the old kind
—(2) Flat Panel Detectors (F.P.D) — the new kind

*We discussed the I.I. — Now lets talk about the F.P.D

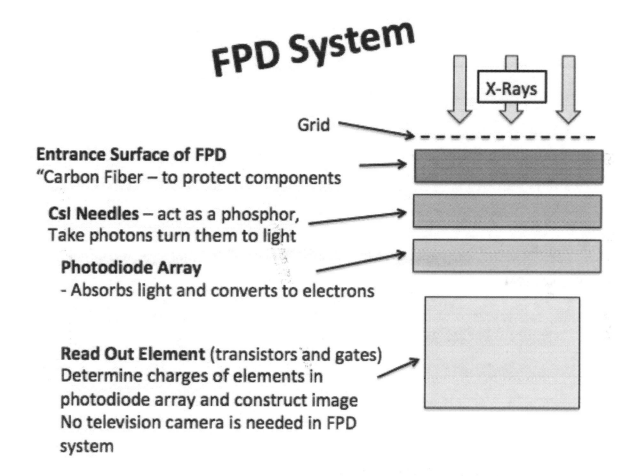

As you can see all that I.I. stuff doesn't happen with the modern system (oh, don't worry you will still get tested on it). There is some general vocab that I want to discuss, then the differences in artifacts between the two systems, then I'm going to end on spatial resolution - a high yield topic.

Vocab:

"Pitch" There is a thing called pitch. Essentially it is the ~~linear dimension of a detector element~~. This is different than the "pitch" you think about with CT (more on that later).

"Fill Factor" There is a thing called fill factor. The system isn't 100% efficient, only a portion is actual sensitive to light. The ratio of the sensitive area over total area is the fill factor.

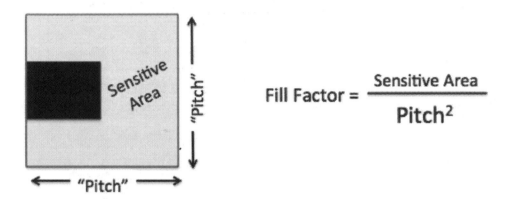

As the detector element gets smaller you get better spatial resolution, but the "fill factor" decreases. In other words, ~~a smaller detector element will have superior resolution but will require more radiation~~.

"Matrix" - The matrix is the number of detector elements (or pixels) on the surface of the FPD - in each dimension (horizontal and vertical).

1 Detector Element = 1 Pixel

Math problem: If the matrix size is 1100 x 1100, and the FOV is 25cm, what is the pixel size (or detector element)?

the formula is: ~~Pixel = FOV / Matrix.~~
But, I was trying to get sneaky with the units (a very common trick): 25cm = 250mm.

250 / 1100 = 0.23mm

Binning: There is a thing called binning. Taking several detector elements (DELs) and making a large DEL. The idea is the you reduce the amount of data (and reduce Quantum Mottle – less variation in x-ray photons from pixel to pixel).

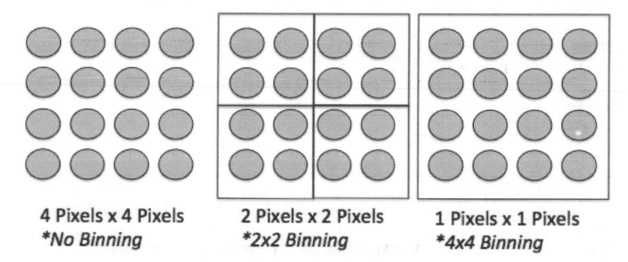

4 Pixels x 4 Pixels
***No Binning**

2 Pixels x 2 Pixels
***2x2 Binning**

1 Pixels x 1 Pixels
***4x4 Binning**

- Less Mottle means you can reduce radiation and keep the same noise.
- Larger DEL does reduce the spatial resolution

When is "Binning" especially useful? –With ~~large FOV~~ (when there are too many pixels in the image)

If there is no "binning" the spatial resolution changes in what way from different fields of view (in a FPD system)? No change. If you have binning, large FOVs will have less spatial resolution (but can use less radiation to maintain the noise level). Remember "binning" is a FPD thing, not an I.I. thing

What usually happens (without employing binning) with smaller FOVs? ~~Dose is increased to reduce quantum mottle.~~ If you employ binning, dose can be reduced. For example, If you combine 4 DEL you can reduce dose by 50%

"~~Frame Averaging (Recursive Filtration)~~)" - This is an image process feature that adds several images together with different weight factors.

> **Pro:** It's done to ~~reduce quantum mottle and increase the signal.~~ SNR improves.

> **Cons:** It ~~increases the susceptibility to motion artifact and ghosting~~.

Artifacts (FPD):

Are artifacts seen with I.I.s the same as FPDs? Nope. **FPDs do NOT have pincushion, S distortions, vignette, glare, or saturation artifacts**

Bad Pixel – appear as either white or black spots. One method to correct for this (often built into the system) is to interpolate in order to fill the data.

Lag Artifact (Ghosting) can also occur with FPD. This tends to occur if the exposure uses very high radiation.

Spatial Resolution:

What limits of spatial resolution of an I.I. fluoro system? –The television display system. The resolution of a TV depends on raster (scan) lines, the bandwidth, and the FOV.

Does the display limit the spatial resolution of a FPD system? Nope, FPDs usually have displays with the same matrix as the image receptor

Vertical Resolution is limited by? The number of raster lines that the display monitor uses. You have to alternate white and black to reproduce a line pair image on the I.I. or FPD, so the max number of line pairs in the vertical direction is half the number of actual lines used. Because the bars in the line pair pattern may not totally line up with the raster lines, it's less than that so you need to correct with the Kell Factor (Kell Factor is some derived factor: 0.7).

$$\text{Vertical Resolution} = \frac{\text{Raster Lines x Kell Factor}}{2 \times \text{FOV (mm)}}$$

So decreasing the FOV (mag mode) improves spatial resolution

How is horizontal resolution different than vertical resolution? The number of dots per line must be calculated indirectly from the bandwidth. The number of line pairs along the horizontal direction is half the dots in a raster line

If you measure spatial resolution at a diagonal (45 degrees to the raster lines) does it get better or worse? Better – spatial resolution improves by a factor of $\sqrt{2}$ over the vertical or horizontal resolution

Better pure spatial resolution FPD vs I.I ? I.I. systems are better, and change with FOV.

Spatial Resolution is Limited By:

FPD systems are limited by? – Detector element size (around 2.5-3.0 lp/mm)

I.I systems are limited by? TV systems (1.0-2.0 lp/mm for GI, and 2.0-4.0 lp/mm for angio)

8 Factors Affecting Spatial Resolution:

FOV – smaller FOV better resolution

Focal Sport Size – usually not an issue unless you get the anatomy away from the image receptor

Image Receptor Limitations – detector element for FPD and television for I.I

Motion and Temporal Factors – motion creates ghosting

Dynamic Range – This is only an issue for I.I systems – with variability in very dense or very transparent stuff

Pixel Binning – Binning increases pixel size – reduced spatial resolution (but improves SNR)

Frame Averaging – increases SNR (less mottle), more susceptible to blur

Pulsed Fluoro – Dose is administered in pulses, instead of continuously. You get less motion artifact (better spatial resolution in moving objects) and overall less dose.

QA

How is spatial resolution tested for? – Lead bar pattern

How is distortion checked for? - Use a mesh screen or plate. Look for straight lines (not pincushion or S distortion).

Fluoro in IR

Focal Spot: You are trying to visualize small things (tiny vessels in real time) – this means you need a small focal spot + large number of x-rays. To deal with this small focal spot, local heat exchanges must be added to avoid melting the whole unit. The anode angle is smaller when compared to conventional x-ray. The smaller angle leads to an increased heel effect. Fortunately, in IR the heel effect remains zero because you use a small field of view and small image detector (only allows the central portion of the x-ray beam to be imaged). Focal spots can be exchanged (large, small, micro) – depending on the need for resolution.

kVp: The best kVp to use with contrast is between 60-80 kVp (average beams hit that k-edge nicely). A higher kVp loses iodine contrast.

Filter: There is a thing called an "equalization filter" or a "soft filter." These reduce intensity but do NOT completely block the beam. They are used to "taper" the radiation profile, and are often employed when imaging the leg, arm, or pediatric patients.

Grid: Since grids are usually used, the testable trivia is that they are often NOT used on extremities or peds.

Digital Subtraction Angiography (DSA) – This system works by taking a single frame mask image and subtracting it from another single frame contrast image – with the goal of removing anything that is not moving. This leaves the stuff that is moving (blood).

Patient Dose
- Most IR systems use a pulsed fluoro (helps reduce dose).
- 50% of the dose is delivered in the superficial 3-5 cm of skin/fat
- The depth of this 50% depends on the kVp and filtration *(higher kVp + Copper Filtration = more penetration)*
- For a body (or body part) measuring less than 10cm (a baby for example) – the grid should be off
- A thicker (fatter) patient gets more skin dose. This is because automatic brightness control sees less penetration – then cranks up the dose (higher kVp).
- Additional high dose situations: lateral and oblique views
- Patient and operator dose doubles with a lateral view (compared to PA)
- The typical dose is about 0.3 – 0.5 mGy per frame at the entrance skin position (10x – 20x more per image than fluoro)
- Total Dose = (dose per frame) x (frame rate) x (duration x number of runs)

"Source to Skin Distance" (SSD) = how close the patient is relative to the x-ray source. If you are using under the table positioning the SSD depends on table height.

Small SSD = High Dose

Short Angiographers should stand on a platform (or be carried by a trainee) so that the source to image receptor distance is kept at 100cm or more.

"Dose Spreading" The idea here is to change the angle of the gantry (especially in a long case) in order to spread the skin dose over a broader area – decreasing the skin dose to any specific location.

"Best Place to Stand" You should try and stand / work on the image receptor side of the patient. You are trying to avoid the large amount of Compton scatter radiation produced where the beam enters the patient.

Dose Area Product (Kerma Area Product) This measures the radiation dose to air in mGy – multiplied by the collimator area – then reported in mGy·cm. **The measurement is independent of beam location.** It's true that as you move the beam away from the patient the intensity decreases- BUT, the beam spreads out more. These two things occur in equal amounts so the DAP (KAP) is NOT dependent on location.

DAP (KAP): Low Dose to Large Skin Area = High Dose to Small Skin Area
Magnification – will increase Air Kerma, but NOT KAP

Obviously this doesn't help you grade risk of a skin burn. Instead it is used to estimate total energy deposited in patient, effective dose, and cancer risk. If something reduces the DAP (KAP) it probably also reduces the scatter and the patient's dose.

Interventional Reference Point (IRP)- This describes the use of an ionization chamber with a set reference point *(15cm closer to the source than the isocenter of the IR system)* to measure radiation emitted from the source. Skin dose can be above or below this point.

Because IRP ignores geometry, table attenuation, and back scatter, it probably over or underestimates patient's skin dose every time – but it is currently the best thing available.

Testable Trivia: The dose (outside lead) standing 1 meter from the patient is about 1/1000 of the dose received by the patient.

Regulatory Doses:

- No High Level Control (HLC) Present = 10 R / min (**87mGy**/min)
- HLC on = 20 R/ min (176 mGy/min)
- During Image recording = no limit if pulsed

Skin Doses:

- Below 2 Gy – No action needed
- 2-5 Gy – advise patient to watch for burns – especially 10 days post procedure
- Above 5 Gy – procedure and dose should be reviewed by physics

- 2 Gy – Early Transient Erythema
- 3 Gy – Temporary Epilation (hair loss)
- 6 Gy – Chronic Erythema / "Main Erythema"
- 7 Gy – Permanent Epilation (hair loss)
- 10 Gy - Telangiectasia
- 13 Gy – Dry Desquamation
- 18 Gy – Moist Desquamation / Ulceration
- 24 Gy – Secondary ulceration

Operator Doses:

- You get about 0.1% of what the patient gets – at 1 meter
- In 1 year – you typically get about 5 mSv
- Regulatory dose limit is 50mSv per year
- Conceptus dose limit is 0.5mSv per month

High Level Control

The maximum entrance exposure is 10 R/min in a conventional setting.

An option for high dose is "specially activated fluoro" or "high dose control", where you can have rates up to 20R/min.

The trick is an audible alarm must be on when this is used.

High Yield Points:

- The tube goes under the patient, as far away as possible (largest SSD possible)
- The receptor goes as close to the patient as possible
- Use pulsed fluoro and collimate when possible
- Move the beam around as much as possible (don't just burn up the dudes skin in the same spot)
- Avoid electronic magnification as much as possible
- No grid on babies or extremities

Calmer than you are dude

Section 6: CT

How does the CT scanner work:

Most CT scanners today are "3rd generation" – which means the x-ray tube and the detectors spin around the patient in synchrony. CT X-ray tubes use tungsten alloy targets placed on high speed rotating anodes. CT tubes are designed to operate at reasonable voltages (between 80 -140 kV) with very high tube currents up to 1000mA. The typical focal spot is "large" measuring 0.6mm to 1.2mm. You need a large focal spot to handle all that power – 100kW.

The x-rays are filtered to remove low energy x-rays that would only increase dose.

Filtration Mechanisms:
- Copper or Aluminum (6mm) is used to filter the x-ray beam
- Heavily filtered beam can have a half value thickness of up to 10 mm Al
- Bow Tie filters are used compensate for uneven attenuation of the beam by the patient. These filters attenuate less in the center and more on the edges. Bow Tie Filters are made of low Z materials – like Teflon (to reduce hardening differences).
- The x-ray tube anode-cathode axis is positioned perpendicular to the imaging plane to reduce the heel effect.

> **Bow Tie Filters:**
> - Compensate for uneven filtration
> - Reduce Scatter
> - Reduce Dose

Scatter Reduction:
- A collimator is used both at the x-ray tube, as well as the detector, with the purpose of shaping the x-ray beam ("*Defines the section thickness on a single slice*"). The collimator also reduces some scatter.
- Additional scatter reduction is further accomplished with "anti-scatter septa." Which are grids, but you can't call them grids – they are "septa!"

The CT fires off x-rays as it spins. The table moves the patient through. The detectors (highly efficient scintillation detectors) have a lot of information – which looks like a wavy mess (Sinogram). Then a bunch of math takes place (filter back projection), and you get a picture.

> **"Filtered"** in Filtered Back Projection refers to "Sharpening of the projection data prior to back projection."

Modern set ups use an "iterative reconstruction" math program that allows more noise, so you can have less dose at the same diagnostic quality… or at least thats the idea.

Detector Types:
There are two types of detectors; Scintillation Detectors (the modern type), and Gas Filled Detectors (the ones used back when dinosaurs roamed the earth). The Scintillator detectors are way more efficient and easier to produce.

3rd Generation Multi-slice vs Single Slice:
The number of detectors in the axial direction determines the number of slices that can be simultaneously acquired. The MDCT can acquire images with "isotropic resolution," – which means they can do non-axial reconstructions without stretching pixels.

High Yield Point: Minimal slice thickness is determined by detector element aperture width in a modern CT.

Vocabulary:

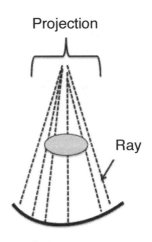

What is this "Ray" – A "ray" is a measure of total x-ray attenuation along a line from the focal point to a single detector

What is this "Projection" – A "projection" is all rays at a given angle of the x-ray tube. In other words, it's a "series of rays that pass through the patient – at the same orientation.

What is this "Sinogram" – A "sinogram" is a bunch of squiggly lines that represent the data from all the projections of all the tube angles (0-360).

What kind of x-rays are used with CT? Highly filtered, High kV (average energy 75 keV)

How is the image actually produced? Generating an image from the acquired data involves figuring out the linear attenuation coefficients of each pixel in the image matrix.

    Back Projection – This was the original way. Equal attenuation was given to all pixels along a ray.

    Filter Back Projection – This is the more modern way. By multiplying projections with a "mathematical filter" you make a better picture.

    Adaptive Statistical Iterative Reconstruction (ASIR) - "Forwarded" information is compared to actual information and differences are used to correct the image. What you need to know is (a) it **can correct for noise**, so you can (b) **use a lower dose**. It requires some major computer power, that's why older systems couldn't use it.

What is the matrix size for CT? Each Pixel is ? The matrix is 512 x 512, with each pixel representing 4096 possible shades of gray (12 bits).

Wait? How did you get that? $2^{12} = 4096$

What is the relationship between pixel width and height to voxels? They are the same. *Pixel W x H = Voxel W x H.* The difference is a voxel has a 3rd dimension (depth), which represents the slice thickness. A voxel is a cube, a pixel is a square.

How do you calculate pixel size ? You divide the Field of View / Matrix Size

How do you improve spatial resolution ? You need to make the pixels smaller (matrix larger). Remember that Pixel Size = FOV/ Matrix

Is mAs the same on CT as it is on plain film? The conventional definition of radiographic mAs is not useful in spiral CT. You have to use "effective mAs". Tube Current (mA) x Length of time that a given point in the patient is in the beam. Basically, the exposure time. Obviously the exposure time is going to be related to the collimated beam width and table speed.

If you turn down the mAs, what happens to your images? Less mAs = More Noise

What is this "Pitch" ?

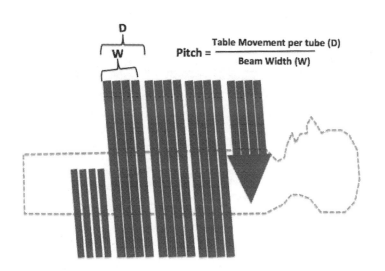

$$\text{Pitch} = \frac{\text{Table Movement per tube (D)}}{\text{Beam Width (W)}}$$

Understanding Pitch:

In this example, the pitch is greater than 1 because there is a gap between slices.

If the pitch is 1 the beam = the distance the table turns in one revolution (no gap).

If the pitch < 1 than you have overlap (which increases dose).

Practice Math Problem. (Beam Width – Slice Thickness)

- Calculate Pitch: Table Moves 12mm, Beam Width is 8mm; 12 / 8 = 1.5

- ***All things being equal – increasing the pitch does what to the radiation dose?*** Reduces it (less overlap)

The Hounsfield Unit: The attenuation of other tissues is a "relative attenuation" - based on a comparison to water. Water is always "0". The formula used to calculate HU is:

~~HU = 1000 x (attenuation of material - attenuation of water) / attenuation of water.~~

What is the relationship between HU and X-ray attenuation? When ~~HU increases by 10 HU~~ x ray attenuation increases by 1%.

Increasing the Beam Width Through the Collimator:

•Reduces Scan Time (larger coverage with 1 turn)
•Reduces Motion Artifact (less scan time)
•Increases Partial Volume (more divergent beam)
•~~Does NOT change the radiation dose~~ (mAs in unchanged, even though the scan time is less, a larger area of tissue is scanned at the same time).

Axial vs Helical Modes

Axial

The table is stationary. The tube comes on and takes a picture. The tube shuts off and the table moves up a slice. The tube comes back on and takes another picture

Advantages:

- ~~Better spatial resolution on the z-dimension~~ since full images sets are taken. No partial volume effect along the long axis.

- The artifacts of partial volume with helical CT are noticed more along a curved surface. *Classic example = skull.*

Helical

The table moves at constant speed. The tube is on the entire time.

Advantages:

- Primary Advantage = ~~Way faster~~

- Secondary Advantage = Post acquisition flexibility in the selection of slice location and lower probability of anatomic discontinuities between adjacent slices containing moving anatomy in the chest/abdomen scans

Fixed and Variable mA

Old scanners had fixed kvp and mA

New scanners can adjust via two methods

- (1) Scout image – to estimate density

- (2) on the fly with continuous modulation

Advantages are reduced radiation and more uniform signal to noise

Spatial Resolution

Spatial Resolution -This is the ability to distinguish small objects that are close together (tell that they are separate). Practically a bar pattern is used to measure this (line pairs per cm).

Spatial Frequency – number of line pairs per cm. This is inverse to the object size. Small objects have high spatial frequency, large objects have low spatial frequency.

Factors that affect spatial resolution:

Focal Spot Size

- A larger focal spot, means the object details are spread out over several detectors. This degrades and blurs the image

- Smaller focal spot = better spatial resolution

Magnification

- More magnification blurs the image

Detector Aperture Size

- As the detector size is reduced the cranial-caudal resolution increases

- The in plane "x-y axis" is NOT affected by aperture size.

Number of Projections

- More projections, more data. Better Resolution

Reconstruction Slice Thickness

- The thinner the detector element aperture, the better the spatial resolution in the Z direction

Spatial Resolution as a function of pixel size and display field of view:

- "Display Field of View" (DFOV) = Space defined by the user based on the anatomy size to be displayed. It is always less than (or equal to) scan field of view.

- Remember that Pixel Size = DFOV / Matrix Size. So increasing the matrix size or decreasing the DFOV will make your pixel size smaller. Smaller pixels = Better Spatial Resolution.

Spatial Resolution as a function of Pitch:

- As pitch increases, so does the width of the slice sensitivity profile (SSP).

- As the SSP widens the slice thickness increases. Thicker slices = Less Spatial Resolution.

Patient Motion

- Voluntary and involuntary movement leads to blurring. Blurring = reduced image resolution

---

Which Vessel is on Top?

At the institution I trained at, a popular quiz was to show a first year resident a MIP CTA of the brain and then say "which is on top, the basal vein of Rosenthal or the PCA?"

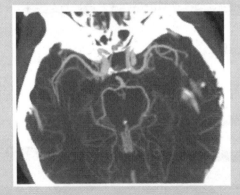

The question was a trick to illustrate that MIPs (maximum intensity projections) don't give you depth, they give you attenuation information. A vessel with a higher attenuation will appear continuous crossing a lower attenuation vessel (making it appear more superficial).

Contrast Resolution

Contrast resolution can be defined as the ability to discriminate small differences in object density from its surroundings for a specific target size and radiation dose (noise).

Dose: As the number of x-ray photons increases, the signal detected by the scanner increases, improving contrast resolution. However, radiation dose increases in proportion with photon flux.

Quantum Noise: Directly dependent on the number of x-ray photons. As the number of x-ray photons doubles, then, the signal increases by a factor of two, while the noise increases by a factor of $\sqrt{2}$.

- X-Ray Double = Signal Double

- X-Ray Double = Noise Increases by factor of $\sqrt{2}$

> **Example:**
>
> If mA goes from 200 -> 400 mA, SNR increases 1.4x (2/root 2)

Signal-to-Noise: Contrast resolution improves with SNR. If the number of x-ray photons is doubled the signal doubles. If the x-rays double the noise increases by a factor of $\sqrt{2}$. So you have an increase of $2/\sqrt{2}$. In other words, as the signal (and proportionately the dose) increases, contrast resolution increases, but at a lesser rate.

Slice Thickness: Small slices = less photons per slice = less contrast resolution (the image is noisier). However, smaller slices = less partial volume averaging = improved spatial resolution.

Pixel Size *(Spatial Resolution vs Contrast Resolution):*

- Holding matrix size constant and decreasing FOV will decrease pixel size. This increases spatial resolution but decreases contrast resolution (less photons per box)

- Holding matrix size constant and increasing FOV will increase pixel size. This decreases spatial resolution but increases contrast resolution (more photons per box).

Factors That Affect Spatial Resolution	Factors That Affect Contrast Resolution
Focal Spot (smaller spot = better)	Number of X-Rays (mAs, kV, pitch). More dose (less mottle) will improve contrast resolution.
Detector Width (smaller detector = better)	Slice Thickness (thicker = more x-ray quanta = less noise).
Nyquist Limitations "Sampling" (Oversampling = better)	Reconstruction Method (Iterative > Filtered Back)
Reconstruction Filter (example – bone algorithm gives a higher spatial resolution)	Reconstruction Filter (Soft tissue > Bone)

- Most CTs have a kVp of 120.
- Peds and Skinny people have kVp of around 80 *(reduces dose and increases image contrast).*
- Fat people need higher kVp.

Cardiac Imaging

Cardiac imaging is best performed during diastole. There are two main methods; prospective and retrospective – I'm certain the differences in the two would make good multiple choice questions.

–Prospective: "Step and Shoot" – R-R interval

- Pro: There is reduced radiation b/c the scanner isn't on the whole time

- Con: No functional imaging

- Trivia: Always axial, not helical

–Retrospective: Scans the whole time, then back calculates

- Pro: Can do functional imaging

- Con: Higher radiation (use of low pitch – increases dose)

- Trivia: this is helical

CT Fluoro

- Near real time imaging, with the CT image constantly updated (6 per second).

- Low tube currents (20-50 mA) are used to minimize radiation doses.

Dual Energy

At a single photon energy is it possible to tell two different materials apart? Nope

How does dual energy CT Work? –Scan is acquired using both 140 and 80kvp (instead of just 120). The H.U. of each pixel is obtained at both energies. The image is dirtier, but you can do all kinds of stuff like characterize the material *(what is the renal stone made of?),* or do a virtual non con. It all has to do with different atomic numbers absorbing photons differently.

T Window Width and Level:

It's a basic concept that is highly testable. The "Level" is the midpoint of the gray scale display (the "center"). You want your level at the attenuation of the thing you are interested in. For example, if you are interested in bone – you want a high level. The width is selected based on what you are comparing. If you are comparing things with very different densities you want a wide width. If you are comparing things with very similar densities (example white and gray matter), you want a very narrow window width.

How this concept can be tested? Really there are two main ways: (1) you can ask a typical window for lung, bone, liver etc… This is partly memorization (see chart) but you can sorta figure it out based on the principals I mentioned above. (2) They can ask you below or above what level will give you a white or black reading.

This kind of question is easiest to solve if you draw it out. For example, if your level is set at 100 and you width is 300, you will have 150 above and 150 below at some gray scale (150 is half of 300). In this case, above 250 will be seen as solid white and below a -50 will be seen as black. A second example shows the same thing using a more narrow window of 150.

Window , Level in HU	
Brain	W 80, L +40
Lung	W 1500, L -400
Abdomen	W 400, L +50
Bone	W 1600, L +500

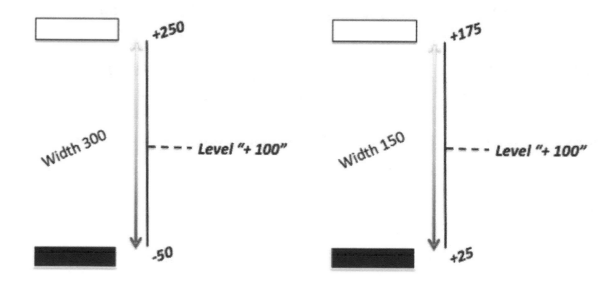

Radiation Dose Measures: CT Specific

"Variation within the Scan Plane" – In regular Dx imaging, the entrance skin dose is much larger than the exit skin dose. In CT, because the scanner spins 360 degrees – the dose is symmetrically distributed. Obviously, the center is still gonna get less (body phantoms show it to be about 50% less in the middle – compared to the edge). When you compare a head to a body phantom the center dose is similar to the skin (smaller diameter).

Head Scans: Central and Surface are very similar

Body Scans: Surface is about twice the central dose.

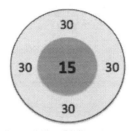
Body CT – Middle is Less

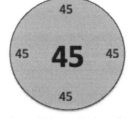
Head CT – Middle is Same

"Z Axis Variation" – There are often "tails" of radiation along the edge of the area being scanned. As a result, the profile of radiation is not limited to the primary area being imaged. If multiple scans are performed these tails add up with the original scan.

"CTDI" – *CT Dose Index* - This is the radiation dose, normalized to beam width. There are subtypes - the difference of which could easily be tested on a multiple choice test.

- "Weighted CTDI" – This is 1/3 the central CTDI + 2/3 the Peripheral CTDI (expressed in mGy)

- "Volume CTDI" – This is obtained by dividing weighted CTDI by the Pitch. Remember that Weighted CTDI is the intensity being used and can relate to mottle.

Quick Review of Pitch

• Doses in helical scanning with a pitch of 1.0 are similar to those from axial scanning.

• If the pitch is < 1.0 then the dose increases because the slices overlap.

• If the pitch is > 1.0 then the dose decreases because energy is more spread out.

• The relationship is proportional. A pitch of 2 halfs the dose. A pitch of 0.5 doubles the dose.

"DLP" – Dose Length Product – This value is simply the CTDI – Vol x the length of the scan in cm.

"Effective Dose" for CT : Effective Dose = k x DLP. Remember that "k" is a body part constant. Effective dose is going to be in Sv.

Phantom Size – These CTDI numbers are based on phantoms. The body phantom is 32 cm in diameter. If the patient is larger than the phantom, then dose is over estimated. If the patient is smaller than the phantom, then dose is under estimated.

Average Dose (CTDI – in mGy) *Corrected effective dose is different*

- Adult Head = 58 (effective dose 1-2 mSv)

- Adult Abd = 18 (effective dose 8-11 mSv)

- Peds Abdomen = 15

There is a "Reference dose" set by the ACR at 75 percentile – doses above that should be "investigated" and reduced if possible.

ACR Established Diagnostic CT Reference Values.

CTDI vol:

- *75mGy for Head,*

- *25 mGy for Adult Abd,*

- *20 mGy for Peds Abd (5 year old)*

Risk of radiation induced cancer per dose?

- 5% per Sv = Adult

- Up to 15% per Sv for Child

- About 1/10th that for someone older than 50

Pediatric Considerations:

- It's recommended that you reduce mAs.

- Reduced techniques are possible because x-ray penetration is greater in children

- Dose Reduction in head CT are more modest than peds belly

Strategies to reduce dose to the breast:

- Do the scan at reduced mA (problem is the images look like shit)

- Use a milliampere modulation (adjust based on density) * this is the preferred method

- Shield the breasts with bismuth – you get artifact and a degraded image (beam hardening can falsely elevate H.U. directly deep to the shield.

Dose Related Trivia:

•Dose of 1 Chest CT is about equal to 100 PA + Lateral CXRs

•CT of the extremities has a very low effective dose (< 1 mSv) because they don't contain any radiosensitive organs.

•Embryo dose in CT A&P is around 30 mGy.

Individual dose monitoring is mandated if the occupational dose is favored to be greater than 10% the annual dose limit (500 mrem).

Gamesmanship: *What if you monkey with the kVp???*

(1) Dose Goes Up: Unlike conventional radiography with automated exposure control, increasing kVp in CT will increase radiation dose to the patient.
(2) Image noise will decrease.
(3) Iodinated contrast will be more conspicuous at lower kVp (such as 80 kVp), as the average energy of the x-ray beam will be closer to the k-edge of iodine.

CT Artifacts:

Beam Hardening- As the x-ray beam passes through an object the lower energy photons are removed preferentially, leaving a "harder beam" with an increased average energy. There are two artifacts associated with this.

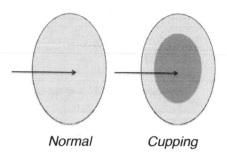

Cupping - The x-rays passing through the middle of a uniform shape (like a head) are hardened more than those traveling through the periphery (a shorter path). The harder the beam the slower the rate of attenuation. The manifestation is the center of the image appears darker than the peripheral portions.

Dark Bands / Streak - This occurs in the setting of two dense objects. X-rays that pass through one are less attenuated than those that pass through both. The result is dark bands and streaks between those two objects. The classic location is bone or where a dense contrast was used.

Fixing Beam Hardening:

(1) Filtration - Pre hardening of the beam, to remove lower energy components before it hits the patient, and/or the addition of a bow-tie filter.

(2) Calibration Correction - Using a phantom to allow the detector to compensate for hardening effects.

(3) Correct Software - An iterative correction algorithm can be used.

(4) Avoidance - Tilt the gantry or position the patient to avoid areas the cause hardening.

Partial Volume: This can occur in two main ways.

Pattern 1 ("Partial Volume Effect"): A dense object protrudes partially into the width of an x-ray beam. This results in divergence of the beam and manifests as shading artifacts adjacent to said object.

Pattern 2: CT voxels are 3D cubes. If you have a dense thing taking up half the cube, and a sparse (low attenuating) thing in the other half of the cube the machine will average the two together giving you something that has intermediate density. The classic location is the skull base averaging with CSF or brain to sorta look like blood.

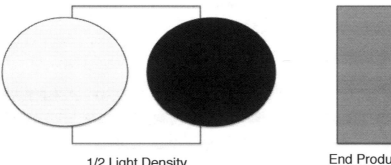

1/2 Light Density
1/2 Dark Density
Both Overlapping in a Single Voxel

End Product will be an
average of the two

Fixing partial volume: Make your slices thinner. If the noise is a problem, acquire thin slices then generate thicker slices by adding them together.

Photon Starvation: High attenuating areas (classically the shoulders) can result in photon starvation manifesting as streaking. It's seen when the beam travels horizontally - through the greatest area of attenuation.

Fixing Photon Starvation: There are two main ways to fix this. (1) Automatic tube current modulation. If you increase the dose through the area of greater attenuation you can add enough photons to overcome this effect. (2) Adaptive filtration can be performed to correct the attenuation profile "smooth the data" in the high attenuation portions.

Under Sampling: An insufficient number of projections used to reconstruct the CT can diminish quality, and result in mis-registration artifacts. There are two main types.

View Aliasing: This is when you have under sampling between projections. You see fine stripes radiating from the edge (but at a distance from) a dense object. This is fixed by acquiring the largest possible number of projects per rotation - slowing the rotation speed.

Ray Aliasing: This is when you have under sampling within a projection. You see strips appearing close to the structure. This is fixed by using specialized high resolution techniques - manufacturer employed.

Metal Artifact: Metal causes streak artifact. It does this through several mechanisms: beam hardening, partial volume, aliasing, and having density ranges higher than what can be handled by the computer. Testable trivia is that metals with high Z (Iron, Platinum) tend to have more artifacts than those with lower Z (Titanium).

Fixing Metal Artifact: Tell the patient to remove it. Increase the kVp (sometimes works). Use thinner slices. Certain interpolation software can help.

Patient Motion: Motion can cause misregistration - which manifests as shading or streaking, especially on reconstructions.

Fixing Motion Artifact: Tie the crazy patients down. Use a modern (fast) scanner. Align the scanner in the primary direction of motion (vertically above or below a chest scan - for breathing). "Over scanning" an extra 10% on the 360 rotation, with the repeated portion averaged. Gating - like in cardiac.

> **Over-Scanning vs Over-Ranging**
>
> *Over-Scanning* - Essentially having a pitch < 1.
>
> *Over-Ranging* - Scanning above and below the target, to collect additional data for a helical scan.

Incomplete Projection - If parts of the patient are hanging outside the field, but still attenuating x-rays this messes with the computer's math. Examples include, arms hanging down or having the IV contrast on or near the patient.

Fixing incomplete projections: Position the patient correctly.

Ring Artifact: A calibration error or defective detector on a third generation scanner will cause errors in angular position - resulting in a circular artifact.

Fixing Ring Artifact - Recalibrate your dinosaur detector, or replace the broken part.

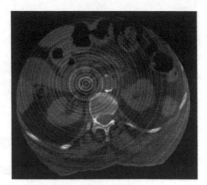

Ring Artifact

Helical Artifact in the Axial Plane: Single Section

You get the same artifacts with helical scanning modes plus you get some additional artifact from helical interpolation. The main place you see this is around the top of the skull (**anatomy changing rapidly in the Z direction**). The higher the pitch the worse this is. To minimize these artifacts you have to reduce the variation in the Z direction - use a low pitch, use 180 degree instead of 360 when possible, and using thin sections instead of thick. Testable trivia - this is why head CTs are still commonly done with axial scanning over helical.

Helical Artifact in Multi-Section

Distortion is more complicated on multi-section scanners, with a classic "windmill" appearance where several rows of detectors intersect. It worsens with increased helical pitch. A "Z-Filter" is done to reduce the severity of windmill artifacts.

Stair Step Artifact: This is seen as a "stair step" on the edges of a multi-planar reformatted image, when you have a wide collimation of non-overlapping intervals. It's less severe with a helical scanner - where you are getting some overlap. It's fixed by making thin slices.

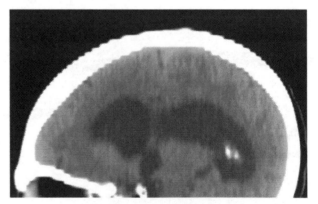

Stair Step Artifact

Zebra Artifact: This is another reformat artifact, which can occur from helical data - secondary to the helical interpolation process (increases noise along the Z axis). The effect manifests as stripes (like a zebra) most pronounced on a 3D image. The effect is most significant away from the axis of rotation - noise is worst off axis.

It's a league game, Smokey

Section 7: Ultrasound

Sound is not light. Sound requires a medium to travel in. It's best to think of sound as a mechanical energy that produces vibrations when propagating through material. These vibrations produce alternating areas of:

- High Pressure (Compression) and
- Low Pressure (Rarefaction)

Frequency: This is the rate of change between compression and rarefaction - given in Hertz. In other words, its the number of times the wave oscillates through a cycle each second.

Wavelength: The distance between areas of compression.

Remember this from general chemistry? *Speed = Wavelength x Frequency*

Speed is thought of as being constant (in a particular medium), so that an increase in frequency decreases the wavelength - and vice versa.

Speed in Different Materials: This is based on the compressibility of something. Things that are very compressible (air) will have a very low speed. Things that are not very compressible (bone) will have a very fast speed. **The ultrasound machine is stupid - and just assumes everything travels at 1540 m/s in tissue.** The fact that the machine thinks speed is constant is a source of artifacts (discussed later).

Speeds effect on frequency – None. The frequency is the same, irrelevant of the sound speed in various media. Therefore the **wavelength changes in media**.

Wave Interference Patterns: Modern ultrasound machines make a bunch of different sound beams. These sound beams can either have "constructive effects" and help each other – increase the amplitude, "destructive effects" and hurt each other – decrease the amplitude, or complex effects and be complex. These interactions are important in shaping and steering the beam.

Relative Intensity – The dB. A change of 10 in the dB scale corresponds to two orders of magnitude (100 times) and so forth. The dB is based on a log 10 scale.

- Reducing the sound intensity to 10% is -10 dB
- Reducing to 1% is - 20 dB
- Reducing to 0.1% is – 30 dB

Testable Point: A loss of 3 dB (-3 dB) represents a 50% loss of signal intensity (power).

Testable Point: The tissue thickness that reduces the ultrasound intensity by 3 dB is considered the "half-value" thickness.

Interactions of Ultrasound with Matter

Ultrasound interacts with matter by:
- Reflection
- Refraction
- Scattering
- Absorption

Reflection: Ultrasound energy gets reflected at a boundary between two tissues because of the differences in the acoustic impedances of the two tissues. A large difference in "stiffness" results in a large reflection of energy.

Impedance: This is defined as: Z = Density x speed of sound. People like to compare this to the compressibility of a spring.

At a muscle-air interface, nearly 100% of incident intensity is reflected, ever noticed how air has some serious shadowing? *This is why gel must be used between the transducer and the skin to eliminate air pockets.*

Refraction: This is the change in direction of transmitted ultrasound energy at a tissue boundary when the beam is not perpendicular to said boundary. Remember the frequency doesn't change, but the speed might.

What influences refraction ? Two Things: (1) Speed Change – which is based on tissue compression, and (2) the Angle of Incidence.

This was described by some dude named Snell:

$$\frac{\text{Sin Angle 1}}{\text{Sin Angle 2}} = \frac{\text{Speed 2}}{\text{Speed 1}}$$

transmission

No refraction occurs if the sound is the same in the two media or with perpendicular incidence.

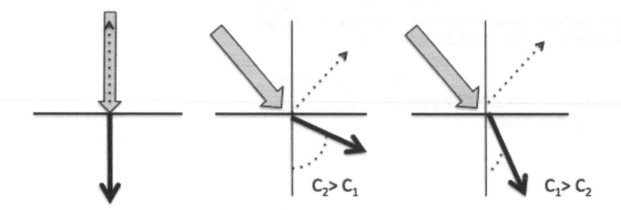

$c_2 > c_1$ $c_1 > c_2$

If it hits straight on, part of the beam will bounce straight back and part of it goes straight through. If it strikes at an angle, part will be reflected and the other part will be refracted - with the severity of this refraction depending on the speed difference of the two media.

Refraction is the cause of the shadows seen at the edges of a fluid filled structure (most commonly the gallbladder), as sound passes from tissue to fluid - altered from it's original path.

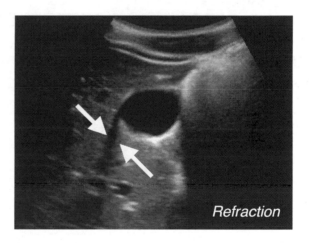

Refraction

Total Reflection: It is possible to have complete reflection if the speed difference, and angle of incidence is great enough (exceeds the "Critical Angle").

Scattering: There are two main categories of reflectors:

- **Specular (smooth)** – The reflector dimensions are much larger than the wavelength of the incident. *Strength of reflection is highly angule dependent.*

- **Non-specular (diffuse)** – The scattering surfaces are about the size of a wavelength or smaller. *Angle has no effect on strength*

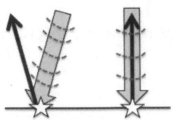

Smooth Reflectors:
will reflect depending on the angle of incidence

With higher frequency ultrasound beams, the wavelength becomes smaller and the boundary no longer appears smooth from the prospective of the small wavelength. In this case, returning echoes are diffusely scattered leaving only a small fraction of the incident intensity returning to the source. Truly smooth reflections are relatively independent of frequency.

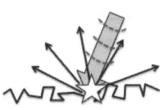

Non-Specular:
Will scatter everywhere – angle doesn't matter

In other words: High Frequency = Small wavelength = Surfaces appear more rough = More Scatter. So **Higher Frequency = More Scatter.**

Differences in Scatter Amplitude: The difference in amplitude of the returning echoes from one region to another corresponds with brightness changes on the ultrasound display (essentially the number of scatterers per unit volume).

- Hyperechoic = High Scatter Amplitude – relative to average background
- Hypoechoic = Lower Scatter Amplitude – relative to average background

Absorption: Sound energy gets turned into heat. This increases with frequency.

"Attenuation" is the loss of intensity of the ultrasound beam from both absorption and scattering in the medium. The degree of attenuation varies widely depending on the type of tissue involved. To quantify the degree of attenuation, people who like math decided to express it in dB as proportional to frequency.

If you are forced into a math problem, the rule of thumb for "soft tissue" is 0.5 dB per cm per MHz or 0.5 (dB/cm)/MHz.

It is proportional:
- A 2-MHz ultrasound beam will have twice the attenuation of a 1-MHz beam;
- A 10-MHz beam will have ten times the attenuation per unit distance.

It is logarithmic:
- The beam intensity is exponentially attenuated with distance.

Testable Point: Half value thickness (HVT): This is the thickness of tissue necessary to attenuate the incident intensity by 50%, which is equal to a 3-dB reduction in intensity. As the frequency increases, the HVT decreases.

Think it Through: You always use the high frequency probe for superficial stuff right? This is why. The higher the frequency the more the sound gets attenuated, so the depth sucks. If you need to see a deeper structure then you have to use a lower frequency probe.

Review Time	
What determines the strength of the echoes?	Angle and Impedance
What is Impedance?	The degree of stiffness in a tissue. The differences in tissue impedance (stiffness) determines the strength of surface reflection.
What is the unit used for impedance?	The Rayl
The speed of sound is assumed to be?	1540 m / s
Attenuation is increased with?	Higher frequency ultrasound waves

Ultrasound Transducers and Related Trivia

Ultrasound is produced and received with a transducer. The device works by taking electricity and running it through a crystal (which vibrates) for conversion into mechanical energy (ultrasound waves). On the way back, the waves (mechanical energy) vibrate the crystal turning back into electricity so they can be recorded. Or something like that… close enough for what you need to know.

Back in the stone ages these things had a single element resonance crystal, now they have a broadband transducer array of hundreds of individual elements.

Piezoelectric Materials: This is a crystal (or ceramic) and is the functional component of the transducer. It could be quartz, but is usually lead-zinc-titanate (PZT). The magic to the material is a well-defined molecular arrangement of electrical dipoles. When mechanically compressed their normally organized alignment gets disturbed from equilibrium; this can be measured and recorded.

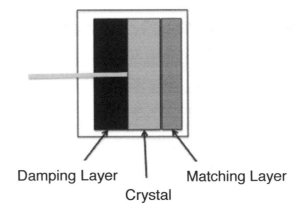

Damping Layer   Crystal   Matching Layer

Resonance Transducers: These are made to operate in a "resonance" mode, where ~~short durations of voltage (usually 150 V) are applied~~, causing the PZT to vibrate at a natural resonance frequency.

High Yield Trivia: The operating frequency is determined from the ~~speed of sound in and the thickness of the piezoelectric material~~. ~~The only way to change frequency is to change the probe~~. *Wavelength changes to accommodate changing velocity in different media.*

High Yield Trivia: ~~*The thickness of the transducer is equal to ½ the wavelength.*~~ Lower frequency is seen with thicker crystals and higher frequency is seen with thinner crystals.

Dampening Block: This thing sits behind the crystal and ~~absorbs the backward directed US energy~~. It also dampens the transducer vibration to create a pulse with a short spatial pulse length – needed to preserve detail along the beam axis (axial resolution). The process of dampening introduces a broadband frequency spectrum.

What you need to know about dampening blocks:

The differences in a thin block and a fat block easily lend themselves to multiple choice questions.

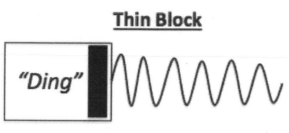
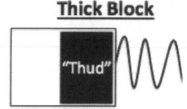

Thin Block

- Called a "**Light Damping**"
- Called a "**High Q**"
- Has a **Long** Spatial Pulse Length
- Has a **Narrow Bandwidth**

Thick Block

- Called a "**Heavy Damping**"
- Called a "**Low Q**"
- Has a **Short** Spatial Pulse Length
- Has a **Broad Bandwidth**

High Yield Trivia:
- Low Damping (high Q) – Narrow Bandwidth – *For Doppler, to preserve velocity information.*
- Heavy Damping (low Q) – Broad Bandwidth – Gives you high spatial (axial) resolution *fewer interference effects and therefore more uniformity*

Matching Layer - The matching layer gives the transducer an interface between the transducer element and the tissue. The key testable point is that it - minimizes the acoustic impedance differences between the transducer and the patient. It's made of stuff that has an acoustic impedance intermediate to soft tissue and the transducer material.

Testable Point: *The optimal matching layer thickness is equal to 1/4th the wavelength*

Transducer Arrays

You can have Linear (which include curved) or Phased Arrays. Linear arrays are sequential, where as phased arrays are "activation / reactivation" types.

Linear	Phased
256-512 Elements	64-128 Elements
Large	Small
Simultaneous Firing of small group of adjacent elements (20ish)	Elements are activated sequentially
A rectangular field of view is produced *(trapezoidal with curved)*.	Time delays in electrical activation can make it possible to steer and focus, without moving the probe

Why is a curved array curved? – Scan lines diverge deeper into the image. This gives you a wider field of view for deeper structures. Used in ABD imaging and OB.

Linear - This type of probe fires all elements simultaneously. This means the width of the transducer is equal to the width of the individual elements.

Phased - This type of probe fires elements at different times. The individual waves firing times can be changed to cause constructive and destructive wave summations - this steers and focuses the beam.

Beam Properties

There are two distinct beam components: a converging beam, which narrows out to a distance determined by the geometry and frequency of the transducer (near field), and a diverging beam (far field).

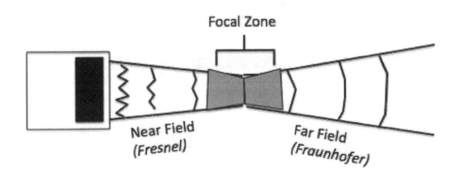

The Near Field (Fresnel Zone): The convergence of the near field occurs because of the multiple constructive and destructive interference patterns.

Beam intensity varies from: MAX-to-min-to-MAX in a converging beam.

The near field length is dependent on: Transducer Frequency and Transducer Diameter.

Testable Point:

- Higher Transducer Frequency = Longer Near Field
- Larger Diameter Element = Longer Near Field

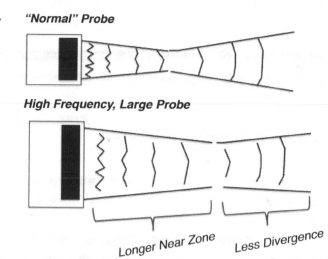

"Normal" Probe

High Frequency, Large Probe

Longer Near Zone Less Divergence

The Far Field (Fraunhofer Zone) - This is where the beam diverges. As the beam diverges the ability to distinguish two objects close to one another is reduced. The divergence is less with a high frequency big probe and more with a low frequency small probe. Ultrasound intensity in the far field gradually decreases with distance.

Intensity – The intensity of the beam is the power (measured in watts) flowing through a unit area. The power of the beam is not uniform along its length or width. This is caused by a variety of factors.

- The beam lacks clearly defined edges and the intensity will decrease from the center ⟶ outward - sometimes called "beam spread"
- The maximum sound pressure is always found along the acoustic axis (centerline)
- Divergence of the beam in the far field causes the power to be spread over a larger area.
- Interference occurs from numerous point sources interacting in the near field. *Less with a broadband transducer

Focal Zone – The point at which the beam is at its narrowest and the area of maximum intensity. You get your best echoes here and you get your ~~best lateral resolution here~~.

"Transmit Focusing" – There are several ways to do this, with the idea being to converge the beam (narrowing it) on the area you want to look at. Understand that the ~~focal distance is a function of the transducer diameter (or width of group of simultaneously fired elements)~~, the ~~presence of any acoustic lenses and the center operating frequency~~.

- *Shallow Focus* – achieved by firing ~~outer transducers in the array, before the inner transducers in a symmetrical pattern~~

- *Longer Focus* – achieved by ~~reducing the delay time differences among the transducer elements~~. This results in ~~more distal beam convergence~~

- *Multiple* – ~~Multiple focal zones can be created by repeatedly acquiring data over the same volume, but with changes in the phase timing of the array elements~~. Because of the fact that each focal zone requires independent set of pulses, increasing the number of focal zones will decrease the frame rate and temporal resolution.

"Receive Focusing" - When using a ~~phased array~~ transducer, ~~all the echoes received by the individual transducer elements are added together~~ to create the signal from a given depth. Echoes received at the perimeter of the array travel from a longer distance than those received at the center of the array. To correct for this, the ~~signals from individual transducer elements must be rephased to avoid a loss of resolution when the individual signals are brought together~~ into an image.

Time Gain Compensation (TGC) – This is the button you push to make the image look better. What it actually does is ~~progressively increase the amount of amplification~~ applied with depth. The man who lives in the ultrasound machine ("computer" I call it), is trying to make the top and bottom uniform. This used to require manual manipulation of buttons, but it is now automated.

What can you do to make this image better? - Answer is probably hit the TGC button.

Dimensions -

There are three dimensions in US:
* Axial
* Lateral
* Elevation (Slice Thickness)

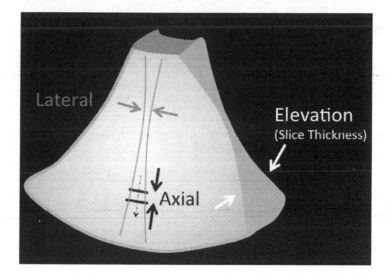

Axial Resolution: The ability to tell two closely spaced objects apart in the direction of the beam. For optimal axial resolution you need the returning echoes to be separate and not overlap. The minimum required separation between two reflectors is ½ the spatial pulse length (SPL), otherwise the returning echoes will overlap.

What is this "Spatial pulse length" ? This is the number of cycles emitted per pulse by the transducer multiplied by the wavelength.

Objects closer than ½ Spatial Pulse Length will NOT be resolved.

Lateral Resolution: The ability of the system to resolve objects in a direction perpendicular to the beam direction. If you want to tell things apart, they must fit into separate beams. The thinner the beam, the more likely that each will fall into a separate beam. You can reason, that improving lateral resolution has a lot to do with making your beam thinner. The beam is most skinny at the end of the near field (at the focal zone). Lateral resolution is worst in areas close to and far from the transducer surface (away from the focal zone).

Is lateral resolution constant at different depths? No , Since the beam diameter varies with the distance from the transducer in the near and far field, the lateral resolution is depth dependent. The best lateral resolution occurs at the focal zone (the interface of the near field and far field interface). **Lateral resolution worsens in the deeper field.**

Is axial resolution constant at different depths? - Yep

Will cranking up the gain help? No - Gain widens the beam. You want a nice narrow beam. So, try and use the minimal necessary gain.

Elevation Resolution (Slice Thickness) – It's the same as lateral resolution but is measured in the plane orthogonal to the image plane. This is usually the worst measure of resolution. It depends on the transducer element height. This type of resolution is why you can get volume averaging of acoustic details in regions that are close to the transducer and in the far field.

Improving Axial Resolution	Improving Lateral Resolution	Improving Elevation Resolution
Shorter Pulses	Narrowing the beam in the proximal field (adding an acoustic lens). Minimal necessary gain (gain widens the beam).	Use a fixed focal length across the entire surface of the array (downside is partial volume effects)
Greater Damping (shorter pulses)	Phased array with multiple focal zones	Minimize slice thickness - done by phase excitation of the outer to inner arrays
Higher Frequency (shorter wavelength)	Increasing the "line density" or lines per cm.	

Dependent On	
Axial Resolution	Spatial Pulse Length
Lateral Resolution	Transducer Element Width
Elevation Resolution	Transducer Element Height

Artifacts:

Ultrasound display equipment relies on multiple assumptions to assign the location and intensity of each received echo. When these assumptions are violated you get an artifact.

Assumptions:
- All echoes originate from within the main beam
- All echoes return to the transducer after a single reflection
- The amount of time an echo takes to return to the probe directly reflects on the object depth.
- The speed of sound in human tissue is constant - 1540 m/s
- The sound beam and its echo travel in a straight path
- Acoustic energy is uniformly attenuated

Beam Related Artifacts:

As stated above, there is an assumption that the detected echoes originate from within the main US beam.

Side Lobe Artifact: The ~~normal US beam looks like a bowtie~~, with a central main beam and off axis low energy beams on the side. These off axis beams are the "side lobes." You get these side lobes from radial expansion of piezoelectric crystals, which ~~happens more in linear arrays~~. If you have a strong enough reflector it could bounce back this low energy side lobe, which will be received by the transducer. This will violate the assumption that echoes originate from the main beam – and it will be incorrectly placed as if it did. This artifact is typically seen when the ~~incorrectly placed echoes overlap an anechoic structure (Bladder or GB)~~. Some people refer to this as "~~pseudo sludge~~" ~~when it's seen over the gallbladder~~.

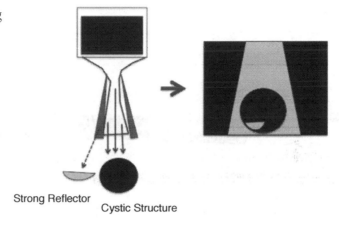

Strong Reflector   Cystic Structure

Testable Point: Side lobe energy is seen more with linear array transducers.

Beam Width Artifact: The US beam first exits the transducer with the same width as the transducer. It then narrows to the focal zone and then begins to diverge in the far field. The beam will eventually diverge out past the original margins of the transducer. ~~If this diverged beam encounters a strong reflector, it could send a signal back~~ – which will be assumed to be from the main beam (within the normal width of the transducer) and will be erroneously displaced as such.

The *bladder is the classic place to show this*, with ~~peripheral echoes~~. A good "next step" question would be to show this artifact and have you improve it by (1) ~~adjusting the focal zone to the level of interest and~~ (2) *placing the transducer at the center of the image*.

Artifacts Associated with Multiple Echoes:

These artifacts violate the assumption that an echo returns to the transducer after a single reflection and that the depth of the object is related to the time for the round trip.

Reverberation Artifact: If the sound wave encounters two parallel highly reflective surfaces, the echoes generated from a primary ultrasound beam may be repeatedly reflected back and forth (like a game of pong) before eventually returning to the transducer for detection. This is recorded and displayed as multiple echoes, with the echoes that return after   a single reflection being displayed appropriately and sequential echoes (which take longer to return to the transducer), erroneously placed at an increased distance from the transducer. This looks like multiple equidistantly spaced linear reflections.

Comet Tail Artifact: A form of reverberation. This time our two parallel highly reflective surfaces are closer together which means the sequential echoes are closely spaced. The space between them may be less than ½ the spatial pulse length (SPL) - which as mentioned above was the minimal distance needed for axial resolution. As a result, the displayed echoes will look like a triangle, instead of linear lines.

Why a triangle and not a square ? The later echoes get attenuated and have decreased amplitude. This decreased amplitude is manifested on the display as decreased width. So you get a tapering triangle (or comet tail).

Ring Down Artifact: The mechanism for this one is slightly different. Instead of encountering two parallel highly reflective surfaces, our sound wave encounters fluid trapped between a tetrahedron of air bubbles. The vibrations create a nearly continuous sound wave transmitted back to the probe. You see this as a line or series of parallel bands extending posterior to a collection of gas.

Mirror Image Artifact: Like other artifact in this category, this is created by the false assumption that an echo returns to the transducer after a single reflection. In this situation the ultrasound beam passes through a highly reflective surface, then gets repeatedly reflected between the back side of the reflector, and the adjacent structure. This is displayed as a duplication equidistant from but deep to the strongly reflective interface.

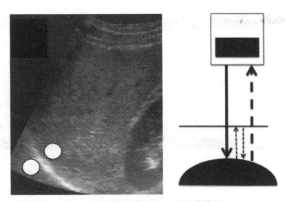

Mirror Image Artifact

The classic location is along the liver / lung interface as shown - with liver parenchyma where you should have lung.

460

Artifacts from Multiple Echoes		
Reverberation	Two parallel highly reflective surfaces -	Multiple equidistantly spaced linear reflections.
Comet Tail	Two parallel highly reflective surfaces - closer together (< 1/2 SPL)	Triangle (comet) shaped
Ring Down Artifact	Fluid trapped between a tetrahedron of air bubbles	Parallel band extending posterior to a collection of gas
Mirror Image	Trapped behind a strong reflector	This is almost always shown with the liver on lung.

Artifacts Related to Velocity Errors:

The assumption is that the speed of sound is 1540 m/sec in human tissue. Sometimes the beam encounters media (air, fluid , fat, bone) where this doesn't hold up exactly. If it travels slower– it takes longer to return and the machine thinks the depth is more. If it travels faster, it comes back to the monitor faster and the machine thinks the depth is less.

Speed Displacement Artifact: The speed of sound slows down in fat, relative to liver. This means the beam takes longer to return and is perceived by the machine as being further away. This creates the appearance of a discontinuous and focally displaced liver border.

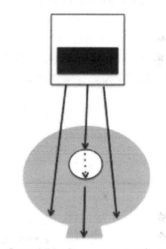

Speed Displacement Artifact

Refraction Artifact: As discussed earlier in the US section, speed difference in tissues causes refraction (as described by Snell). This change in the direction of the sound wave violates the idea that the beam is going straight and can cause three things: (1) the object can appear wider than it actually is, (2) object can be misplaced to the side of the returning echo, or (3) object can appear duplicated.

The classic look (and location) for this is deep to the rectus muscles and midline fat. The so called "duplicated SMA," occurs secondary to symmetry of the geometry. The SMA will become a normal single vessel if you move the transducer to the side (removes symmetry of refraction).

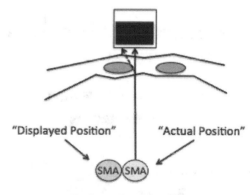

"Displayed Position"   "Actual Position"

SMA SMA

Refraction Artifact

Artifacts Related to Attenuation Errors:

Ultrasound beams are attenuated as they travel through the body (from scatter and absorption). The longer the echo travels the more it will be attenuated (relative to an echo which traveled a shorter distance).

"Compensation Amplification" – This is a type of processing ultrasound machines use on echoes that take longer to return to the transducer. Essentially, the echoes that return later are amplified more than echoes that return earlier. The end result is an image that appears more uniform in the deep field.

Shadowing - If the ultrasound beam runs into a material that attenuates sound to a larger degree than the surrounding tissue, the strength of the beam distal to this structure appears weaker (darker) than in the surrounding field.

Increased Through Transmission - This is the opposite of shadowing. Instead the beam runs into material that attenuates sound less than the surrounding tissue, the strength of the beam distal to the structure appears stronger (brighter) than the surrounding field.

Modes / Misc

A Mode, B Mode, M Mode

A Mode - "A" stands for amplitude. This is of historical context – and only used now by optho to take eye measurements. This gives you processed information from the receiver versus time. An echoe's return from tissue boundaries and reflectors creates a digital signal proportional to echo. "A"mplitude is produced as a function of time.

B Mode – "B" stands for brightness. Basically this is the conversion of A line information to brightness-modulated dots on a display. There is a proportional relationship of brightness to the echo signal amplitude.

M Mode – "M" stands for motion. Essentially, B-mode information is used to display the echoes from a moving organ (like heart valves) from a fixed transducer and beam position on the patient.

Trivia - M mode is 4x greater than B mode
Trivia – Pulsed Doppler is 20x greater than B mode

Harmonics

As the ultrasound beam travels into the patient's tissues the transmitted pulse is progressively distorted. However this occurs primarily in the central zone of the main beam where the intensity is high. A distorted pulse will give rise to distorted echoes and these have significant energy at harmonic frequencies. Tissue harmonics are made using the second harmonic component of the echo signal, with the fundamental frequency excluded. Undistorted echoes coming from lower intensity areas (fringes of the beam, side lobes, superficial tissues) are not seen.

Advantages	Disadvantages
Improved lateral spatial resolution	Being at a high frequency, the second harmonic attenuates far more rapidly than the fundamental, so the depth of penetration is reduced
Reduced Side Lobe Artifact	
Removal of Multiple Reverberation Artifact – from adjacent anatomy	The processing used to remove the fundamental frequency generally requires that two transmitted pulses are used for each line of sight in the image. This reduces the frame rate by a factor of two.
	Hypoechoic masses look like cysts
Cysts look clearer.	

Mammo Ultrasound - Special Topic

Compound Imaging - Having the electronic steering of the ultrasound beams from the transducer image an object in multiple different directions. This will sharpen the edges and cause loss of posterior shadowing (can make a cyst look solid).

Compare and contrast normal settings, harmonics, and compound imaging of a

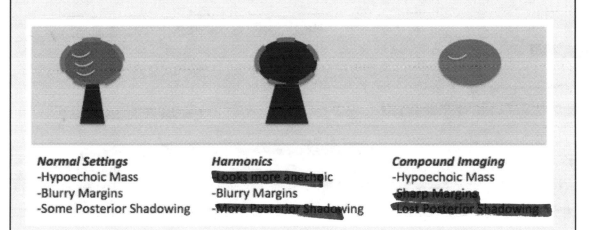

Normal Settings
-Hypoechoic Mass
-Blurry Margins
-Some Posterior Shadowing

Harmonics
-Looks more anechoic
-Blurry Margins
-More Posterior Shadowing

Compound Imaging
-Hypoechoic Mass
-Sharp Margins
-Lost Posterior Shadowing

Doppler

Doppler Shift: When sound is reflected from a moving object and the frequency of the reflected sound changes - PhDs call that a "Doppler Shift."   With some math, this change in frequency can be used to determine the speed and direction of blood.

Doppler Angle: In an ideal world, the sample volume would be placed in the mid-part of the lumen, with an angle of incidence parallel to the vessel. If this angle is placed incorrectly the velocity calculation will be incorrect (especially if the angle is greater than 60).

The angle should be between 30- 60.

Why less than 60? Because of the formula for calculating it.   Notice that the cosign of the angle is on the bottom.

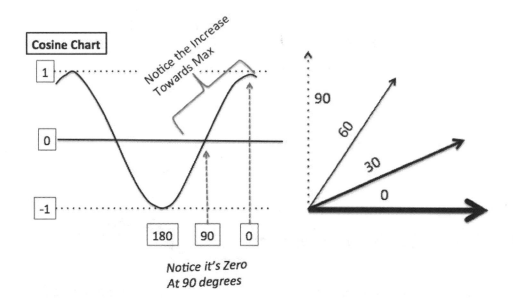

Looks like zero is best. So why more than 30? – Angles less than 20 degrees cause refraction and loss of signal. Aliasing also becomes an issue.

Why Not Perpendicular ?– If you placed the probe perpendicular to the vessel, it can give a false impression of no flow (occlusion). The other thing it can do is create a mirror image.

Pulsed Wave (Spectral) Doppler- This utilizes a single transducer for both reception and transmission. Blood flow velocity varies yielding a spectrum of doppler shifts instead of a single frequency. You can obtain the direction of blood flow (plotted above and below the baseline) and velocity.

Color Doppler: This uses the gray scale image with a superimposed color blood flow image. Gives the direction of flow, this time with colors (red and blue). Color intensity varies depending on the flow intensity (things holding still are gray). This type of doppler obtains samples of each pixel multiple times then displays the average shift.

Testable Trivia: The spatial resolution is less compared to gray scale imaging (although smaller vessels are better seen).

Testable Trivia: The doppler angle is not as important since the information is semi-quantitative.

Power Doppler: Power doppler is different because it gives you a very sensitive look for the presence of flow without information on direction. You still get color but instead each pixel registers the total number of "frequency shifts".

Testable Trivia: Power Doppler does NOT exhibit aliasing *(both color and spectral can)*.

Testable Trivia: Power Doppler has NO dependence on the Doppler Angle - *you can measure doppler totally perpendicular to the vessel.*

Testable Trivia: Power Doppler is extremely sensitive to flow *(even very slow flow)*

Doppler Artifacts:

Aliasing - Super high velocities are displayed as low (negative). On a spectral system it looks like the spectrum is cut off and "wrapped around the baseline", reappearing on the opposite end.

Testable Trivia: This artifact occurs when the doppler shift is greater than a threshold called the "Nyquist frequency"

$$\text{Nyquist limit (kHz)} = 1/2 \times \text{pulse repetition frequency (PRF)}$$

Example: A frequency shift of 3.5 kHz requires a PRF of 7 kHz to avoid aliasing.

Aliasing can be reduced or eliminated by:
- Decreasing Doppler shift – by either using a lower frequency transducer or using a doppler angle closer to 90 (increasing the angle)
- Increasing the Pulse Repetition Frequency (which will increase your Nyquist) or selecting a sample volume at a lesser depth or increasing the scale.

Tissue Vibration: This occurs secondary to turbulent blood flow. The doppler shows a mixture of red and blue colors. The classic example is a A-V fistula in a kidney post biopsy.

Mirror Image: Just like the gray scale version, this occurs secondary to a vessel adjacent to a highly reflective surface, such as the lung. This results in the duplication of the structure being evaluated. The classic locations are the subdiaphragmatic region of the liver and the supraclavicular region.

Twinkle Artifact: This occurs behind strongly reflecting surfaces such as calcifications. It manifests as a noisy spectrum with rapid fluctuation of red and blue colors.

Testable Trivia: This artifact has a greater sensitivity for detection of small stones than acoustic shadowing.

Testable Trivia: This is highly dependent on machine settings and how round the reflecting surface is (more rough = more twinkle).

Pseudoflow (Pseudoblood) Artifact: Things that move like blood but aren't. The classic example is ureteral jets.

Flash Artifact: This is a burst of color filling the screen. It's secondary to transducer or patient motion. The classic example is the **"fetal kick!"**

Color Bleed - This looks like color extending beyond the vessel wall. It can decrease sensitivity to thrombus or stenosis.

Making it better: Decrease the color gain.

Power and Gain - Some Quick Points:

- Increasing power increases your penetration depth.
- Gain only changes the brightness on the imaging monitor, but has no affect on the actual ultrasound output.
- If you crank up the power too much, you can create an artifactual image.

Safety

Two acoustic output parameters are used as indicators of the potential for biologic effect.

- **Thermal Index** – this is the maximum temperature rise in tissue secondary to energy absorption. This is based on a homogeneous tissue model with certain instrument parameters.

- **Mechanical Index** –this is how likely it is that cavitation will occur considering peak rarefaction pressure and frequency. This index is the indicator of mechanical bioeffects (streaming and cavitation). **This matters the most with contrast enhanced US.**

Cavitation - Sonically generated activity in compressible bodies composed of gas and/or vapor. This can be sub-classified as either stable or transient.

- **Stable Cavitation** - Micro bubbles are already present in the media. They expand and contract as the waves cycle (responding to pressure). This occurs at low and intermediate ultrasound intensities (as used clinically). The MI is an estimate for producing cavitation.

- **Transient Cavitation** – "The violent one" – Bubble oscillations become so large that the bubbles collapse. This collapse results in shock waves rippling through tissue planes causing tissue damage.

Testable Trivia: The rate of energy absorption increases with frequency. Eventually the rise in temperature slows secondary to conduction and perfusion with an eventual steady state.

Testable Trivia: Thermal induced damage is a threshold phenomenon (you get no tissue damage until a certain temperature is reached).

Testable Trivia: Cavitation is most likely to occur with low frequency and high pressure.

Testable Trivia: Spectral Doppler deposits more heat compared to gray-scale ultrasound.

Testable Trivia: Per the NCRP - a risk-benefit decision when the TI exceeds a value of 1.0 and the MI exceeds a value of 0.5.

Obstetrics:

The bottom line is ultrasound has been around for fucking ever, and there has never ever ever been a single case of a human fetus injured by it. Having said that, Radiologists are massive cowards so caution is still advised.

Since temperature rises are most likely at bone surfaces and adjacent soft tissues, a baby with increasing mineralization (2nd and 3rd trimester) has the theoretical risk of the possibility of heating sensitive tissues such as brain and spinal cord.

Testable Trivia: The Thermal Index for Bone "TIB" applies to an ultrasound beam passing through soft tissue then hitting bone (the scenario for 2nd and 3rd Trimester).

General Recommendations (not at all evidenced based) for 1st Trimester:
- Pulsed doppler (spectral, power, and color) should NOT be routinely used
- Keep the TI under 1.0 (some sources say 0.7).
- Scanning maternal uterine arteries with doppler is probably ok (as long as the fetus is outside the beam)

Thermal Index:
- Below 0.7 - for OB imaging
- Between 1.0 - 1.5 - US should NOT exceed 30 mins
- Between 2.5 - 3.0 - US should NOT exceed 1 min
- Greater than 3.0 - US should NOT be used.

You mark that frame an 8, and you're entering a world of pain

SECTION 8: NUKES

Nuclear medicine is unique in that instead of passing a beam of energy through the patient, you are injecting a tracer into the patient and observing a normal or abnormal distribution of that tracer.

Stability / Decay: Everyone wants to be happy. I want to be happy, you want to be happy, and even isotopes want to be happy. We seek it in different ways. Some of us incorrectly thought that going to medical school would make us happy. Isotopes seek happiness through stability. In general, what makes an isotope stable is a balanced number of protons and neutrons. The process of emitting energy or particles is an attempt to become more stable.

Some Vocab: *"Transmutation"* – A change in the number of protons, which by definition changes the element.

Subtypes of Transmutation:

- *Alpha Decay* = This tends to occur in heavier unstable atoms. Alpha particles are basically Helium nuclei (2 protons, 2 neutrons). Alpha particles are slow and fat. They can't even penetrate a piece of paper, and are worthless for imaging.

- *Beta Minus Decay* = **Seen with Neutron Excess**. A neutron is converted to a proton, then emits an electron *(beta particle)* and antineutrino. The range of these dudes is about 1cm, so they are also worthless for imaging. They do have the potential to harm DNA and form the basis of radionucleotide therapy with ^{32}P, ^{89}Sr, ^{90}Y, ^{131}I, and ^{153}Sm

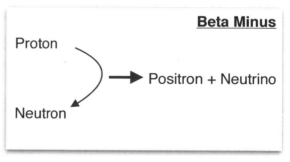

- *Beta Plus Decay* = **Seen with Proton Excess** *(Neutron Deficiency)*. A proton is "transformed" into a neutron. *(**Trivia to know**= **you need 1.02MeV for this to occur**)* A positron *(beta particle)* is then emitted which travels a short distance before colliding into a real electron and then destroying each other. The mutual destruction emits **two 511 keV photons which come out 180 degrees apart.** Beta plus and Electron capture both occur in the setting of proton excess (neutron deficiency) and therefore compete with each other.

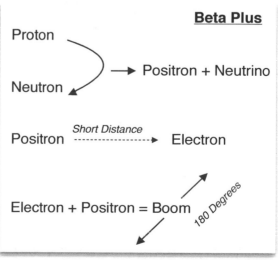

- *Electron Capture* = Also **Seen with Proton Excess** *(Neutron Deficiency)*. This occurs in the setting of insufficient energy *(remember beta plus needs 1.02MeV)*. A proton eats (captures) an electron and then turns into a neutron. The neutron *(formerly a proton)* then burps *(emits)* characteristic radiation

Alpha Decay	Heavy Unstable Atoms	Lots of tissue damage
Beta (-)	**Neutron Excess** *(Proton Deficiency)*	Electron Emission Can Damage DNA (basis of Radionucleotide Therapy)
Beta (+) –*Rival Of Electron Capture*	**Proton Excess** *(Neutron Deficiency)* *Has at least 1.02MeV*	Positron Emission , leading to two 511 keV photons which fly 180 degrees apart
Electron Capture –*Rival Of Beta (+)*	**Proton Excess** *(Neutron Deficiency)* *Does NOT require 1.02MeV*	Leads to gamma emission (sometimes) and characteristic radiation, both of which may be used in imaging

High Yield Trivia: Particle emissions cause more problems than photon emissions. What do I mean problems? Even though Beta (-) and Beta (+) don't travel far, they can damage DNA. So plastic should be used to shield against them (NOT LEAD because it will create Bremmstahlung x-rays). So just remember **B emission = Plastic Shield (NOT LEAD).**

Rivals
- *Isometric Transition* – **"The Good Guy"** Any process that gives off gamma radiation but Protons and Neutrons don't change.

- *Internal Conversion* – **"The Bad Guy"** Excess Energy Exceeds Binding Energy so you get an Ejected Electron plus some characteristic radiation.

These two dudes compete with each other and their ratio is termed the "Alpha." The lower the alpha the more useful radiation you get and the less harmful radiation you produce.

Low Alpha = Good.   *Tc has a low Alpha.*

More Vocab:

Metastable: If you have some decay between particle delay and gamma emission then you can call it

"Metastable." The classic example (and probably only one you need to know) is the metastable Tc99.

— Isomers are nuclides that contain the same number of protons and the same number of neutrons but the isomer exists in an excited energy state.
— Tc-99m decaying to Tc-99 through the emission of a 140 keV photon is an example of an isomer undergoing an ISOMERIC transition.

142.7 KeV Tc99M (half life 6 hours)

↓

140.5 KeV

↓   ┊
↓   ↓

Summary Chart:

Here are some classic diagrams that illustrate the different processes of decay.

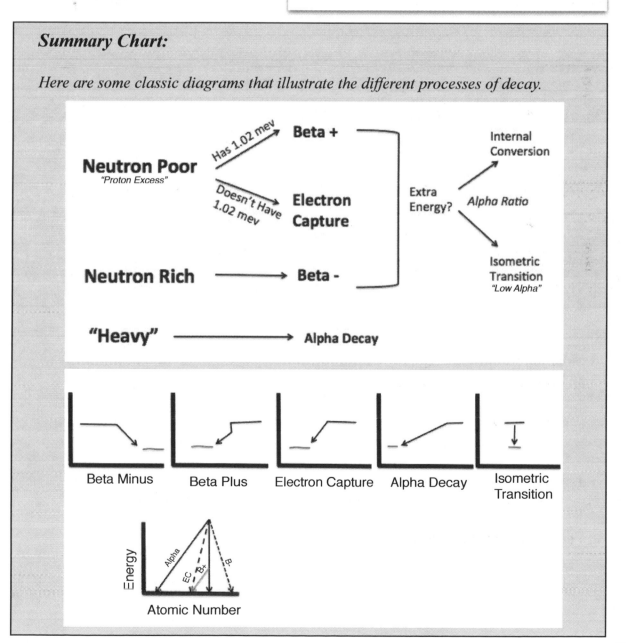

Production

There are two main ways you can create tracers, both of which alter the Neutron/Proton ratio to make them unstable:

(1) Bombardment (in a nuclear reactor or cyclotron)

(2) Fission

Bombardment: This is basically striking target elements with either neutrons (in a nuclear reactor), or with charged particles (alpha particles, protons, or deuterons) in a cyclotron. The downside to the nuclear reactor method is that you have to clean up the left over parent element. This is referred to as not being carrier free. The cyclotron has the advantage of producing elements via transmutation, therefore you don't have any parents to clean up "Carrier Free."

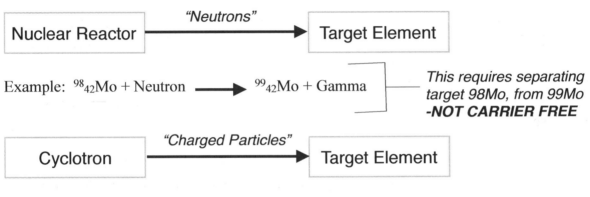

Nuclear Reactor ——"Neutrons"——▶ Target Element

Example: $^{98}_{42}Mo$ + Neutron ——▶ $^{99}_{42}Mo$ + Gamma — This requires separating target 98Mo, from 99Mo **-NOT CARRIER FREE**

Cyclotron ——"Charged Particles"——▶ Target Element

This usually results in transmutation, so you don't have to clean up the parent.
-CARRIER FREE

Fission: Neutrons are fired into large atoms (like Uranium and Plutonium) and split them into pieces. Basically just results in a bunch of random crap being made; Iodine-131, Xenon-133, Strontium-90m Molybdenum-99, Cesium-137. Obviously the desired isotope also has a bunch of fission products (contaminants) which have to be separated out - can be done with chemistry. These guys demonstrate a bunch of different decay methods.

Neutron Activation: Target atoms eat up neutrons to form a new isotope. These neutrons don't really even need to be accelerated. Because the products are isotopes of the target atoms they cannot easily be separated from each other. As a result these are NOT carrier free. These neutron rich products tend to decay via beta emission.

- *Neutron Bombardment and Nuclear Fission -> Elements with Neutron Excess (will decay via beta emission)*
- *Cyclotron -> Elements with Neutron Deficiency (will decay by electron capture or positron emission)*

Neutron Bombardment	68-Ga, 82-Rb, 99m-Tc, 113m-In
Cyclotron	11-C, 13-N, 15-O, 18-F, 111-In, 123-I, 67-Ga, 201-TI
Fission	99-Mo, 131-I, 133-Xe, 137-Cs

Radioactive Decay

"Activity" is defined by the amount of disintegrations per second. Historically this was measured in Curie (Ci) which is 3.7×10^{10} disintegrations per second. **The new SI unit is the Becquerel (Bq), which is one disintegration per second.**

"Specific Activity" is defined as the activity per unit of mass (Bq/g). The longer the half-life, the lower its specific activity.

"Half Life" – The physical half-life. The amount of time necessary for a radionuclide to be reduced to half of its existing activity. In addition to **physical half life**, you have **biologic half life**. The biologic half life is basically how long it takes to shit or piss half the tracer out. The **"effective half life"** takes both of these things into consideration.

1/Te = 1/Physical + 1/Biologic
   Example: I-131 has a T ½ -Biologic of 24 days

   1/Te = 1/8 + 1/24 = 1/6 , so 6 days

Now having said that – if you have a large mismatch with biological and physical half life, effective half life basically becomes the short one. In other words, if you breath the Xe out in 15 seconds it doesn't matter what the physical half-life is. On the other hand, if your biological half-life is 10,000 years then you are 100% counting on physical half-life to clear it.

How long do you have to keep radioactive material? The general rule is 10 half lives.

The Perfect Tracer:

- Ideally photons need to be emitted within a range that can be detected by a camera. Ideally between 100-200 keV.
- Ideally the tracer should have no particle emissions *(this increases the dose, without making the image better).*
- The half life needs to be long enough to be imaged, but not too long that you are getting extra dose.

How the Gamma Camera Works:

A gamma camera takes photons emitted from the radionuclide, turns it into a light pulse, and then takes that light pulse and makes some voltage. The voltage makes a picture.

Collimator: There are a lot of unwanted photons (background, off-axis, Compton scatter, etc…). The purpose of the collimator is to reduce scatter and allow for correct localization of radionuclide events. It works by discriminating based on direction of travel. It can NOT tell the difference in photon energy (that's done by the photon height analyzer).

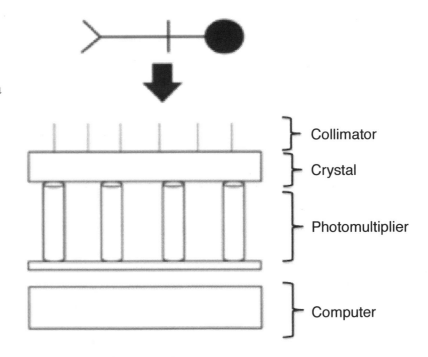

Parallel Hole Collimator: "The Work Horse" This can be modified based on the energy of the tracer being used.

- Low Energy (1-200keV)- Thinner Plates: ^{99m}Tc , ^{123}I, ^{133}Xe, ^{201}Tl

- Medium Energy (200-400keV): ^{67}Ga, ^{111}In

- High Energy (> 400keV) – Thicker Plates: ^{131}I *(technically most energy peaks are medium)*

•*Sensitivity vs Resolution:* **These two guys have an inverse relationship.** As one goes up the other goes down. A high sensitivity collimator will allow twice as many counts to be imaged but will degrade the spacial resolution. High sensitivity collimators are important with dynamic imaging (like the flow phase of a bonc scan).

•*Effects of Distance on Sensitivity and Resolution*: **Distance has NO effect on Sensitivity** (increased distance reduce counts by inverse square, but the increased distance allows for a greater field of view. NO change occurs in the net counts). **Distance DOES affect Resolution** (septa are no longer able to eliminate photons from oblique angles as distance increases).

•*Septal Length (collimator depth):* Short septa give a crappy spatial resolution, but better sensitivity. Long septa give excellent spatial resolution, but crappy sensitivity (noisier image).

•*Hole Diameter:* Wide holes = Highly sensitive, low resolution. Narrow holes = low sensitivity, high resolution.

Parallel Hole Factor		
Septa Length	Long Septa: - Low Sensitivity (Noisy) - High Spatial Resolution	Short Septa: - High Sensitivity - Low Spatial Resolution
Hole Diameter	Wider Hole: - High Sensitivity - Low Resolution	Narrow Hole: - Low Sensitivity - High Resolution
Septa Thickness	Thick Septa: - Less Penetration - Less Available space for holes (Less Sensitivity)	Thin Septa - More Penetration (Blur) - More Available space for holes (More sensitivity)

In General:
- *You want to use long thick septa + wide holes for high energy*
- *You want to use short thin septa + narrow holes for lower energy*

Pinhole Collimator: Magnifies and inverts image. Used for thyroids and other small parts. It's usually cone shaped.

Magnification occurs at a ratio of: pinhole to detector "f" / pinhole to patient "b"

- If F = B there is no magnification
- If F > B = there is magnification
- If F < B = object gets smaller.

In other words, if you move it far enough back it will make the image smaller. Magnification at the front is greater than the back (objects are 3D), this is why large objects get distorted and pinholes work best on small things. Sensitivity for pinhole cameras is garbage.

Converging Hole Collimator (Cone Beam): Holes are close together on the object side and far apart on the crystal/camera side. **Magnifies WITHOUT inverting the image**.

Diverging Collimator: The opposite of converging. Holes are far apart on the object side, and close together on crystal/camera side. This **takes a large object and minimizes it**. The result is that you can image a large part of the body on a small crystal. So increased area, decreased sensitivity and resolution.

Collimator Type	
Parallel Hole	"The work horse." You want the collimator and detector as close as possible to the patient for the best spatial resolution (this is affected by distance). Sensitivity is NOT affected by distance.
Pinhole	Magnifies and inverts image - used for thyroids and other small parts. Large objects get distorted (front is magnified more than back). Sensitivity is garbage.
Converging	Magnifies without inverting
Diverging	Takes a large object and makes it small.

Resolution Pearls:

- An increase in object-to-collimator distance degrades the system spatial resolution. The practical application is patient positing.
- The closer the detector is to the patient, the better the resolution of the images.

Scintillation Crystal- Once the photon emerges from the collimator, it impacts on the crystal. The crystal is made of sodium iodine doped with thallium. The crystal has the property that when struck with a photon it produces a pulse of light.

The thicker the crystal the less photons will be wasted (just pass through). On this same principal, thin crystals will let more photons through (without generating light). Energy of the photons themselves also plays a similar role. Higher energy photons will pass right through the crystal (lower ones won't). A thicker crystal is obviously better for high energy photons. So why not just make all the crystals super thick? Apparently you sacrifice spatial resolution with a thick crystal, because with a thinner crystal the photomultiplier tubes can sit closer to the event and more accurately localize it.

- *Thick crystal = Better Sensitivity, But Worse Spatial Resolution*

- *Thin crystal = Better Spatial Resolution, but Worse Sensitivity*

Photomultiplier Tubes (PMT) – The PMTs detect the light and convert it into an electric signal or measurable magnitude. The more PMTs you have, the more light you pick up and the greater the resolution. The PMTs record two things: (a) location – on x and y axis, and (b) signal intensity "Z." The X and Y coordinates go straight to the computer. The Signal Intensity (Z) goes to this gadget called a pulse height analyzer (discussed next).

Pulse Height Analyzer – The function of this thing is to discard background crap, and only look at the photons from the tracer you are looking for. The background crap can come from multiple sources (compton scatter, iodine escape from the crystal itself, backscatter).

The texts make a point in distinguishing the difference of background from a point source versus background from a person. Basically you should know that the Compton scatter in a person is a lot closer to the energy you want to image, but really degrades the images.

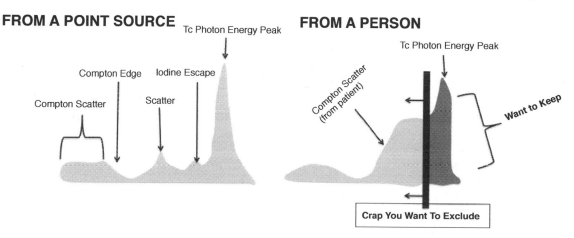

You can set a window that will exclude all that crap higher or lower to the desired peak. Some cameras allow you to record multiple peaks (great for things like ^{67}Ga and ^{111}In which have multiple peaks or dual tracer studies).

Key Concept: "Downscatter"- There is a thing called downscatter, which is super super high yield. Essentially high energy photons can spill into the window of a low energy emitter, mainly resulting from Compton scatter effects.

Example 1: You are doing a V/Q scan using ^{133}Xe and ^{99m}Tc. Xe has an energy of 81keV, whereas Tc has an energy of 140keV. The Tc Compton scatter is gonna range down from about 135 to 90 (as in the above diagram "from a person"). So if you inject the Tc first and image that will turn out just fine. But when you give the patient the Xe they will still have the Tc on board so you will be getting Xe peaks at 81, with a bunch of Tc Compton scatter all over it. So you totally hosed yourself, because the Pulse Height Analyzer can't tell what is Compton scatter from the Tc and what is signal from the Xe. The solution is to image with the Xe first, because the 81 keV and downstream Compton effects from the Xe would not affect the peak at Tc (140) at all. Hopefully that makes sense. Otherwise just remember, **LOWER PHOTON ENERGY TRACERS MUST BE USED FIRST.**

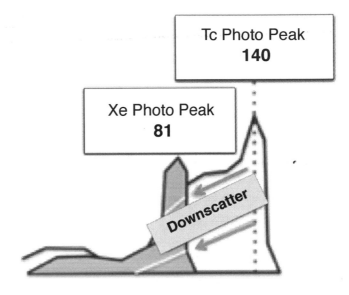

Example 2: If you are using ^{99m}Tc and ^{67}Ga for a bone scan of the spine looking for osteomyelitis. Gallium has a bunch of photopeaks (93, 184, 300, 393) and an effective half life of 50 hours. You have to give the Tc first and image, otherwise you'd end up waiting 50 hours.

SPECT and Matrix:

Gamma camera imaging can be "static" or "dynamic." When improved spatial resolution is needed "SPECT" can be performed by rotating a camera 180 or 360 degrees around the patient. The longer you image on SPECT the better it looks, but patients just can't hold still forever – and movement degrades the images. Another thing to consider is matrix size.

Matrix size: Size matters in most things in life, matrix being no different. A matrix size of 128x128 has superior resolution to 64x64. However, a larger matrix size means longer acquisition time (which patients hate), and reduced count density per pixel (which impacts image contrast)

Star Artifact:

If you have very focal intense energy you can sometimes see a star artifact, **caused by septal penetration of the hexagonal collimator holes.** This is typically seen in the thyroid bed after a high therapeutic dose (using a medium energy collimator, instead of high).

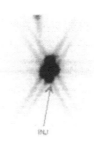
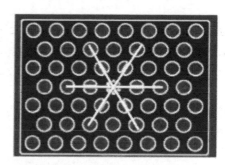

Star Artifact - From Septal Penetration
Star Pattern is seen if collimator holes are arranges in a hexagonal pattern

Quality Control for Gamma Cameras

Possibly the most dreaded portion of radiology multiple choice exams (*right up there with safety, and mammo MQSA*). Daily, weekly, and quarterly tests are done on the camera (*BY A TECH! NOT A RADIOLOGIST!!!*) to make sure it's functioning properly. Four parameters are usually tested for: field uniformity, window setting, image linearity and spatial resolution, and Center of Rotation (COR).

Field Uniformity: So the photo multiplier tubes can have subtle variability in what voltage they assign to a given photon of light. Additionally, the crystal isn't totally uniform, and has subtle variations in thickness. For exam purposes, you want to try and keep these two things as uniform as possible. A 2%-5% non-uniformity is allowed (1% if SPECT).

The **test is known as a "Flood", and is used to see if the camera can produce a uniform image along the entire crystal surface**. It's done two ways: (1) extrinsically (with a collimator), and (2) intrinsically (with NO collimator). You can use either a $Na^{99m}TcO_4$ source or a Co^{57} source to perform the flood. The **recommended counts for both extrinsic and intrinsic range somewhere between 5-10 Million** (*Siemens recommends 10 Million*).

- Extrinsic (WITH Collimator) – is done daily. This tests the collimator and crystals.

- Intrinsic (WITHOUT Collimator) – is done weekly.

A computer will check to make sure the field is uniform. You can also visually inspect the test images, to see if there is an obvious problem like a bunch of bullseyes, or a segmental region of failed PMTs.

Normal
-"Flood" - For Field

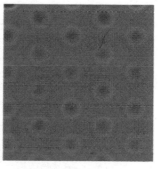

Bull's Eye
Appearance of Tubes
Indicates a Problem

Energy Window: The correct window needs to be used prior to each study, therefore this test **should be performed daily**. The most common approach to testing this is to use a symmetric window centered at the peak energy used in the imaging test. The source can be a syringe, a vial, or if absolutely necessary the patient. For Tc you would use a 20% window centered at 140keV.

Image Linearity and Spatial Resolution: Lead bar phantoms with parallel lines, placed between the collimator and a ^{57}Co sheet, are used to test image resolution and linearity. This only needs to be **done weekly**. Resolution is defined by the ability to differentiate between two distinct points (can you tell the bars are separate). Linearity is tested by looking to see if all the bars are straight (some distortion at the edges is ok). The bars should NOT look wavy.

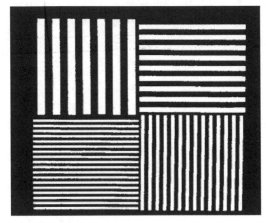

Bar Phantom
– Lines should be straight (not wavy)

Center of Rotation: Gamma cameras that are used for SPECT have to be routinely monitored for alignment offset at the COR (Center of Rotation). The test is **done with** 5 small ^{99m}Tc **point sources** along the axis of rotation. The **axis should be straight**, with minimal deviation. This is **performed weekly**.

Lead Aprons / Film Badges / Ring Badges

Why don't nuclear medicine techs were lead?

Two reasons: (1) Thin lead doesn't stop gamma rays. To stop them it would have to be so heavy you couldn't move. (2) When high energy gamma rays collide with a dense material that is not thick enough to stop them (lead apron) they rapidly slow down and lose energy which turns them into deeply penetrating Bremsstrahlung x-rays – which actually makes the dose worse.

Correct Positioning on the Film Badge and Ring Badge
- *Film Badge:* Should be worn on the collar at the chest / neck level
- *Ring Badge:* Worn on **dominant hand, index finger, label in towards source *(usually this means towards the palm),* under a glove (to avoid contamination)**

Safety:

This is also an excruciating topic for Radiologists to learn about. As previously stated nukes is full of random trivia, and let's be honest academic nuclear medicine tends to attract eccentric personalities... and they are writing the questions.

Instruments:

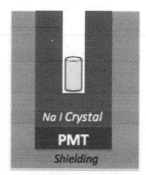

Well Counter

- **Sodium Iodine Well Counter** – This is basically a small gamma camera, with just one PMT. There is a hole in the block of NaI crystal into which the sample is placed (so it's surrounding the sample). So this gives you great efficiency in detection, but has a problem with being overwhelmed. If the sample exceeds 5000 counts per second (a lot less than a micro curie), it will be under reported. It's good for in-vitro blood or urine samples. It's good for "wipe test" samples.

- **Thyroid Probe** – This is a modified version of the NaI well counter. Its primary use is to calculate thyroid uptake values. The device has shielding, with a small opening that is pointed at the patient, at a precise distance. Dose is compared to a calibrated capsule of the same radionuclide.

- **Geiger –Muller Counter** – this is a device used to detect small amounts of radioactive contamination. The device has a gas filled chamber, which when it comes in contact with radiation becomes ionized and creates some voltage between a cathode and an anode - lots of beeping and clicking occurs. There are two ways that questions about this device are classically asked; (1) by just showing you a picture of one and saying "what is this", (2) by testing the concept of **"dead time."**

  What is this "dead time" ? Although the device is very sensitive, it is also vulnerable to being overloaded by a large dose of radiation. Then you have **"dead time"** as the ionization must dissipate before it can respond again. **The maximum dose it can handle is about 100mR/h.** So if the device clicks once and stops it might be because of "dead time" (it might also be "dead time" for you).

  Trivia - The GM Counter can NOT provide info on radiation type

- **Ion Chamber** – This is what is **used when higher doses are expected**. You don't have the dead time problem, for reasons that don't matter. Ion chambers can be used to detect exposure rates from **0.1 to 100R/h** (*note the unit change*). The dose calibrator used in most nuclear medicine departments is actually an ionizing chamber.

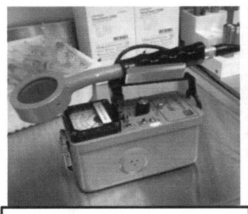 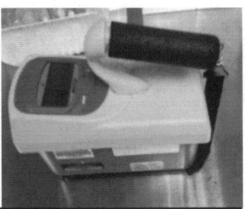

Geiger Muller
- With pancake probe
– Detects ionizing radiation
(alpha, beta, and gamma)

Ion Chamber
– For measuring dose rate
- Used with higher rates

Geiger - Muller Counter	Ionizing Chamber
Very Sensitive	Lower Sensitivity
Great for Low-Level Radioactive Survey	Stable across a wide voltage range - Excellent for accurate estimates (or exposure).
Terrible for Very High Radiation Fields ("Dead Time")	

Device	Trivia
Personal Dosimeters	*"Pocket Ionization Detector"* - uses a miniature ionization chamber. They give you real-time estimated dose, but must be charged and zero'd prior to use. These are not used anymore - which makes them high yield. *"Solid State Dosimeter"* - Accumulated dose or rate can be read real time with LCD display. *"Film Badge"* - Uses a thin metallic filter with a radiosensitive film. The degree of darkening (relative optic density) corresponds with dose. They can be damaged by temperature, humidity, etc... *"Optically Stimulated Dosimeter"* - Replaced the film badge. Chips / Strips are placed under a filter. *"Thermo-luminescent Dosimeter"* - The ring badge. Should be worn under a glove, with the label facing the palm (target).
Survey Meters	G-M and Ionization Detectors - discussed above
Well Counter	Basically a small gamma camera, with one PMT. Susceptible to "dead time" at counts over 5000 per second. Good for urine and blood samples. Good for "wipe test" samples.
Dose Calibration and Automated Dose Injection Systems	Used to measure radiopharmaceuticals.
Thyroid Uptake Probe	Compares counts from region over the thyroid to a calibrated capsule of the same radionuclide. The probe is a cylindrical scintillator detector attached to a PMT. A positioning guide keeps the distance constant
Intra-operative Probes	Used for lymphoscintigraphy

Q/A on the Dose Calibrator (Ionizing Chamber): Readout of activity is made in mCi. The range of most devices is 30 microCi to 2 Ci. Dose **should be within 5% of computed activity**, and this **should be checked daily**.

- *Consistency* – should be within 5% of computed activity. Checked with reference sources (checked **Daily**)

- *Linearity* – accurate readout for activities over the whole range of potentially encountered activities – checked with a large activity of Tc (around 200mCi) and decaying it down to less than the smallest activity you would measure for use. Or – the easy way – use a Calicheck© or Lineator© kit (which contains sheets of varied thickness of lead, simulating decay over time). (checked **quarterly**).

- *Accuracy* – Standard measurements of radiotracers measured and compared to what the activity should be (performed **at installation of the device and annually**). ·

- *Geometry* – Correction for different positioning and size (different volumes of liquids) of the sample (performed at **installation and any time you move the device**)

Regulations:

No bureaucracy is complete without lots of rules and regulations (and of course agencies to police such regulations). The Code of Federal Regulations (CFR) is where you will want to look for all your rules and regulations. Specifically part 19 (inspections), part 20 (radiation protection), and part 35 (human use of radioisotopes) . The "NRC" is the governing body that has been charged with the task of enforcing all these various directives. It is possible for individual states to reach an agreement with the Federal Government to enforce these rules on their own. These are called **"Agreement States"**, and the main thing to know is that **they can be more strict, but not less strict than the national agency.**

Radiation Safety / Contamination

Accidents happen. Rules to know for answering questions about spills:
First Things First – is it a MAJOR spill or a MINOR spill ? **(HIGH YIELD SECTION)**

Major Spills
- Activity level greater than **100 mCi of Tc-99m** is considered a major spill.
- Activity level greater than **100 mCi of Tl-201** is considered a major spill.
- Activity level greater than **10 mCi of In-111,** is considered to represent a major spill. ·
- Activity level greater than **10 mCi of Ga-67,** is considered to represent a major spill.
- Activity level greater than **1 mCi of I-131** is considered to constitute a major spill.

Radiation Safety Officer needs to be notified immediately when a major spill occurs, to direct the decontamination process.

Minor Spill = You Clean It Up
Major Spill = Don't Clean it Up, Call the Radiation Safety Officer

Minor Spills

(1) **Protect the Patient:** If a spill occurs while a patient is in distress, address the patient first. Once he/she is stable then address the spill.

(2) **Confine the Spill / Limit the Spread:** Secure the area and make sure people aren't tracking it all over the place.

(3) **Clean Up the Spill:** Use gloves (wear shoes), and all other personal protective equipment including a radiation badge. If possible tongs or forceps are even better for grabbing stuff. Use a damp absorbent material to clean the spill (working from the outside to the center).

(4) **Survey Cleanup Items:** Anything used in the clean up needs to be surveyed or presumed contaminated (held until they decay to safe levels – rule is 10 half lives).

(5) **Survey Cleanup People:** People also need to be surveyed by the radiation safety officer (in a different area – to avoid count interference).

Major Spill – what do I do ???

1. Clear area.
2. Cover spill with absorbent paper. **Do NOT clean it up.**
3. Clearly indicate boundaries of spill area. Limit movement of contaminated persons
4. Shield source if possible
5. Notify the Radiation Safety Officer immediately
6. Decontaminate persons

What ifs:

- *What if it gets on my clothes ? Take them off – they are contaminated. Clothes will be held by the RSO until activity has decayed to safe levels.*
- *What if it gets on my skin ? Wash with soap and water (don't scrub so hard you break your skin).*
- *What if there is a Xenon leak?*
    - Without alarming the patient, instruct all individuals to leave room as quickly as possible. Close the door.
    - Testable Trivia = The wipe test does NOT work on xenon contamination.

Obviously it is best if the Radiation Safety Officer (RSO) is involved and doing all that stuff. In the real world that is what will happen. But the ABR feels that on an intermediate level test you should be able to perform the tasks of doctor, tech, radiation safety officer, and janitor (while receiving the salary equivalent of the janitor).

Regulations Affecting the General Public

Regulations demand the following:
- Annual Dose limit of 100mrem to the public
- Not greater than 2mrem per hour – in an "unrestricted area"
- "Restricted Area" = Any place that receives a dose greater than 2 mrem/h

Signs must be placed with the following slogans:
- *Radiation Area:* Any place you could get 0.005 rem (0.05mSv) in 1 hour at 30cm
- *High Radiation Area:* Any place you could get 0.1rem (1mSv) in 1 hour at 30cm
- *Very High Radiation Area:* Any place you could get 500 rads (5 gray) in 1 hour at 1 meter

Occupational Exposure Dose Limits

The following are the rules:
- Total Body Dose per Year = 5 rem (50 mSv)
- Dose to the Ocular Lens per year = 2 rem (20mSv)
- Total equivalent organ dose (skin is also an organ) per year = 50 rem (500mSv)
- Total equivalent extremity dose per year = 50 rem (500mSv)
- Total Dose to Embryo/fetus over entire 9 months – 0.5rem (5mSv)

> **Unit Mischief - Expect Fuckery**
>
> 1 rad = 1 rem, 1 rad = 0.01 Gy
> 1mSv = 100 mrem = 0.1 rem

NRC Trivia:
- 10 CFR part 19: Notices, instructions, and reports to workers.
- 10 CFR part 20: Standards for protection against radiation.
- 10 CFR part 35: Medical use of by-product material.

Recordable and Reportable Events

The dose you order should be the dose the patient gets (sorta). The limit is 20% from the dose via the NRC (and 10% in some agreement states). You want to be a Radiologist? You better get your vocab straight on this stuff. Bean counters take this stuff pretty seriously:

When does **a medical event** occur??? Well you have to meet two criteria:
- (1) You have to "F" it up:
    - Wrong drug, Wrong route, Wrong patient, or Wrong dose (more than 20%).
    - OR Patient receives a dose to a part of the body other than the intended treatment site that exceeds by 50% or more the dose expected by proper administration and prescription
- (2) You have to harm the patient
    - Defined as either: (a) whole body dose > 5 rem, or (b) single organ dose > 50 rem

Watch out for unit fuckery: 5 rem = 0.05 Sv = 50mSv

Recordable Event	Diagnostic Medical Event
Whole Body Dose < 5 rem	Whole Body Dose > 5 rem
Single Organ Dose < 50 rem	Single Organ Dose > 50 rem

Medical Events require you to call the doctor who ordered it, patient, and NRC/State and explain what happen and if anything needs to be done about it.

Recordable events have to be documented (recorded) and kept for safe keeping – for 3 years.

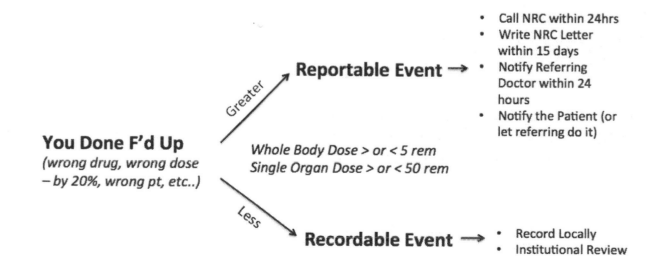

You Done F'd Up
(wrong drug, wrong dose – by 20%, wrong pt, etc..)

Greater → **Reportable Event** →
- Call NRC within 24hrs
- Write NRC Letter within 15 days
- Notify Referring Doctor within 24 hours
- Notify the Patient (or let referring do it)

Whole Body Dose > or < 5 rem
Single Organ Dose > or < 50 rem

Less → **Recordable Event** →
- Record Locally
- Institutional Review

Receiving, Storing, and Disposing of Radioactive Material

Within 3 hours of receipt (3 working hours) you (the tech) has to survey packages when they arrive. This process involves a GM counter test at the surface and 1 meter from the package, as well as wipes of all surfaces of the package (>6600 dpm/300 cm2 is not allowed). Keep the package in a controlled area, like the hot lab (just in case Al Qaeda invades your hospital). Contact shipper and the NRC if beyond allowable limits.

Package labels and allowable limits
White 1: No special handling, surface dose rate < 0.5 mrem/hr, 1 meter 0 mrem/hr
Yellow 2: Special handling required, surface dose rate < 50 mrmem/hr, 1 meter < 1 mrem/hr
Yellow 3: Special handling required, surface dose rate < 200 mrem/hr, 1 meter < 10 mrem/hr
these assholes couldn't pick another color? - instead they choose "yellow 3"

"Transport Index" – "T.I." – This is the measured max dose at 1 meter. This is an actual dose rate measured at 1 meter (not an allowable dose rate), at the time of shipping.

- *Radioactive Label 1:* White 1 – There is no T.I. because the rate at 1 meter will be so low.

- *Radioactive Label 2:* Yellow 2 – The T.I. is < 1.0 mR per hour.

- *Radioactive Label 3:* Yellow 3 – The T.I. is > 1.0 mR per hour.

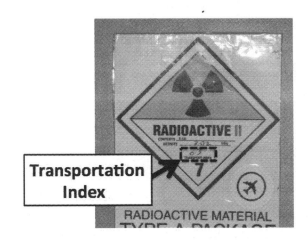

Transportation Index

Trivia:
5 mRem/hr (0.05mSv) is a "Radiation Area" and 100 mRem/hr = "High Radiation" Area

"Common Carriers" – A truck that carries regular packages and radioactive material the T.I. should not exceed 10 mR / per hour. The surface rate should not be more than 200mRem.

"Multiple Packages" – Those shipped together; the sum should NOT exceed 50 mR.

--- *(switching gears gracefully)* ---

Tc-99

I now want to transition into discussing Tc-99. It's the workhorse of nuclear medicine, and its production / purity is likely high yield for multiple choice.

First let's talk about talk about how Tc is made.

Step 1 _^{99}Mo / ^{99M}Tc Generation_

Because Molybdenum's half life is longer than Tc _(Mo = 67 hours, Tc = 6 hours)_, it can be made and shipped in a Tc generator. Mo adheres to the aluminum column tightly. As it decays it does not stick as tightly and can be washed off with saline across the column. When it comes out the Tc is stuck to Na ($Na^{99m}TcO_4$). The piece of trivia to know, is that it's in a +7 valence state, and must be reduced to be used. This is accomplished with stannous ions.

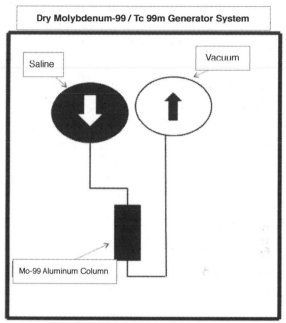

Dry Molybdenum-99 / Tc 99m Generator System

Saline — Vacuum — Mo-99 Aluminum Column

Step 2: _Radionuclide Purity_

You want to make sure you just have Tc, and you didn't wash any Mo off as well. Mo that is in the sample is called _"break through."_ The basis for the test is to look for the different photo peaks of the radionuclides. The sample is placed behind a lead shield. Mo is assayed for first. The basis of the test is that the high energy photons of Mo (like 740 keV) will NOT be attenuated by the shield, but the 140 keV Tc photons will be.

- NRC allows **no more than 0.15 micro Ci of Mo per 1 milli Ci of Tc, at the time of administration**.

    - _Few pitfalls here: (1) note the unit change from micro to milli, (2) note the "time of administration"_

- _If ratio is less than 0.038 at the time of elution, the material will be suitable for injection for a least 12 hours._

Step 3: _Chemical Purity_

Remember that the column is made of Aluminum Oxide, and that can wash off, clump up with the Tc and show up as liver activity, or cause sulfur colloid aggregation and show up in the lungs on liver spleen scan. **The test for purity is performed with pH paper. The allowed amount is < 10 microgram Al per 1 ml**

Step 4: _Radiochemical Purity_

As mentioned above Tc comes out of the generator as $Na^{99m}TcO_4$. So, to use it for anything useful it needs to be reduced (accomplished by adding it to $SnCl_2$). Thin layer chromatography is used to assess for purity.

Limits for Free Tc
- _95% $Na^{99m}TcO_4$_
- _92% for ^{99m}Tc sulfur colloid (MAA)_
- _91% for all other Tc radiopharmaceuticals_

Some Sneaky Sinister Stuff:

They can ask questions in a variety of ways about this stuff but here are a couple of key points:
- When you check the radiochemical Purity of 99mTc-MAA you are checking for free pertechnetate
- Testing for Chemical Purity is NOT mandatory in NRC States
- The 99Mo and 99mTc ratio must be known at **the time of ADMINISTRATION**, not elution
- When you are checking for Radionuclide Purity (breakthrough Mo), you have **to assay for Mo FIRST**, before the Tc (to prevent issues with residual charge).
- Technically ^{99m}Tc made in a generator is not considered carrier free because of the presence of ^{99}Tc which is technically a radionuclide (but essentially stable since it's half life is 200,000 years).

Free Tc

Free Tc can occur from a lack of stannous ions (reducing agents), or accidental air injection into the vial or syringe (which oxidizes). The way it's shown on images is Tc scan with **gastric uptake, salivary glands, and thyroid.**

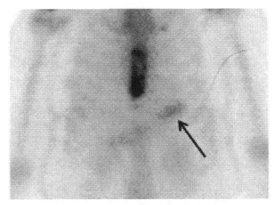

Free Tc: - Gastric Uptake on bone scan
*incidental note of sternal met from breast ca

Vocab	What is it?	Tested?	Limit?
Radionuclide Purity	How much Mo in the Tc ?	Tested in a dose calibrator with lead shields;	0.15 microcuries of Mo per 1 millicurie of Tc
Chemical Purity	How much Al in the Tc ?	Tested with pH paper	< 10 micrograms Al per 1ml
Radiochemical Purity	How much Free Tc?	Tested with Thin Layer Chromotography	• 95% $Na^{99m}TcO_4$ • 92% for ^{99m}Tc sulfur colloid (MAA) • 91% for all other Tc radiopharmaceuticals

Equilibria

Equilibrium: Concentration of parent and daughter isotopes are equal.

Transient Equilibrium: This type of equilibrium occurs when the half life of the daughter is shorter than the parent (but not by a lot). The **classic example is the Moly-99 generator making Tc-99**. A transient equilibrium occurs after 4 half lives (usually).

Secular Equilibrium: This type of equilibrium occurs when the half life of the daughter is way way way shorter than the parent.

Critical Organ

I want to define two frequently used terms:

- *"Critical Organ"* – An organ that limits the dose of the radiopharmaceutical due to the increased susceptibility of the critical organ for cancer. This may or may not be the "Target Organ."

- *"Target Organ"*- This is the organ you want the tracer to accumulate in. It's your organ of interest.

A few **generalizations on Critical Organs:** If you are trying to figure it out, it's the organ that the tracer is going to spend the most time in. For example Gallium ends up in the bowel. Tc RBC scans are going to end up passing through the heart a lot, unless they are heat treated then the spleen eats them. Tc-MAG3s and DTPA is going to be the bladder, but **DMSA (which sticks to the kidney) is going to be the kidney**. For anything that uses free Tc (meckels scan), it's going to be the thyroid. MIBG scans are going to hit the bladder (or thyroid if it's not blocked).

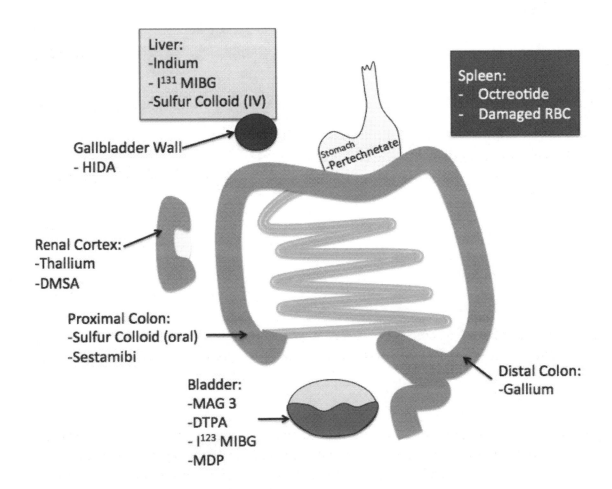

SPECT

SPECT provides a 3D look at isotopes in the body. SPECT uses a mounted parallel hole collimator that rotates around the patient. Each projection takes like 30 seconds and the total scan is around 15 mins. The matrix size is usually around 128 x 128 (for things that are not cardiac). The scan uses iterative reconstruction to make a picture. Because the data is isotropic volume, reconstruction in 3 planes is possible. Sensitivity is depth dependent, with radiation from different tissue origins attenuated to different degrees. Special collimators with longer holes are used to help improve the collection of photons.

Testable Point: The big advantage SPECT has over planar is improved contrast from overlapping structures.

Testable Point: SPECT is depth dependent (PET is not).

Tuning Fork Artifact: Cardiac SPECT uses a 180 orbit. When a point source is imaged, it should look like a point source. If there is an error with the center of rotation (misregistration error) then is will look like a tuning fork (two lines in one direction and one line in the other). The same appearance can be seen with motion.

PET

As mentioned previously beta plus decay results in a proton being "transformed" into a neutron. This transformation requires *1.02MeV for this to occur.* A positron is then emitted which travels a short distance before colliding into a real electron, whereupon the electron and positron destroy one another. The mutual destruction emits **two 511 keV photons which come out 180 degrees apart**.

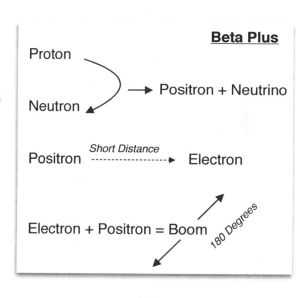

Detector System:

You can't use the normal NaI crystals for a 511 keV energy photon, they aren't strong enough. Instead Lutetium Oxyorthosilicate (LSO) and Gadolinium oxyorthosilicate (GSO) are used.

Coincidence Timing:

The positrons shoot out in opposite directions (180 degrees) and collide on the detector at the same time. If they don't land at the same time (within nanoseconds) they are not counted. This is called "*coincidence timing.*" This provides a type of virtual electronic collimation - giving PET an advantage over SPECT (which uses parallel hole collimators).

Spatial Resolution:

Spatial resolution in PET depends on (1) detector resolution and (2) positron range / angulation. Range is determined by photon energy and is characteristic of what they came from (F^{18} is 2.8mm, C^{11} is 3.8mm). Scatter and random coincidences cause degradation of image quality.

Scatter - There are three types of events detected by a PET scanner: (1) True, (2) Scattered, and (3) Random.

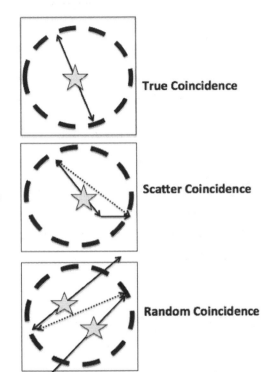

True Coincidence - Two 511 photons resulting from an annihilation reaction are detected in the same coincident window.

Scatter Coincidence - One of the photons has a compton interaction and is deflected, but still hits the detector within the coincident time window (just not in the calculated location).

Random Coincidence: Two photons, from different annihilation reactions just so happen to land within the same coincident window - creating the false calculation that they occurred from the same event.

Rejecting Scatter:

As mentioned above, you can reject scatter based on the incident time on the detector. Another way you can also reject scatter is based on photon energy. In the perfect world, both photons should measure 511. If the photon undergoes scatter it will lose energy, so you can exclude scatter by saying you will only keep a photon at 510 kev or above. However, if you exclude things that are just barely off of the 511 mark you will exclude a ton of true events as well. So, it turns into a balance of sensitivity and specificity. A tighter window gives you a more specific exam, but you are going to lose a lot of normal counts (and decrease your sensitivity). The opposite is obviously true as well.

2D vs 3D PET:

The modern scanners are "3D" and use the incident time to exclude scatter. Older scanners are "2D" and use septa to deal with scatter. This is the main difference, and only thing I can imagine could be tested.

Time of Flight PET
By measuring the difference in arrival times between the two photons from an annihilation event, a Time of Flight image can be created. TOF *can enhance spatial resolution and image contrast.*

Attenuation Correction:

The CT part of PET-CT is performed for two main reasons: (1) so that you can see where things are and (2) for attenuation correction.

Attenuation correction is a correction for the different levels of attenuation a photon might undergo as it tries to get out of the body to the detector. Think about traveling through bone vs traveling through lung. The classic trick is the pacemaker (metal) making something appear really really hot – when attenuation is corrected for. This is why you always look at the uncorrected data, when reading a PET.

Which one is the uncorrected?

A sneaky trick is to ask you to distinguish between corrected and uncorrected PET. The secret is to look at (1) the skin – which will be hot on uncorrected, and (2) the lungs – which will also be hot on uncorrected.

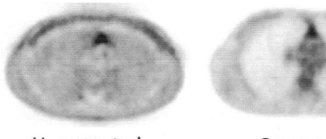

Uncorrected
- Dark Skin
- Dark Lungs

Corrected
- Light Skin
- Light Lungs

Testable Point: Attenuation in PET is depth independent.

Calculation of Standard Uptake Value (SUV):

SUVs are not like H.U. (calibrated to water). There are multiple factors which go into the calculation of the SUVs, and essentially make it highly variable from institution to institution and even patient to patient.

The calculation is this:

$$SUV = \frac{\text{Tissue Radioactivity Concentration at Time Point 1 x Patient Weight}}{\text{injected dose activity}}$$

Fat vs Skinny: Fat has a low FDG uptake. So, it's actually more accurate to use the patients lean body mass instead of weight (this is why the value is different from patient to patient). **SUVs in fat people are overestimated** (there is more sugar around for the tumor) – this can be corrected for my using lean body mass.

Timing: The longer you wait between FDG administration and imaging the more FDG uptake you get. At first the uptake of FDG in the tumor is rapid (rapid in first 2 hours), then it goes up slower. In other words, if you did "delays" you would get higher FDG values. Another point is that if scan (1) is done after an hour, and scan (2) is done after 2 hours, then scan 2 will falsely appear to have increased SUV. Basically, you need to do the scan at the same time interval after FDG administration if you want to compare apples to apples.

Glucose Levels: This is one of those competitive kinetics things. The more non-labeled glucose is floating around, the less FDG the tumor can drink. **High glucose = Lower SUV.**

Size Matters: There is a size threshold for PET (usually 1cm). Anything smaller than 1cm, will be subjected to partial volume effects, and give a false low SUV. **Smaller than 1cm = Lower SUV.**

Dose Extravasation: FDG is given IV (most things are – except xenon you breath and Iodine you eat). If you put all your FDG in the soft tissues of the arm, you have less circulating and get lower SUV. **Dose Extravasation = Lower SUV.**

Reconstruction Type: Iterative reconstruction can mess with the SUVs. The more iterations the higher the SUV.

Attenuation Correction: Attenuation correction with CT, also makes an adjustment for SUVs (the positrons have to go through denser stuff too). The method used for the computer to calculate attenuation correction also varies and can make comparing SUVs difficult.

Truncation Artifact:

This has to do with differences in FOV from PET and CT. The classic example is a giant monster fat person who is so fat that they have several feet of blubber outside the FOV (and therefore not providing data for attenuation correction). Bottom line = Giant Fat People can have artificially lower SUV…. Although the presence of fat may elevate SUV (as described above). So, maybe it will cancel out and be normal. **Just say Truncation Artifact = Falsely Lower SUV.**

Pre FDG PET prep:

Diet – Fasting for 4 hours prior to the test is the typical recommendation. If they just ate, they will spike their insulin and drive all the FDG into their muscles. Minimizing cardiac activity (you might want to do if you have a thoracic cancer) can be done with a 12 hour fast, and a low carb/ high protein & fat diet for 24 hours.

Hydration – Oral hydration, and frequent voiding decreases the dose to the bladder and improves urinary visualization.

Muscle Uptake – There are a couple of causes for diffuse muscle uptake; exercise (most places discourage this for 24-48 hours prior to the exam), eating or insulin use. More focal uptake (classic forearms from stress gripping) can also be seen.

Insulin – If you have to have insulin, long acting insulins are better to avoid diffuse muscle uptake. Metformin is ok – it won't mess with the muscles.

Brown Fat – Excessive brown fat uptake can be distracting. You can decrease it by (1) making the room warm, (2) giving drugs – with the big two being propranolol and diazepam (valium).

PET QA

Just like there is QA on all the other pieces of equipment in nuclear medicine, PET also has a whole bunch of QA. I've chosen two QA tests which I think are the most high yield. I believe they are high yield because their names sound similar and that means they'd make good distractors for each other on multiple choice.

Normalization Scan - This corrects for discrepancies in the thousands of detector elements. You scan a calibrated position source placed *in the FOV*. The scan serves to "normalize" the detection lines. This should be done once a month ("N-M" Normal Month).

Blank Scan - This is done to help keep the attenuation correction data accurate. This is done with *nothing in the FOV*. You simply use the systems transmission radiation source. I think about this as "zeroing" the scanner, or setting it as a "blank slate." It's done daily (you want to start each day with a blank slate).

High Yield Summary Chart

Tracer	Analog	Energy	Physical Half Life
Tc – 99m		"Low" – 140	6 hours
Iodine -123	Iodine	"Low" – 159	13 hours
Xenon - 133		"Low" – 81	125 hours (biologic t1/2 30 seconds)
Thallium - 201	Potassium	"Low" – 135 (2%), 167 (8%), use 71 ^{201}Hg daughter x-rays	73 hours
Indium -111		"Medium" – 173 (89%), 247 (94%)	67 hours
Gallium - 67	Iron	Multiple; 93 (40%), 184 (20%), 300 (20%), 393 (5%)	78 hours
Iodine -131	Iodine	"High" - 365	8 days
Fluorine -18	Sugar	"High" - 511	110 mins

Treatment Radionuclides Half Life	
Strontium 89	50.5 DAYS (14 days in bone)
Samarium 153	46 Hours
Yttrium 90	64 Hours
Radium 223	11.4 DAYS

"Hell, I can get you a toe by 3 o'clock this afternoon..... with nail polish"

SECTION 9: MRI

Although you can use other types of atoms, for the most part Hydrogen atoms (the proton) are what is being manipulated with MRI. Your body is full of water and fat, and therefore full of lots of hydrogen atoms (protons) thats spins can be manipulated. Some people think about these protons as little tiny magnets.

How does MRI work?

The very basic answer is that you have a magnetic field - that is always on. Protons are normally randomly aligned, about half up and half down. When you stick someone in the magnet slightly more than half of them will align with the direction of the magnetic field. You can then slap them down with an RF pulse, and then watch how fast they bounce back up. The difference between how fast different protons bounce up is the "contrast" used to tell things apart - and make a pretty picture.

What is this "coordinate system" ?

Real quick basic point, is that when you see an arrow pointing up or down or sideways - this does not represent a single proton, but instead the addition of all the protons as a vector. Protons aligned in the direction of the external magnet field are called "longitudinal magnetization." This is the "default setting" when someone is in the magnet. If they are aligned perpendicular to the Z axis, then they are considered "transverse magnetization."

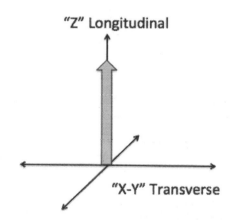

What is this "RF Pulse" ?

The RF pulse is a radio wave used to "knock the protons down." To do this it has to push them. Pushing protons that are spinning in a magnet is a lot like trying to push your 5 year old on a swing. You have to wait until he's swinging back at you and you push him as he is moving forward. In other words, you have to time it just right. Another way to think about this is if you wanted to hand someone something but they were running. You would need to run at the same speed as them to be able to hand it to them.

So how do you know how "fast to run" , or "when to push" ? There is this thing called the **Larmor Equation**.

$$\omega_0 = \gamma B_0$$

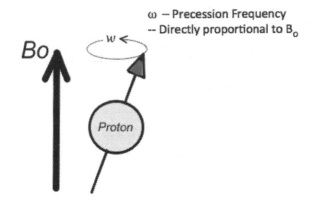

- ω_0 is the precession frequency
- B_0 is the external magnetic field strength given in Tesla.
- γ is a proportionality constant called the gyromagnetic ratio

The Larmor equation describes the precession frequency of a nuclear magnetic moment and resonant frequency of a nucleus, and relates these aspects to the magnetic field strength. It basically says the precession frequency gets higher as the field strength increases.

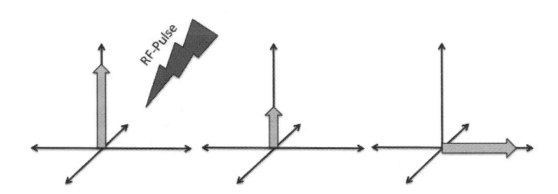

The RF pulse actually does two things: (1) it decreases the longitudinal magnetization, and (2) it causes the protons to synch up and precess in-phase (which establishes a transverse magnetization).

When can you measure signal?

Signal can only be measured when it is **NOT in the longitudinal direction.** If you are running next to someone at the same speed, you can't really measure how fast they are going (it's like an Einstein relativity thing). But, if they turn and run away from you, then you can measure that. It's sorta like that.

What is this T1?

After you knock the protons down with an RF pulse, they will grow back up to normal size (their spin magnitude will re-orient in the direction of Bo). The time it takes for this to happen is different in different tissues "called longitudinal relaxation".

Some people call this "spin-lattice relaxation" because energy from the RF pulse is handed over to the surrounding lattice. The "1" of T1 resembles a thermometer - which is useful in remembering that T1 relaxation involves the exchange of thermal energy.

Plotting the time vs longitudinal magnetization creates the T1 curve.

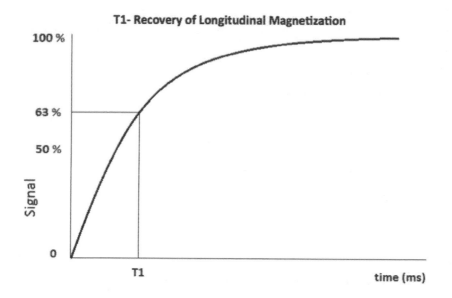

The return to longitudinal relaxation follows an exponential curve approaching 100% over time. T1 is defined as the time at which longitudinal magnetization is **63% of its final value**. Each tissue has a different T1 and the **greater the field strength the longer the T1** (because net magnetization is greater in a larger field).

Things with short T1 signals are bright. Hence the phrase "intrinsic T1 shortening" is something that is bright on T1. Things that have long T1s are dark.

Is T1 different in a stronger magnet? A stronger magnet makes T1 longer. Protons in this stronger magnetic field have more energy (they precess faster), and therefore it takes longer to hand that over to the lattice.

What is this T2?

Remember I said the RF pulse caused the protons to synch up and precess in phase (which establishes a transverse magnetization). As time progresses the protons will slowly fall out of synch and start doing their own thing again. This is the T2 Transverse relaxation.

Plotting the time vs transverse magnetization creates the T2 curve - which resembles the downward portion of a ski slope. I like this analogy because it helps me remember that T2 is shorter than T1 (takes less time to go down a hill than up it).

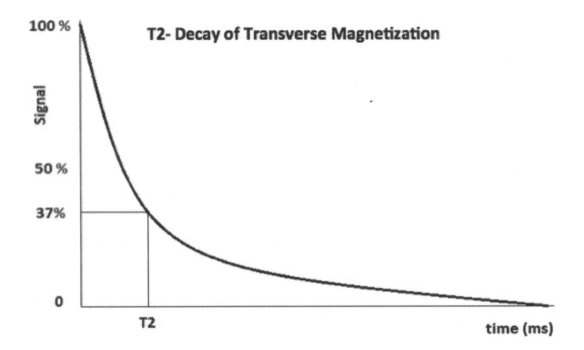

Transverse magnetization decay is also described by an exponential curve with T2 representing the time at which the signal has decayed to 37% of its original value of transverse magnetization (63% of it has decayed). Another term often used to describe T2 is "spin-spin relaxation."

What causes protons to lose their transverse sync (T2 relaxation) ?

There are two main reasons (1) inhomogeneities in the external field, and (2) inhomogeneities in the local magnetic filed - within the actual tissues. Pure things (water) with less inhomogeneities take longer to decay their transverse magnetization, and are therefore bright (the opposite is true of impure liquids).

T2 vs T2 ?*

The signal of T2 decays faster than various PhDs would predict based on tissue spin interactions alone. The reason for this is that math falsely assumes the main external field is absolutely homogeneous --- it is not. This heterogeneous field creates additional interaction which further speeds decay. It is because of this that **T2* decay is ALWAYS faster than T2.**

- T2* = Tissue Spin Interaction + Field Inhomogeneity; *"random + fixed causes"*
- T2 = Tissue Spin Interaction ; *"random causes only"*

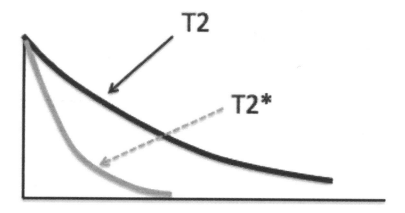

"Free Induction Decay" ? Without any magnetic gradient the received signal is called free induction decay.

Fixing T2 and making it T2 ?* At 1/2 the time of TE a 180 pulse can be given to refocus ("turn around") the signal which helps remove the fixed field Inhomogeneity.

What is this Proton Density?

If you choose a long TR and a short TE the difference in magnetization recovery and in signal decay between fat and water is essentially nothing. In this situation the contrast is the result of differences in proton density. Tissues with more protons will have high signal. Tissues with fewer protons will have low signal.

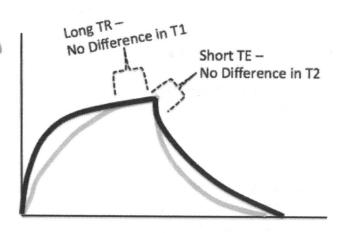

What is this TR ? Repetition time (TR) – is the time between the initiation of two successive RF pulses

What is this TE ? The time between the middle of the 90° RF pulse and the peak of the detected echo.

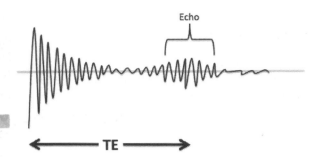

T1	T2	Proton Density
Short TR	Long TR	Long TR
Short TE	Long TE	Short TE

The Longer the TE, the Greater the T2 Effects.
MRCP has a very long TE

	Short TR	Long TR	Short TE	Long TE
Spin Echo	250-700 ms	>2000 ms	10-25 ms	>60 ms
GRadient Echo	< 50 ms	>100 ms	1-5 ms	>10 ms

What is this k-Space and Image Matrix ?

First let me introduce this thing called a "Fourier Transform." A fourier transform is a mathematical technique for converting data from the time domain to data in the frequency domain.

K-space is a Fourier plane (like an x-y axis coordinate system) in which MR signal is stored. Turning K-space into an image requires an inverse two dimensional Fourier Transform (lots of math... which computers are good at).

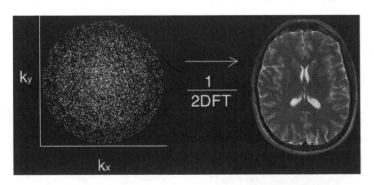

Testable Point:
- The center of K-space is made from the information about gross form and tissue contrast.
- The periphery of K-Space is made up of information about spatial resolution.

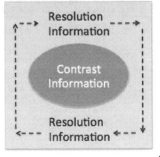

Spatial Encoding

Localization of signal requires three steps:
(1) Select the desired slice
(2) Encode spatial information along the rows
(3) Encode spatial information along the columns

This vs That
Gradient can be turned on or off.
Superconducting magnet is always on.

The localizing gradients have identical properties they are just applied at different times and different directions. Because you have three gradients in three planes you can localize anything in the body.

(1) Selecting the Desired Slice: The use of a slice selection gradient (SSG) is used to select the area of interest. This gradient is placed perpendicular to the desired slice plane. The slice selection gradient determines the view (axial, coronal, sagittal, even oblique).

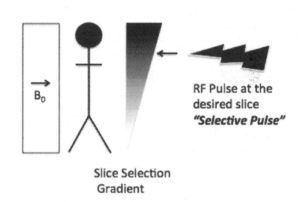

$\vec{B_0}$

RF Pulse at the desired slice
"Selective Pulse"

Slice Selection Gradient

Selective Pulse: On top of this gradient, an RF pulse is applied - at the same frequency as the protons in the slice plane you want to sample. That way only the protons in this plane will be affected. This pulse is called a selective pulse.

Dealing with the 180 degree refocusing pulse: In a spin echo sequence you apply a 180 RF pulse after your 90 degree pulse. Apparently this jacks up your nice field (especially along the edges). To deal with this, before and after the 180 degree RF you place two identical gradients (which cancel each other out) and correct for errors around the edges.

(2) Encoding Spatial Information in Vertical Direction (Phase Encoding): This is the second step in the process. This gradient is applied causing protons in the same row perpendicular to the gradient to have the same phase. All protons at this point will have the same frequency.

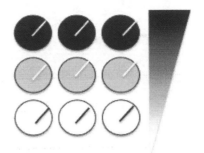

Phase Encoding Gradient

Phase encoding is much longer than frequency encoding - this is why it's done on the thinner portion. They don't want to lose time including the tip of the nose on phase encoding - this is why it's side to side in the head. The opposite is true in the abdomen, where it's front to back. Breast is an exception to this rule (I'll touch on that later).

Contribution to duration of study: The number of phase encoding steps contributes to the duration of a 2D imaging sequence.

Duration = TR x Npy x Nex

TR = Repetition Time
NPy = Number of phase encoding steps
Nex = Number of excitations

(3) Encoding Spatial Information in the horizontal direction (Frequency Encoding): This gradient is applied perpendicular to the phase-enc direction, which results in the modification of Larmor freqs over the duration of its application. The end result is column of protons which have identical frequencies.

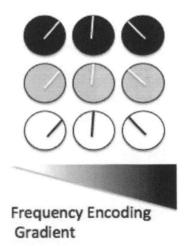

Testable Trivia: This is encoding gradient is applied at the same time as the readout.

Frequency Encoding Gradient

Lets walk through the Spin Echo Diagram to help solidify this process:

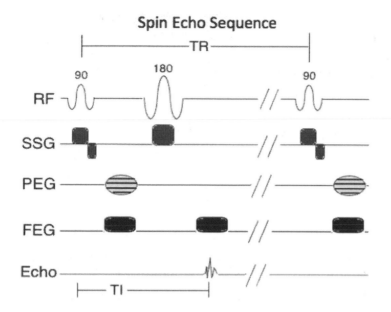

(1) Slice Selection: This SSG is applied the same time as the 90 degree RF pulse (called a selective pulse).

(2) Phase encoding and frequency encoding gradients are applied.

(3) Next a 180 refocusing RF pulse is given. Before and after this 180 pulse two identical SS gradient lobes are applied to help correct undesired spin on the edge of the slice.

(4) Lastly a second FEG is applied at the same time as the read out echo.

This process is repeated for as many phase encoding steps you do.

Slice Thickness:

Slice thickness is manipulated adjusting both the bandwidth of the selective pulse and the amplitude of the slice selection gradient.

Slice thickness is governed by the following equation:

$$\text{Slice Thickness} = \frac{\text{Transmitted RF Bandwidth}}{\text{Slice Selection Gradient x Some Random Constant}}$$

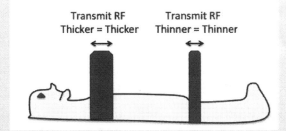

Transmit RF Bandwidth *- Increasing the transmit RF bandwidth gives you a thicker slice.*

Slice Selection Gradient - Decreasing the slice selection gradient gives you a thicker slice.

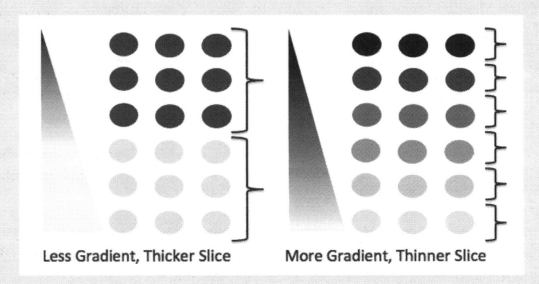

Less Gradient, Thicker Slice   More Gradient, Thinner Slice

"Less is More" - Using a narrower RF pulse bandwidth will take longer to excite, resulting in a longer scan time. Thinner Slices = Longer Study.

3D Spatial Encoding:

Pulse sequences are either two dimensional or three dimensional. The three dimensional ones acquire volume from multiple sections in a single acquisition.

Spatial Resolution and Other Image Characteristics

Factors affecting spatial resolution: Spatial resolution is governed by the size of a voxel. The voxel size is determined by the matrix, field of view, and slice thickness.

$$\textbf{Voxel} = \text{Slice Thickness} \times \left\{ \frac{FOV_{Phase}}{Matrix\ Size_{Phase}} \times \frac{FOV_{Read}}{Matrix\ Size_{Read}} \right\}$$

Field of View: The smaller the field of view the better the spatial resolution. So, why not make the FOV super super small? Because you will get aliasing or wrap around artifacts from signal outside the FOV.

Matrix Size: Unfortunately, no one can be told what the matrix is, you have to see it for yourself. OK, fine the matrix size corresponds to the image width and height (in pixels). The larger the matrix the smaller the pixels. (pixel = FOV / Matrix)

Gradient: A gradient with higher amplitude (more intense) or one applied for a longer period of time results in better spatial resolution. Makes sense since the point of a gradient is to localize stuff.

Slice Thickness: For a thicker slice you can either increase the Transmit RF pulse (the slice selection pulse) or you can decrease the slice selection gradient. For a thinner slice you would do the opposite. The thinner the slice, the better the spatial resolution.

Factors affecting signal to noise ratio (SNR): Noise is random variation in the signal that leads to its degradation. In MRI the primary source of this noise is the patient's body. Overall the SNR depends on voxel size (bigger is better), field strength, and some random sequence parameters.

Voxel Size: Anything that makes your voxel bigger improves your SNR (the opposite of spatial resolution).

- Thicker slices = Higher SNR
  - Increased Transmit RF Pulse
  - Decreased Slice Selection Gradient
- Larger FOV = More SNR
- Smaller Matrix = More SNR

Field Strength: A stronger field gets you more signal. Greater Field Strength = Greater SNR.

RF Coils: Smaller surface coils improve your signal (increased SNR) compared to a coil within the scanner.

Number of Excitations per Slice (number of averages): The more excitation you perform the more signal you get (increased SNR). The main trade off is a prolonged imaging time.

Longer TR, Shorter TE = Better SNR

Receiver Bandwidth: A fat bandwidth gives you a rapid sampling of data, a narrow bandwidth gives you slow sampling of data. Since noise is constant, the fatter band will pick up more noise. So, fat bandwidth = decrease SNR, narrow bandwidth = increased SNR.

Bigger Bandwidth isn't All Bad
As an aside, the larger receiver bandwidths allow for a higher frequency bandwidth per pixel which decreases mismatch artifacts like chemical shift or magnetic susceptibility.

Tradeoffs among spatial resolution, SNR, and acquisition time: In summary, each of these entities is affected by attempts to optimize the other.

For example, SNR can be increased by increasing field strength, but this increases tissue T1 times (and thus acquisition time). Spatial resolution can be increased by smaller voxel size, but this creates a noisier image.

Extremely High Yield Summary Table

Modification	Signal to Noise	Spatial Resolution	Duration of D...
Thicker Slices	Increased	Decreased	No effect
Larger Field of View	Increased	Decreased	No effect
Larger Matrix	Decreased	Increased	Increased
Greater Field Strength	Increased	No effect	No effect
Greater Receiver Bandwidth	Decreased	No effect	Decreased
More Excitations per Slice	Increased	No effect	Increased
Utilizing Partial K Space Sampling	Decreased	No effect	Decreased

MRI Sequences

There are a bunch of sequences, but two general categories:

- Spin Echo - which uses a 180 degree rephasing RF pulse
- Gradient Echo

Spin Echo:

Spin echo is composed of a 90 RF pulse followed by an 180 rephasing pulse. This rephasing pulse is done at 1/2 the time of echo (TE). The sequence is repeated (TR) until k space is filled.

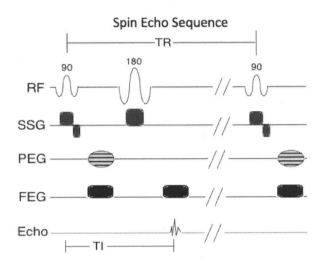

Why do you give this 180 pulse? In an ideal world the magnetic field is homogeneous, but we don't live in an ideal world. The pulse is **given to try and improve the heterogeneous nature of the field** and this is the reason spin echoes give us T2 and not T2*.

As discussed in the spatial encoding section, the slice selection gradient is applied with the 90 degree RF pulse. Then you have the Phase encoding and the frequency encoding gradients. The 180 degree pulse is flanked by self canceling slice selection gradients. Lastly the frequency encoding gradient fires again with the read out echo.

High Yield: *Duration = TR x Npy x Nex*

TR = Repetition Time
NPy = Number of phase encoding steps
Nex = Number of excitations

Contrast: The contrast on spin echo sequences is determined by the TR (interval between 90 degree RFs), and the TE (interval between the 90 degree RF and the receipt of the echo). As mentioned above, a short TE and TR gives you T1 weighting, long TE and TR gives you T2 weighting, and long TR & short TE produce a proton density sequence.

High Yield Fact: Because a line in k space is filled at each TR, the TR contributes to the duration of the sequence. So, much so that long TR times are the reason a true spin echo is of historic significance.

Fast Spin Echo

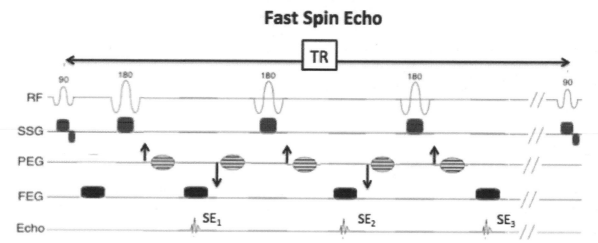

The idea behind the FSE sequence is to reduce the TR, which I already mentioned is a major contribution to the duration of the study. This is done by applying multiple 180 RF pulses each resulting in an echo.

Echo Train Length - Number of echoes in the same TR.

Fat Signal - There is a "normal" phenomenon called **"*J coupling*"** which occurs between the nuclei of lipid molecules, causing intrinsic shortening of T2 signal. The fast repetition of 180 degree pulses mess up the J couples and cause the T2 of fat to lengthen.

Testable Point: T2 fat signal is longer with fast spin echo (interferes with J coupling).

Testable Vocab: With each progressive echo train the transverse signal gradually decreases. This is called *"T2 Blurring"*

Testable Point: Acquisition time is approximately proportional to 1/ETL

Inversion Recovery

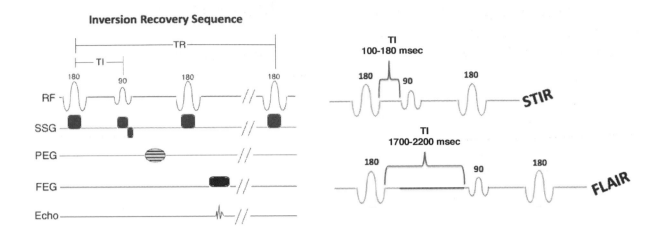

Inversion Recovery Sequence

This time instead of starting with a 90 degree RF pulse, you start with a 180 degree "preparation" pulse. You wait for the relaxation of the thing you want to saturate (water, fat, myocardium) to hit its null point then you slam it with the 90 degree pulse. This way that particular tissue gives no signal.

"TI" - The time between the 180 and 90 pulse.

"STIR" - Short T1 Inversion Recovery, employs a *short* TI (120 – 160 ms) to suppress fat, which is based on the T1 for fat. Often used on MSK imaging to suppress the fat within bone marrow to allow visualization of fluid (edema) within bone.

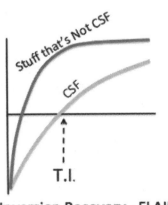

Inversion Recovery - FLAIR

"FLAIR" - Fluid Attenuated Inversion Recovery, employ a TI designed to suppress water signal (approximately 2000 ms). Frequently used in Neuro-imaging to suppress CSF signal (based on the T1 relaxation time of CSF) to allow visualization of edema or inflammation (i.e. in multiple sclerosis).

Testable Point: Relative to other fat suppression techniques - STIR is much less "susceptible" to magnetic susceptibility (metal) and field inhomogeneity

Testable Point: STIR can NOT be used with Gadolinium. Gd+ enhanced tissues have a similar TI as fat, so they may get totally nulled out.

GRE Sequences

Gradient echo sequences are different than spin echo sequences because they (1) use a flip angle less than 90 and (2) do NOT have a 180 pulse.

The advantage to this low flip angle is faster recovery, shorter TR/TE times, and a faster scan. The flip angle is used to determine how much transverse and how much longitudinal magnetization is going to be used.

Testable Point: Because there is no 180 pulse you are dealing with T2* (not T2). For the same reason GRE is more susceptible to susceptibility artifacts.

Gradient Echo

Testable Point: Gradient sequences have a lower Specific Absorption Rate (less heating).

If there is no 180 pulse, how do you create an echo? A bipolar readout gradient (basically a frequency encoding gradient) is used.

Vocab: An echo in gradient is called a "Field Echo"

If gradient is so fast and has a nice low SAR, why don't we use it for everything? The signal to noise ratio isn't that great. Plus, you get more susceptibility artifacts.

"Steady State" Because the TR is shortened in GRE you can get stuck with permanent residual transverse magnetization - where the magnetization never completely goes away. What is often the case is that the TR is shorter than the T1 and T2 of the tissues, so T2* dephasing dominates. The two main flavors in GRE imaging are classified depending on how this residual transverse magnetization is handled.

Spoiled (incoherent) GRE: Gradients and/or RF pulses are used to get rid of the transverse magnetization (T2) that is persisting in the steady state.

Refocused (coherent) GRE: The steady state is preserved by using a "Rewind gradient." Therefore these sequences are T2* weighted. These refocused sequences can be partial or full. An example of the full refocus is the SSFP (steady-state free precession) which is used in cardiac imaging to provide a fast sequence with high signal to noise.

> **Spoiled (Incoherent) = Basically T1**
> **Refocused (Coherent) = Basically T2**

Echo-Plannar Imaging (EPI) "The Noisy One"

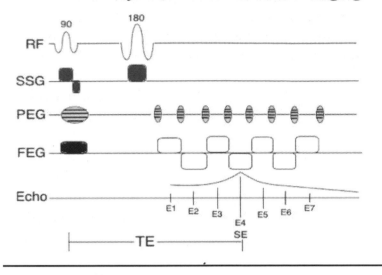

Spin-Echo – Echo Planar Imaging

EPI can be done with spin echo (90 + 180) or gradient echo (90 + a bunch of gradients). EPI is MRI's fastest acquisition method, on the order of 100 ms/slice. One RF pulse is used to acquire data for an image (aka single shot).

The sequence works by turning the phase encoding and frequency encoding gradients on and off very rapidly - causing a very fast filling of k space.

Compared to a regular GRE: The sequence is more vulnerable to magnetic susceptibility, gives you better tissue contrast, and is faster.

Artifacts linked to EPI:
- Magnetic Susceptibility - can be improved with segmented sequences (instead of single shots)
- Ghosting - Gradient imperfections mess with spatial encoding
- Chemical Shift - A narrow readout bandwidth is used. As mentioned before, a fat readout bandwidth improves chemical shift (lets a bigger range in), a narrow one does the opposite.

Testable Trivia:
- Echo-planar is the technique of choice for Diffusion Weighted Imaging
- Echo-planar is highly vulnerable to magnetic susceptibility (even more than normal gradient sequences)

Diffusion

The base sequence is either a fast GRE or an echo planar. Generally speaking, diffusion weighted imaging works by using two very strong and symmetric MR gradients. The acquisition is repeated in each of the 3 dimensions in space with b-factors of 0 and b-factors of 1000. The signal differences are based on mobility and direction of water.

Scenario 1 (no net movement): The first gradient fires dephasing the spins. The molecules do not move. The second gradient fires rephasing the same molecules - giving you high signal.

Scenario 2 (net movement): The first gradient fires dephasing the spins. The molecules move out of the way. The second gradient fires missing the original protons - gives you low signal.

Vocab: The direction of diffusion is described as isotropic (movement in all spatial directions) and anisotropic (movement in a single direction).

"B-Factor" - The higher the "B-Factor" the greater the diffusion weighting. The "factors" of a B-factors include amplitude, duration, and spacing.

ADC (Apparent Diffusion Coefficient); - As I'm sure you know an ADC is needed to read diffusion correctly. The ADC map is calculated by obtaining (a) set of images without a diffusion gradient - poor mans T2, and (b) set of images with the diffusion gradient. A negative logarithm of the ratios is performed. Low signal is true restriction, high signal is T2 shine through.

Additional Sequences - *Mentioned For Completeness:*

Perfusion imaging
*   Perfusion MRI quantitates cerebral micro-vascularization parameters. These parameters include regional blood flow and blood volume and mean transit time.

Functional MRI (fMRI)
*   The basics underlying fMRI are increased blood flow to local vasculature that accompanies neural activity resulting in local reduction of deoxyhemoglobin. Deoxyhemoglobin acts as a contrast agent because it is paramagnetic (thus alters $T2^*$ MR signal).

*   In fMRI procedures: First the patient performs a task, then Blood Oxygen Level Dependent *(BOLD) imaging* is done before and after the task. The pre and post task images are then subtracted and overlaid on a gray-scale brain image to localize the signal origin.

Angiography: *2D time of flight (TOF) MRA, 3D-TOF MRA, Phase contrast MRA*

*   *2D-TOF MRA:* Uses a gradient echo sequence where a saturation pulse is employed to null venous or arterial blood flow. Has a SMALL VOXEL SIZE.

*   *3D-TOF MRA:* Is collected as a 3D volume, as opposed to slices, and allows for smaller voxels than 2D. 3D-TOF is well-suited for high flow arterial systems like the Circle of Willis. Benefits include a higher SNR than 2D, a shorter imaging time, more smooth vessel contours, and better saturation (which limits venous circulation).

*   *Phase contrast MRA:* Uses bipolar gradients to create contrast from flow. High velocity encoding time (VENC) is needed for arterial imaging, and low VENC for veins and sinuses. Phase contrast MRA is a quantitative image and can measure mean blood flow velocity and direction.

*   *In general:* TOF MRA is faster and less sensitive to signal loss from turbulent vessels than Phase Contrast MRA. Phase contrast MRA has advantages in increased background suppression and decreased sensitivity to intravoxel dephasing.

Fat Saturation Techniques

There are two broad categories.
- •Inversion Sequences (STIR) that are based on the T1 of fat
- •Those that exploit the resonance difference between fat and water protons.

STIR - As described above, this is a short inversion sequence (180, followed by a well timed 90). It does great with metal artifact. You can NOT use Gd with it.

Selective Pulse: The protons in water and the protons in fat have different resonance frequencies. This difference can be exploited by delivering a selective RF excitation wave with a narrow bandwidth. The RF will only flip the fat protons, which can then have their magnetization destroyed by a "crusher" or "spoiler" gradient. This requires excellent field homogeneity, and can be used with most sequence types. This is the method used most commonly for contrast enhanced studies.

Selective Water Excitation: An alternative method is to use a combination of RF pulses (instead of just one) so you can flip the protons of water only. This technique also prefers a homogeneous field.

Fat Related Topics:

In Phase and Out of Phase: The chemical environments of fat and water are different for protons. This causes these protons to precess at different rates. A spoiled GRE is performed when the protons are spinning with each other (about 4.4 msec at 1.5T) and directly out of phase of each other (2.2 msec at 1.5 T). Microscopic fat will drop out on the out of phase.

High Yield Topic: Out of phase imaging at 2.2 seconds (on 1.5 T) MUST be done before in phase imaging at 4.4 seconds. If you compare the 6.6 second out of phase you will not be able to tell a fatty liver from an iron filled liver.

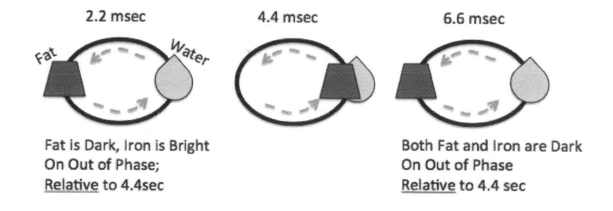

2.2 msec   4.4 msec   6.6 msec

Fat is Dark, Iron is Bright
On Out of Phase;
Relative to 4.4sec

Both Fat and Iron are Dark
On Out of Phase
Relative to 4.4 sec

Chemical Shift Artifact: This will be mentioned again below, but I want to just touch on it briefly as it's related to fat. Again, because of the difference in proton environments between fat and water precession differences cause an artifact in the read out (frequency encoding) direction.

There are two subtypes.

Type 1: This one manifestation is a bright rim on one side and a dark rim on the other. This can occur on either SE or GE sequences.

Testable Trivia: Chemical shift increases with field strength (it's not seen below 1 T)
Testable Trivia: Chemical shift decreases with increased gradient strength
Testable Trivia: Chemical shift decreases with a wider read out bandwidth

· Type 1 Chemical Shift Artifact

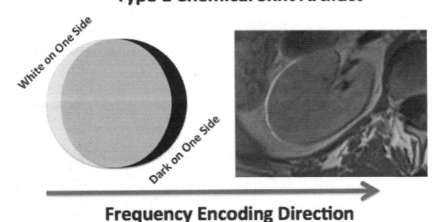

Frequency Encoding Direction

Type 2 Chemical Shift Artifact "India Ink"

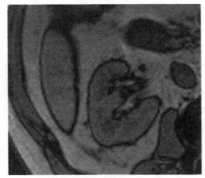

Type 2: India Ink Artifact (Black Boundary) - This type of chemical shift artifact shows a black line in all directions of the fat-water interface. On Gradient Echo sequences, if a voxel has about 50% fat and 50% water the signals will cancel out - leaving this black line.

Testable Trivia: Using SE sequences will get rid of the India Ink, but NOT the Chemical Shift.

MR Contrast (Gd+)

Broadly speaking MRI contrast can be grouped into either "positive agents" which cause bright T1 signal (shortens T1), or "negative agents" which produce magnetic inhomogeneity from susceptibility leading the T2 shortening.

Gadolinium: This is a highly toxic metal that can cause all kinds of badness even in small doses - including liver necrosis. To solve this issue, Gd is complexed with a chelate. The toxicity, clearance routes, bio-distribution, and relaxation properties are all attributes to the chelating agent (DTPA).

How do Gd+3 cause a T1 shortening? Gd^{+3} has seven unpaired electrons, and the interaction of these ELECTRONS causes augmentation of the external magnetic field. The field of the electrons is very short so the contrast agent needs to be right next to the tissue to have an effect on it.

What about T2 effects ? At weak concentration the T2 effect is essentially nothing. However, at **high concentration (classically seen as a "pseudolayer" the bladder) T2 effects dominate**. MRI Perfusion techniques use this T2 effect by using a concentrated bolus in the first intravascular passage - causing a drop in both T2* and T2 signal.

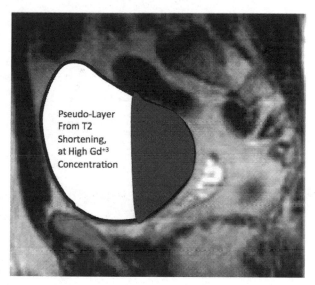

Pseudo-Layer From T2 Shortening, at High Gd^{+3} Concentration

T1 Shortening = Bright
T2 Shortening = Dark

Extracellular Agents: These are the most clinically used agents that have a brief vascular phase, followed by an equilibrium in the extracellular space. *All of these agents are very hydrophilic.*

Blood Pool Agents: Keeping the agent in the blood can be done two ways (1) by using a large Gd ligand, or (2) by binding the Gd to a big sugar or protein molecule

Pharacokinetics:
- Gd cannot pass through a normal (intact) blood brain barrier
- Elimination is primarily renal
- Some agents (Gd-BOPTA and Gd-EOB-DTPA) have more excretion in the bile

MRI Artifacts

Image Process Artifacts: *These include aliasing, chemical shift, truncation, and partial volume.*

Aliasing: This error occurs when an area is under sampled. You get wrapping of anatomy from under sampled portions. This occurs in the phase encoding direction. You can correct for it by (1) increasing the field of view, or (2) changing the phase encoding direction. If you are dealing with aliasing in a 3D sequence then you can add slices or increase coverage to cover your field of view.

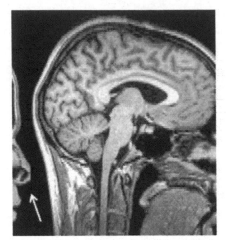

Aliasing - Nose Wrapped Around

Chemical Shift: As discussed above, the protons of different molecules precess at different frequencies. The difference between water and fat is around 220 Hz at 1.5 T (even worse at 3 T). This shift in the Larmor frequency is the so called "chemical shift." The type 1 error occurs in the frequency encoding direction (opposite of most of artifacts which are P.E.).

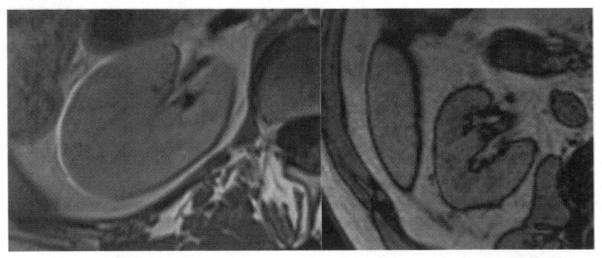

Type 1   Type 2 – India Ink

Truncation / Gibbs: The transformation of K space through inverse fourier transform ideally (but never) resulting in a block of data. Ripples in this data - especially at abrupt intense tissue changes result in the appearance of lines. You classically see these at high contrast interfaces (skull -brain, Cord-CSF, and meniscus/fluid). **The CSF-Cord interface is the most classic - mimicking a syrinx.** If prompted I would say the cause is limited sampling of free induction decay. It *can be seen in both the frequency encoding and phase encoding directions* but is **more commonly seen in the phase encoding** because many times a phase encoding matrix that is smaller than the readout matrix is selected to reduce time.

Gamesmanship: The classic way to show this is sagittal view of the spine - looking like a syrinx.

Making it better: Short answer = **more matrix**. Long answer = Decreasing the bandwidth or decreasing pixel size (more PE steps, less FOV, more matrix).

Improvement penalty: Increased acquisition time and reduced per-pixel signal to noise.

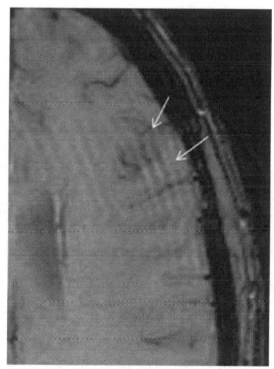

Gibbs at the Skull -Brain

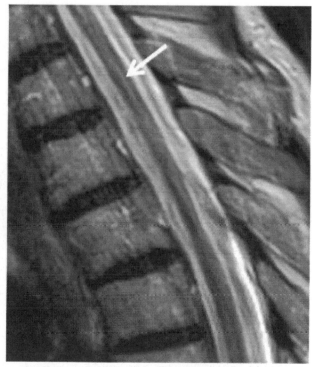

Gibbs – Mimicking a Syrinx

Partial Volume: This is just like in CT. You have different signal intensities in different adjacent structures. If they overlap in a signal voxel - you get averaging. This can result in an intermediate signal from mixing of high and low intensities.

Making it better: Make your pixels smaller. More slices in the z-direction.

Patient Related Artifacts: These include Motion and Magic Angle

Motion: This can be seen with both voluntary and involuntary (cardiac, respiratory) movements. Motion creates difference between frequency encoding (which is fast) and phase encoding (which is slow). You will see ghosting or smearing - primarily in the phase encoding direction. You can also see the classic pulsation artifact from the aorta.

Making it Better:
*   Perform Breath Holding / Having the Patient Hold Still - This is the best method
*   Respiratory Gating (increases acquisition time)
*   ROPE (Respiratory Ordered Phase Encoding) - Phase encoding steps are ordered with respiration
*   Breathing Navigator - An echo from the diagram determines its position, then timing and acquisition are based off this.
*   Apply a fat sat band across the abdomen
*   Switch the phase encoding direction.

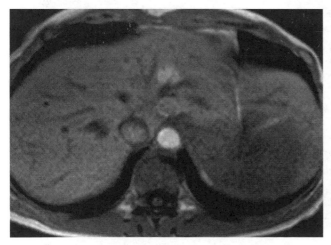
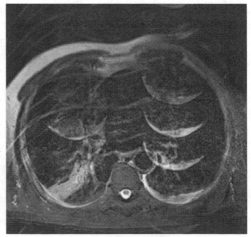

Pulsation - From the Aorta   **Breathing Artifact**

Flow: This is a type of motion artifact, related to blood flow. Blood flow causes ghosting in the phase encoding direction. GRE sequences are more susceptible to this than SE sequences.

SE Sequences - Flow looks **dark**. Moving blood that got hit with the 90 pulse, moves out of the way prior to getting the 180 pulse. Therefore, it doesn't have any signal.

GRE Sequences: In flowing blood looks **bright**.

Making it better:
- Apply a saturation band adjacent to the imaging section - 90 pulse followed by crusher gradient.

What Makes A Flow Void?

The dark hole of a patent vessel is called a "flow void." This is generally a spin echo imaging finding (as stated above - flow looks dark on SE).

Why does this happen? To make an echo, the proton must be exposed to both a 90 pulse and a 180 pulse pulse. If the blood is flowing fast it will get hit with the 90 degree, but then miss the 180 degree pulse. This means no echo, and thus no signal.

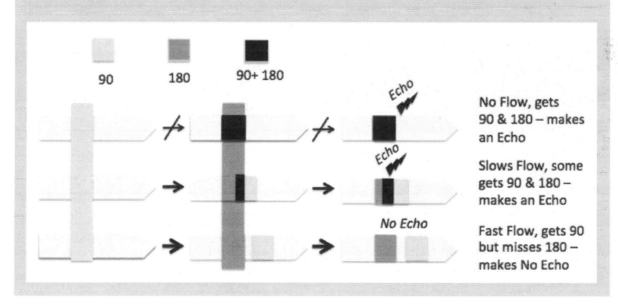

Magic Angle: This is an MSK artifact seen with tendons. You see this with short echo time (TE) sequences where the focus forms **an angle of 55 degrees** with the main magnetic field (magic angle phenomenon). This will NOT be seen in T2 sequences (with long TE). This phenomenon, is reduced at higher field strengths due to greater shortening of T2 relaxation times.

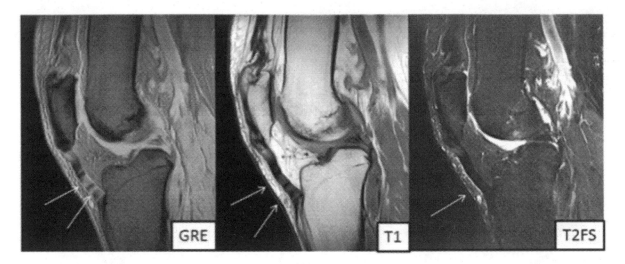

Magic Angle: You see it on short TE sequences (T1, PD, GRE). It goes away on T2.

RF Related: These include Cross talk and Zipper Artifacts

Cross Talk: RF and FT pulses are not perfectly rectangular. So if they are placed close enough together then you get excitation of neighboring section more than once in a single repetition. These lead to partial saturation and lower signal. So all sections (except the ones on the ends will be subjected to this).

Making it better: Increasing the gap between sections. Interleave slices (all odds, then all evens).

Testable Trivia: The 3D images are not susceptible to this artifact because the entire volume undergoes excitation with sections within the volume acquired with gradients.

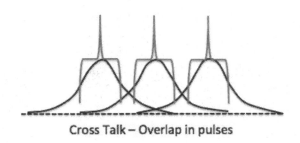

Cross Talk – Overlap in pulses

Zipper Artifact: There are lots of random stray RF signals (radio, tv, etc...). Remember that the RF pulse is a "radio-wave." Anyway, if you have defective or inadequate shielding you can get a "zipper" of high signal - 1-2 pixels in width running across the image. This typically extends in the phase encoding direction.

Gamesmanship: A possible scenario for this is that anesthesia left the pulse ox monitor in the room.

Making it better: Try closing the door (if it's open). Remove all electronic devices from the room. Call the tech people to repair the faulty RF shielding. Alternatively, you could write an email, cc 15 people, and use the phrase "patient care". That will ruffle some feathers.

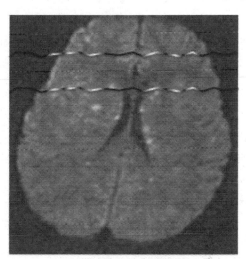

Zipper Artifact

External Field: This is magnetic inhomogeneity:

Inhomogeneous Fat Suppression: If the field is actually homogeneous you get a uniform fat saturation by applying an RF pulse with the resonance of fat protons. In the real world, local field inhomogeneities cause fat protons to precess at difference frequencies. These differences allow certain areas of fat to resist suppression - which can mimic edema.

Making it better: Using an inversion recovery - STIR, especially in the setting of metal.

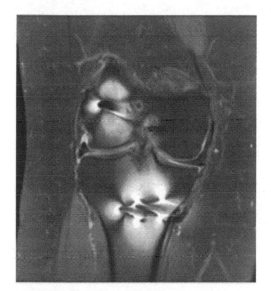

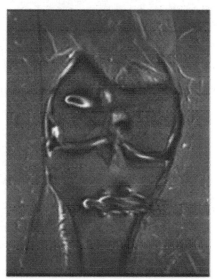

T2FS: Fat Sat in bone marrow is ruined by metal messing with the local field

Improved with STIR Sequence

Magnetic Susceptibility: This includes diamagnetic, paramagnetic, and ferromagnetic

Susceptibility - This refers to the ability of a substance to become magnetized by the external field. Obviously metals have large susceptibility. Calcium hydroxyapatite and accumulations of gadolinium chelate can do the same thing.

Generally speaking, susceptibility affects all pulse sequences, but is most severe with GRE images and least severe with SE (because of the 180 degree refocusing pulse - to lose those T2* effects).

A less prominent version occurs at tissue interfaces (bone and muscle, or air and bone). The classic location for this is the transition from paranasal sinus to skull base.

Making it better: Using SE and FSE instead of GRE. You can swap the phase and frequency, use a wider receiver bandwidth, or align the longitudinal axis of a metal implant with the axis of the main field. STIR does way better than frequency selective fat suppression.

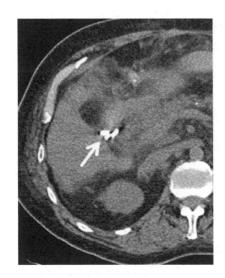 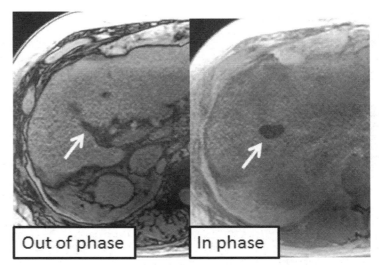

Notice the Blooming Artifact from the
Metal Choley Clips Worsens with Time
(In-phase is done after Out-phase)

A key concept is that susceptibility artifact worsens on in phase imaging relative to out of phase. This has nothing to do with the phase of water and fat. Instead it has everything to do with in phase being done later. The longer TE, the more susceptibility. Remember, air will do the same thing.

Shimming

Shimming is a thing that can be done to improve field homogeneity. When the magnet comes from the manufacturer the field homogeneity is terrible. To correct for this a process called "shimming" is used. There are two types of shimming, passive and active. Most of the time a combination of the two is used; passive to get the thing going in the right direction and active to optimize the field for each patient.

- *Passive Shimming* – A phantom is scanned and the position of the shim plates is adjusted until the field becomes homogeneous (are at least better than it was). This is done at the time of installation.

- *Active Shimming* – This is done by using the electromagnetic coil, and can be done after each patient (or sequence). Essentially, gives you the chance to have a homogeneous field (or nearly) regardless of the size of the patient.

Gradient Related: This includes Eddy Currents

Eddy Current: These things called "Eddy Currents" are generated when gradients are rapidly turned on and off. The actual location of said currents can be in the magnet, the cables, the wires or even in the patient. This looks like distortion (contraction or dilation of the image) or shift/shear.

Testable Trivia: Most severe with DWI pulses.

Making it better: Optimizing the sequence of gradient pulses.

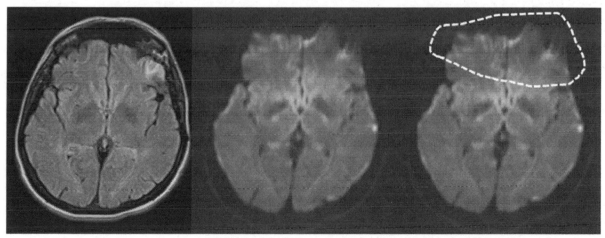

FLAIR – for non-distorted comparison

Diffusion – Notice the stretch / smear at the brain - bone interface. This is from Eddy Currents

Errors in Data: This include dielectric effects and crisscross

Dielectric Effects / Standing Wave effects - Biologic tissues have a dielectric constant that results in reduction of wavelength by the inverse of some constant. Interactions can cause local eddy currents in the imaged tissues. Since RF waves are shorter at 3T - the effects are **worse with a stronger magnet**. You also see this worsen with large bellies, especially if they have **ascites.** Larger body parts (the abdomen) are primarily affected.

Classic Look / Location: Dark signal in the central abdomen over the left lobe of the liver.

Making it better:
•Application of dielectric pads - placed between patient and anterior body array coil
•Parallel RF transmission (SENSE) - RF pulses from a set of coils; each coil sends an independent RF pulse. Gives you a longer pulse.

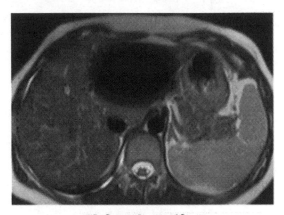

Dielectric Artifact

Crisscross or Herringbone: If you see obliquely oriented stripes throughout the image, you are probably dealing with this artifact. The cause is data processing and/or reconstruction errors.

Making it better: Reconstruct the image again.

Artifact	Direction	Better	Worse	Trivia
Aliasing	Phase Encoding	•Increase the field of view •Change the phase encoding direction	Smaller FOVs	Caused by a small FOV
Chemical Shift	Frequency Encoding	•Bigger Pixels •Fat Suppression •Increase Receiver Bandwidth	•Stronger Magnetic Field •Lower Receiver Bandwidth	Caused by differences in resonance frequencies
Gibbs / Truncation	Both **phase** and frequency	•Bigger Matrix •Decrease Bandwidth •Decrease Pixel Size (increase PE Steps, Decrease FOV)		•Caused by limited sample of FID •Classically seen in the spinal cord
Partial Volume		•Decrease Pixel Size (increase PE Steps, Decrease FOV)	Thicker Slices	
Motion Artifact	Phase Encoding	•Saturation pulses •Respiratory gating •Faster sequences (BLADE, PROPELLER)		
Cross Talk		•Increase slice gap •Interleave slices		Caused by overlap of slices
Zipper	Phase Encoding			Caused by poor shielding
Field Inhomogeneity		•Shimming	GRE Sequences	Caused by geometric distortion
Susceptibility			GRE Sequences	•Caused by augmentation of magnetic field •Very bad in EPI
Eddy Current		•Optimize sequence of gradient pulses	DWI - large gradient changes	•Caused by geometric distortion or non-uniformity
Dielectric Effects		•Parallel Transmit •Use 1.5 T	3 T	•Standing waves created as radiowave approaches length of body part
Magic Angle		•T2	T1, PD	•Occurs at 55 Degrees

531

Special Topic - Cardiac MRI

It's best to think of cardiac imaging in two flavors: (1) Bright Blood, and (2) Dark Blood.

Bright Blood: These are **gradient sequences**, and they make up the majority of the cardiac work load.

Steady State Free Precession "SSFP" – This is a type of gradient sequence that is the primary sequence used for wall motion and volume analysis. If you see a CINE MRI of the heart it is probably a SSFP.

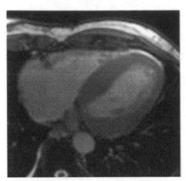

Gradient Echo - Bright Blood

Dark Blood: These are **spin echo** sequences. Remember that spin echo sequences have less susceptibility artifacts, so they can be of benefit when looking at the mediastinum in a patient who has had a prior sternotomy (with metal wires).

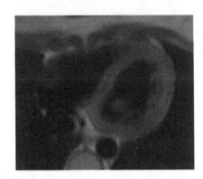

Spin Echo - Dark Blood

Inversion Recovery: Just like STIR nulls fat signal, and FLAIR nulls CSF signal, cardiac MRI uses an inversion technique to null myocardium. The reason you do this is to look for delayed enhancement (scar).

Trivia to know about inversion recovery:

- A "PSIR" or Phase Sensitive Inversion Recovery or a T.I. Scout Series is done to help choose the correct time to use for inversion. This will produce a series of hearts. You want to pick the one with the darkest myocardium. This will give you the correct inversion recovery time.

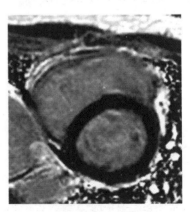

Nulled Myocardium

- *Why not just do it like FLAIR or STIR, with a set time?* Although myocardium usually nulls at around 330 msec, it's highly variable depending on the person

Special Topic - Breast MRI

There are a few artifacts and technical differences specific to breast MRI that are worth knowing about. MRI of the breast is done for several reasons (high risk screening, implant rupture evaluation, surgical planning, etc…). The reason for the exam will dictate sequences.

Testable Trivia: Breast CA screening will have dynamic post contrast sequences

Testable Trivia: Implant Rupture screening will NOT have contrast, but instead have a fat and water saturated sequence (only silicone will be bright).

Testable Trivia: A breast specific coil is used to increase SNR.

Artifacts:

Chemical Shift: You see this all the time in breast MRI, at the fat water interface. Remember this can be corrected by increasing the bandwidth to capture both fat and water in the same phase.

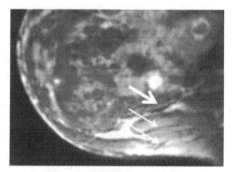

Chemical Shift Artifact

Motion / Breathing / Cardiac: Breathing and the beating of the heart would normally degrade the image on breast MRI. This is corrected for by running the phase encoding direction side to side , instead of front to back (like it is in body imaging).

Phase Encoding Direction:

– Axial: Breast is left to right (Body Imaging is front to back)

– Sagittal: Breast is top to bottom

Signal Flair – If the breast is too close to the coil element, it will not fat sat out correctly (look bright). You can fix this by repositioning the patient in the scanner.

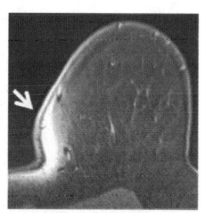

Flair Artifact

Safety, Bioeffects, and FDA limits

Specific Absorption Rate (SAR)

SAR estimates the amount of energy deposited in a patient *(measurement of the rate the RF pulse dissipates in tissue)*. The units of SAR are Watts/Kilogram (energy/mass).

Let's look at the formula - only for understanding some possible questions.

$$SAR = B_0^2 \times Alpha^2 \times Duty\ Cycle$$

Potential ways you could ask a question about this:

(1) *If you double the B_0, you do what to the SAR ?* It **Quadruples**

(2) *If you double the Flip Angle (example 5 to 30), you do what to the SAR ?* It **Quadruples**

(3) *If you double the Duty Cycle (make the TR 1/2), you do what to the SAR?* It **Doubles**

(4) *Which has a higher SAR, Spin Echo or Gradient?* Spin Echo (they have higher flip angles - especially inversions).

(5) *What are the limits?* Standards stipulate that no tissue shall endure a temperature increase of greater than 1 degree C. FDA limits are 4 W/kg over 15 minutes and 3 W/kg over 10 minutes.

body   head

Other Random MRI Safety Concerns:

- Static magnetic field (ferromagnetic materials): ferromagnetic materials present a risk in the presence of a strong magnetic field. Ferromagnetic objects, foreign or surgically placed, are at risk of displacement. Electronic devices such as cardiac pacemakers/ defibrillators, nerve stimulators, etc, may suffer malfunction.

- *Gradient Field (nerve stimulation)*
  - The rapid switching of magnetic field gradients can trigger peripheral nerve and muscular stimulation. EPI sequences are most likely to cause such an effect, as they put the greatest strain on gradients.
- **Contrast agent safety issues**
  - The concern with Gadolinium contrast agents is Nephrogenic Systemic Fibrosis. The answer on the test is: GFR must be > 30 to administer Gadolinium.

Accreditation, quality control (QC) and quality improvement

- Weekly QC for accredited MR scanners (per ACR and performed by MR technologist): Center Frequency, table positioning, setup and scanning, geometric accuracy, high contrast resolution (verified by phantom), low contrast resolution, artifact analysis, film quality control, and visual checklist.
- Annual QC for accredited MR scanners (per ACR and performed by medical physicist or MR scientist) includes: Magnetic field homogeneity, slice position accuracy, slice thickness accuracy, radiofrequency coil check, display monitor check

You're out of your element Donny

Section 10: Radiation Biology

"Exposure" – The ability of x-rays to ionize air, measured in Roentgens (R). This is the concentration, in air, of radiation at a specific point – and is the ionization produced in a specific volume of air.

"Absorbed Radiation Dose" or *"Radiation Dose"* – The amount of energy absorbed per unit mass at a specific point. It is measured in Gy or Rads (1 Gy = 100 rads). This is how much energy from ionizing radiation has been absorbed in a small volume.

"Equivalent Dose" (EqD)– The absorbed dose of different types of radiation creates different levels of biologic damage (thus measured in Sv). A weighting factor is used to adjust the value. For example, an alpha particle can do more damage than an electron.

EqD = Dose x Weight Factor

Weight Factor = for x-rays and gamma rays this is 1, for alpha particles it's 20.

"Effective Dose" (EfD) – This takes into account whether radiation has been absorbed by the specific tissue. In other words you are taking into account the type of radiation and the variable sensitivity of the organ / body part. If all the dose is absorbed then 1 Gy = 1 Sv. If you are dealing with organs or specific body parts you have to use a "tissue weighting" conversion factor.

EfD = EqD x Tissue Factor

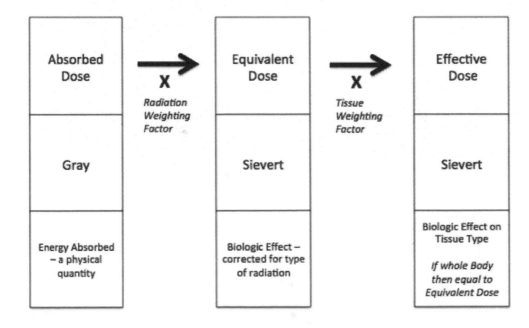

Kerma

Kerma is actually an acronym for "kinetic energy released per unit mass." I want to take a minute and give a basic explanation of how energy is transferred. The process typically has two steps:

(1) Energy is transferred to a charged particle (via Compton, P.E. effect, or whatever).

(2) The now charged particle transfers energy to a medium via excitation and ionization.

Kerma is described step 1 (NOT step 2).

Why do I bother making this point?

- If you are dealing with a low energy photon, then Kerma is going to be the same as the absorbed dose.

- If you are dealing with a high energy photon, then Kerma is going to be MORE than the absorbed dose. This is because some of these secondary electrons are going to escape the area of interest before depositing their energy. These will be counted in Kerma, but not absorbed dose.

- In general, tissue doses are higher than air kerma (usually around 10%).

What is this "Air Kerma" ?

This is the sum of kinetic energy of all charged particles made when an x-ray (or gamma ray) passes through a unit mass of air.

What is this "Entrance Air Kerma"?

This is the air where the x-ray beam would enter the patient (measured without the patient).

What is this "Air Kerma Product" (KAP) ?

This is supposed to account for the total amount of radiation on the patient. It is calculated by summing the Entrance Air Kerma x the Cross Sectional Area. The most important point is that KAP is **independent of the source distance**. This is because changes in beam intensity (from inverse square law) are matched exactly by changes in cross sectional area.

Trivia: SI Unit for Kerma = Gy

Stochastic Effects vs Deterministic Effects:

Deterministic Effects	Stochastic Effects ("Random")
Has a threshold	Has NO threshold
Severity is dose related	Severity is NOT dose related
	Probability of effect increases with dose
Does Not include Cancer Risk	Includes heritable effects and carcinogenesis (NOT cell killing)

Interaction of Radiation with Tissue:

As discussed before you have two primary methods that x-rays interact with matter; the photoelectric effect and compton scatter. The key interaction is the production of a free electron, which can then transfer it's energy to other electrons by ionization and excitation. The actual **damage done is the result of ionization** produced by x-rays / gamma ray photons giving energy to orbital electrons and alpha / beta particles interacting electromagnetically with orbital electrons.

What Determines the Biologic Effects from Ionizing Radiation?

Primary variables include those inherent to the cells and the conditions of the cells at the time of irradiation. There are also variables related to the radiation (absorbed dose, dose rate, type of radiation, and energy of radiation).

Damage to biologic systems occurs in this order:

Molecular -> Cellular -> Organic

Molecular damage is always first. Ionized atoms do not bind properly to other molecules. Loss of function in the molecule leads to loss of cellular function.

Charged Particle Tracks:

When radiation crashes into a biologic material, energy is deposited along the tract. The pattern of this deposited energy depends on the type of radiation involved.

X-Rays / Gamma Rays: X-ray ionization density is low along the track

Neutrons, Protons, and Alpha Particles: Ionization events occur much more frequently.

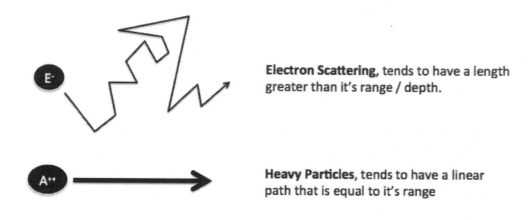

Electron Scattering, tends to have a length greater than it's range / depth.

Heavy Particles, tends to have a linear path that is equal to it's range

Concepts / Vocabulary:

Linear Energy Transfer (LET) - This is the **average amount of energy deposited per unit path** length of the incident radiation. LET is important for assessing the potential tissue and organ damage. LET comes in two flavors:

- *High LET:* Neutrons, Protons, Alpha Particles, and Heavy Ions. These are MUCH MORE DAMAGING ("has a higher quality factor").
- *Low LET:* Photons, Gamma Rays, Electrons, and Positrons

Relative Biologic Effectiveness (RBE) - This is the relative capability of radiation with differing LETs to produce a particular biologic reaction.

RBE = Dose of 250 kV x-rays / Dose in Gy of Test Radiation

Example Problem: A reaction is produced by 5 Gy of test radiation. It takes 10 Gy of 250 kVp x-rays to produce the same reaction. What is the RBE ?

10 / 5 = 2 ; In this example the test radiation is 2 times as effective in producing this biologic reaction than the "standard" 250 kVp x-rays.

The "Kill Effect"
As LET increases, RBE will increase... to a certain point.
Above 100 keV/micrometer of tissue, RBE decreases with increasing LET - because the maximum potential damage has already been done - additional increase in LET is wasted dose.

Oxygen Enhancement Ratio (OER) - This is the relative effectiveness of radiation to produce damage at different oxygen levels. The idea is that biologic tissue is more sensitive to radiation in an oxygenated state. A testable piece of trivia is that OER really only matters for low LET radiation. With high LET radiation the OER is often 1 (biologic damage without oxygen = biologic damage with oxygen).

Direct vs Indirect Ionizing Radiation: Actions, are called "direct" if they act "directly on the DNA." Actions are called "indirect" if they act on water. **The majority of irradiation in living cells is the result of indirect action on water** (your body is 70% water and < 1% DNA). This indirect action on water creates a free radical which then jacks the DNA.

This vs That: Direct vs Indirect Radiation			
Direct Radiation *(minority)*	Acts on DNA	Most likely for High LET Radiation (unusual in x-ray imaging)	
Indirect Radiation *(majority)*	Acts on water in the cytoplasm, creating free radicals - which in turn damage the DNA	More likely for Low LET Radiation	This process is promoted by the presence of oxygen

Effects on DNA

Single Strand Break - Ionizing radiation can cause a break in one of the chemical bonds (point mutation). This is more likely with low - LET radiation. Repair enzymes can move in and fix this.

Double Strand Break - Ionizing radiation can cause a break in multiple chemical bonds. These are more likely with high - LET radiation. These are harder to fix.

Mutation - It's possible for radiation to cause a loss of or change in the nitrogenous base in the DNA chain. If the cell doesn't die from this, this incorrect information will be transferred as the cell divides.

Testable Point: The syndrome with the most sensitivity to x-rays is Ataxia Telangiectasia. Common distractors include Bloom Syndrome and Fanconi Anemia (both of which have genetic instability but no particular relationship with x-rays). Xeroderma pigmentosa is another classic distractor - but it is more sensitive to UV radiation.

Chromosome Anomalies - Two types have been described at metaphase.

Chromosome Aberrations - Damage occurs early in interphase (before DNA synthesis). Both chromatids are broken so each daughter will get a broken copy.

Chromatid Aberrations - Damage occurs later in interphase (after DNA synthesis). Only 1 chromatid is going to have a break (the other one will be fine)

Effect on the Cell:

Testable Point - An x-ray or gamma ray dose of 1000 Gy in a period of second / minutes will cause instant death of a large number of cells.

"Mitotic Death" - This is when a cell dies after 1 or more divisions. A relatively small dose of radiation can cause this.

"Mitotic Delay" - A very small dose (0.01 Gy) just before a cell starts to divide can cause a delay or failure in the timing of the normal dividing.

Cell Cycle Phase - Cells are MOST sensitive during M phase (mitosis). They are more sensitive during late G2 phase. They are less sensitive during G1 phase. There are the LEAST sensitive during late S phase.

Testable Point: In order of sensitivity: M > G2 > G1 > S.

Testable Point: G1 is the part of the cell cycle that is the most variable in length (shorter in cells that turn over quickly).

Surviving Cell Synchronization - If you blast a group of cells with radiation, the ones that survive will have their cell cycles synchronized. The reason is that the most resistent part of the cell cycle is late synthesis. So most of the surviving cells are in this phase.

Law of Bergonie and Tribondeau - Cell sensitivity is directly related to their reproductive activity, and inversely related to their differentiation. So, the more a cell turns over (skin, blood, GI tract lining, reproductive cells) the more sensitive they are. The less cells turn over and more differentiated they are (brain, nerves, muscles) the less sensitive they are.

Testable Point: The small bowel is the most radiosensitive part of the GI tract.

The Survival Curve (possible source of questions).

This is a graph of dose vs cell survival. The point to notice is the **"Quasi-threshold dose"** which is the portion of the graph when repair mechanisms are in there trying to hold the ship together. It is a measure of "sub-lethal" damage to the cell.

A testable point is that this shoulder only exists with low-LET radiation curves.

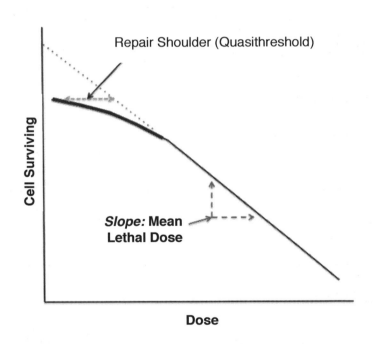

$1 / $ Slope (D_0) describes the linear portion of the curve, and the radio-sensitivity of the cell population. The higher the D_0 the more radio-resistant the cell is.

Key Points:
- Higher Dose Rate makes a smaller shoulder, and steeper drop in the curve
- Low LET will have a shoulder, High LET will NOT have a shoulder
- Oxygen will make a steeper drop in the curve (more pronounced with low LET)

Effect of Ionizing Radiation of Blood:

Lymphocytes are the MOST sensitive blood cells in the body. A dose of 0.25 Gy is enough to depress the amount circulating in the blood.

Lymphocytes can actually be stimulated to divide and you can score the number of chromosomal aberrations at first mitosis to reflect average total body dose.

Acute Radiation Syndrome (ARS):

This is a clinical response when the body is hit with a large amount of radiation. There are 3 subtypes of this syndrome. You typically have 4 phases. You start out feeling terrible (GI flu like symptoms - nausea / vomiting / diarrhea), then you feel better "latent phase," then your syndrome subtype manifests - related to underlying organ system as below, the fourth phase is death/recovery.

Acute Radiation Syndrome	Dose Needed	Latent Period	Outcome
Bone Marrow	> 2 Gy	1-6 Weeks	You do worse with higher doses. It's possible to survive.
GI	> 8 Gy	5-7 Days	Death within 2 weeks
CNS	> 20-50 Gy	4-6 Hours	Death within 3 days *(unless you get to Elysium)*

Testable Point: A total body dose of 0.75 -1.25 Gy will cause nausea about 30% of the time.

For Perspective:

mGy = A dose that is diagnostic. For example, 30mGy is a dose for a CT Abd and Pelvis.

Gy = A dose that makes you sick. For example, 2 Gy is going to mess with your bone marrow.

Triaging Patients with Possible ARS:

This basic idea is that the earlier the symptoms appear the worse they are going to do.

GI	Skin	WB Dose (Gy)	Action
No vomiting	No skin redness	< 1	Surveillance for 5 weeks
Vomiting 2-3 hours after exposure	Skin redness (12-24 hours after exposure)	1-2	Surveillance for 3 weeks, Consider General Hospital
Vomiting 1-2 hours after exposure	Skin redness (8-15 hours after exposure)	2-4	Hospitalize - Burn Center
Vomiting < 1 hour after exposure	Skin redness (1- 6 hours after exposure)	> 4	Hospitalize - Specialized Radiation Center

High Yield Point: *Early Vomiting is a marker of severity / poor prognosis.*

Effect of Ionizing Radiation - Lethal Dose 50/30:

This is the dose which will kill 50% of people within 30 days. **The LD 50/30 for a person is around 3-4 Gy without treatment**. With medical treatment you may be able to tolerate up to 8.5 Gy *(depending on if you ate your wheaties).*

Lethal Dose 50/60 = Lethal dose at 60 days for 50% of the population. This is used for bone marrow failure. This is about 3-4 Gy.

Lethal Dose 50/4 = Lethal dose at 4 days for 50% of the population. This is used for GI failure. This is about 10 Gy.

Genetically Significant Dose (GSD) = This term is used for expressing genetic risk as an index of presumed impact on the entire population. GSD is the dose if received by all members of the population that would result in the same hereditary damage as the actual doses received by the gonads of the people who actually get radiation exposure. This depends on gonadal dose, and child bearing potential (age of patient, sex of patient).

Increased Risk of Cancer: The risk of cancer (estimated by BEIR 5 and UNSCEAR) was 8% / Sv. A reduction factor of 2 is used for low dose and low rate - so the working **population has a risk more like 4%-5% /Sv.** Some people throw around the following calculation:

Risk for Hereditary Effect of Radiation:

    0.2 /100 x Dose

      Example: Women gets CT scan 0.3 Gy then gets pregnant 1 year later. Chance of radiation induced hereditary defect? $0.2 / 100 \times 0.3 = 6 \times 10^{-4}$, or 6 in 10,000

Latency: The time between exposure and appearance of cancer is sometimes called the latency. It's variable for cancers. For example, leukemia has a short latency of 5-7 years, where as solid tumors have a latency as long as 20-50.

Radiation Effect on a Fetus: Teratogenicity of radiation is dose dependent, and timing dependent.

- First two weeks (implantation) = 50-100 mGy may cause fetal loss. If the baby doesn't die from the dose in the first weeks he/she is likely to have no lasting effects (*all or nothing*).

- Between 8-15 weeks = The <u>MOST VULNERABLE TIME</u>. Doses over 100-200 mGy are associated with reduced head diameter and mental retardation.

- After 15 weeks the brain is less sensitive to radiation.

- *Trivia:* IQ is said to drop 30 points per 1 Sv, with the risk of retardation being 40% at 1 Sv.

- *Trivia:* It takes a very low dose (just a few radiographs) to the fetus to increase the risk of childhood leukemia.

- *Trivia:* The fetal thyroid does NOT take up iodine prior to week 8. So, if mom gets I-131 prior to week 8 the fetus will not be hypothyroid (after that it's hosed).

Skin Problem	Dose (Gy)	Onset
Early Transient Erythema	2 Gy skin dose	Hours
Severe "Robust" Erythema	6 Gy skin dose	1 Week
Telangiectasia	10 Gy skin dose	52 Weeks
Dry Desquamation	13 Gy skin dose	4 Weeks
Moist Desquamation / Ulceration	18 Gy skin dose	4 Weeks
Secondary Ulceration	24 Gy skin dose	> 6 weeks

Hair Problem	Dose (Gy)	Onset
Temporary Epilation	3Gy	21 Days
Permanent Epilation	7 Gy	21 Days

I remember this by saying 3 x 7 = 21

Symptom / Issue	Dose
Nausea (30% of people)	0.75-1.25 Gy WB
Depress circulating lymphocytes	0.25 Gy WB
LD 50/60 (Marrow)	3-4 Gy WB
LD 50/4 (GI)	8-10 Gy WB
LD for CNS	> 20 Gy (20-100) WB
Double the natural or spontaneous mutation rate	1 Gy
Effective dose from background radiation in the US	3 mSv per year

Dose Trigger for additional patient care / follow up = 15 Gy to a single exposure field (most places will call this a "Sentinel Event"

Sterility / Infertility

Females: The threshold is age dependent. The younger the patient, the more dose they need. Close to puberty think about 10 Gy, Close to Menopause think about 2 Gy.

Male: Temporary sterility is going to occur somewhere between 0.15- 2.5 Gy. More permanent sterility requires an acute dose around 5 Gy.

Sterility / Infertility	
Male Temporary	0.15- 2.5 Gy
Male Permanent	5 Gy
Female Age 12	10 Gy
Female Age 45	2 Gy
Female - *No age given*	Just say around 6 Gy

Cataracts

Trivia: Senile cataracts tend to involve the anterior lens. Radiation induced cataracts tend to involve the posterior lens.

Trivia: IR people tend to be the ones to get these... sorta makes sense.

The cataract tends to develop years (like 20 years) after exposure. This latent period is inverse to the exposure amount.

The threshold for development from an acute exposure is around 2.5 Gy (some studies go as low as 0.5 Gy.)

Cataract	
Acute Exposure Threshold to Cause Cataract	2.5 Gy
Annual Dose Rate Limit	0.15 Gy/Yr

Exposure Limits	
Occupational Workers (minimal age 18)	
Lens	150 mSv/year *(some new papers say 20 mSv)*
Radiation Worker	50 mSv/year
Extremity	500 mSv/year
Public Exposure	
Infrequent	5 mSv /year
Continuous	1 mSv/year
Embryo/fetus	5 mSv .year
Embryo Fetus (post declared pregnancy)	0.5 mSv/month
Controlled Areas	50 mSv/year
Uncontrolled area	5 mSv year
Genetically Significant Dose	0.25 mSv
Effective dose from background radiation in the US	3 mSv per year

Shield Your Eggs!

Part of the tech's job is placing the gonad shield. Proper placement is critical - mainly because I don't want to see that penis on my pelvis x-ray. Another day of "hog watch" on MSK plain film....

Male: Shield is placed just below the symphysis pubis

Female: Shield is placed 1 inch medial to each palpable anterior superior iliac spine. The coverage is considered adequate if it covers the middle two thirds of the pelvic basin from the sacrum to the symphysis pubis.

MRI Safety Trivia:

Specific Absorption Rate (SAR)
The RF power absorbed per unit mass.
Depends on number of images acquired per unit time, patient dimensions, RF waveform, tip angle, and coil type
The SAR should not exceed 4W/kg for the whole body for 15 mins.
RF heating is considered acceptable if the core temperature increase is < 1 C.

Noise: The noise with MRI is the result of vibrations in the gradient coils. The peak acoustic noise should not exceed 140 dB.

Burns: If you have a "conductive loop" - either from crossed arms, ECG leads, or unconnected surface coil leads in contact with skin it's possible to get a nice thermal injury (and a law suit). If the patient is contacting the inner bore (where high level standing RF waves are highest) there can be a burn (and a law suit). Implanted metal objects can also heat up.

Peripheral Nerve Stimulation: Rapid changing of gradients has the potential to cause peripheral nerve stimulation, and muscle movement.

NSF (Nephrogenic Systemic Fibrosis) - This is a very serious, extremely rare (possible not real) thing that caused fibrosis of skin, joints, and organs. It was seen in end stage renal failure patients (GFR < 30), who got Gd. The risk is related to the chelation structure, not the actual Gd.

- Most Likely To Cause - "Linear Non-Ionic" - Omniscan , Optimark
- Intermediate Risk - "Linear Ionic" - Multihance, Magnevist
- Least Likely to Cause (most safe) - "Cyclic Structure" - Gadovist

Pregnancy - There is NO evidence that MRI is dangerous to the fetus. Having said that, most institutes tend to say no contrast in pregnancy. *Fear of Litigation > Rational Thought*

High Yield Radiation Biology/Safety Blitz:

- The majority of energy received by biologic material from x-rays is transferred by electrons
- Two thirds (around 60%) of x-ray damage to biologic material is mediated by free radicals
- Interaction of two separate chromosomal breaks can lead to aberrations such as dicentrics and rings
- Double stranded DNA breaks are the most important lesions caused by x-rays.
- The final number of double stranded DNA breaks is more important than the initial number of breaks - because some will be repaired.
- You can score whole body radiation exposure by stimulating lymphocytes to divide.
- Risk of Radiation induced CA: 4-5% per Sv = Adult, Up to 15% per Sv for Child , About 1/10th that for someone older than 50
- Transient skin erythema can be seen in hours, with the main wave occurring after 10 days
- Radiation induced sterility in males does NOT affect hormone levels or libido.
- Radiation induced sterility in males has a "latent period" between irradiation and sterility
- Radiation induced sterility in females causes symptoms similar to menopause.
- Carcinogenesis by radiation is stochastic (all or nothing) - based on Beir 5 and UNSCEAR committees
- Sentinel Event = 15 Gy
- The thyroid can have radiation induced benign and malignant nodules
- Radon workers get more lung cancer
- Cataracts caused by radiation start in the back of the lens
- If Al-Qaeda attacks your hospital with a dirty bomb, remember that the causalities may present a risk to medical personnel (because they are contaminated with radionuclides).
- Inhaled Radon (an alpha emitter) contributes about 55% of the effective dose to the US population, and is the largest single contributor to effective dose.
- The greatest source of exposure to ionizing radiation for the general population of the United States from *due to human activity* is medical imaging.
- For MRI; you must have a controlled access so that the fringe field outside the area doesn't exceed 5 Gauss.
- For MRI; there is a thing called "Specific Absorption Ratio" - which is the RF power absorbed per unit mass. The SAR should not exceed 4W/kg for the whole body for 15 mins.

You're killing your father, Larry!

Blank for Notes / Scribbles

Blank for Notes / Scribbles

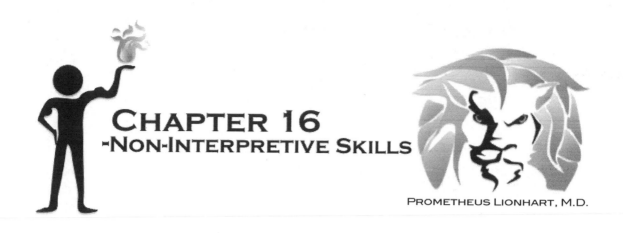

CHAPTER 16
-NON-INTERPRETIVE SKILLS

PROMETHEUS LIONHART, M.D.

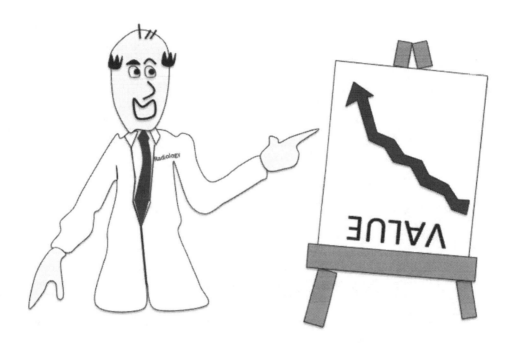

As stated in public interviews, the idea for this portion of the exam is for the 3rd year resident to show that he/she can do more than read studies - but can also "serve and lead." Topics for this chapter were taken from the study guide published on the ABR's website, and the articles references within said study guide. To view that masterpiece for yourself, simply google "ABR non-interpretive skills study guide."

The author advises caution to the reader - the question writer likely does not understand the material in this chapter. Partially because it's made up material. A majority of the material is just words taken out of the dictionary and placed next to each other. It is therefore dangerous to attempt to understand it too well.

Section 1: "Quality" & Other Random Meaningless Buzzwords

QA vs QI

Back in the dark ages Doctors had "QA" or "Quality Assurance" meetings. This is of course a laughable practice that is backward and outdated. "QA meetings" are like using leaches to cure an imbalance of the bodily humors. Now, in the modern age, Doctors (or people who wished they went to business school instead of medical school) use the term "QI" or Quality Improvement. This change in vocabulary has really revolutionized medicine.

QA- old term : reactive, retrospective, punitive or finger pointing.

QI- new term : prospective and retrospective reviews; aimed at improvement.

The "**I**" in QI stands for **I**mprovement. If you want to improve your rank in academic institutions you better learn about QI. This is how you make full professor, so pay close attention.

Various Catchphrases and Buzzwords Invented By Career Administrators

Best Practices: The idea behind "best practices" is that everyone should do things the same way. The "best" way. Of course, if everyone does it that way it just makes it a "mediocre practice."

Dashboard – A visual display of the most valuable information you need to achieve your objective.

Benchmarking – Measuring the quality of organizational policies by comparing them with standard measurements or peers.

TQM: Total Quality Management – When reading about TQM my favorite line is this "there is no widespread agreement as to what TQM is and what actions it requires of organizations." In other words, it's just a made up buzzword. Having said that, I'd remember that quality improvement should be continuous, with responsibility in the top management, and that the definition of quality is defined by what customers require.

CQI: Continuous Quality Improvement – Another meaningless buzzword that is essentially the same thing as TQM.

Key Performance Indicators "KPI": Ideally this is a reproducible measurable thing – like patient safety, customer service satisfaction, or the number of publications a faculty member has. This tool can be used to assess the well-being of the department and need for potential improvement / intervention.

Methods to Improve Quality:

PDSA (Plan-Do-Study Act)

This is a powerful, amazing, and totally original tool that can be used for an action-oriented process. The idea is that you chain the 4 steps together

- **Step 1 "Plan"** : What needs fixed and how should we fix it.

- **Step 2 "Do"** : Do the thing, and record data.

- **Step 3 "Study"** : Did it work? Or Not work?

- **Step 4 "Act"** : If you failed in step 3, then *fix the root cause* and implement a new plan (repeat at step 1).

Lean:

"Lean" is a style of organizing workflow that has two main principals:

(1) Elimination of Waste through standardized workflow (*no unnecessary variation*).

(2) Respect for Long Time Employees, and Customers

There are 4 "tools" that are used to create a Lean workflow. *This is critical knowledge for being an intermediate level radiologist.

- **Value Stream Mapping:** This is a tool to help improve workflow, by creating a "visual map" of the entire process from beginning to end. You can create alternative maps of how things could be done differently for QI projects.

- **Five S:** This is the kind of thing that gets you promoted straight to the top. Take 5 words that all mean something similar and start with the same letter, and give it a catchy name "FIVE S!." Boom , instant promotion. In this case, the 5 words basically mean "organized" or "standardized."

- **Pull Systems:** This is the idea that you don't overwork one guy in the assembly line. You create a system where work flow is constant. Never have one guy making 3 pieces in step 2, while the guy at step 3 only makes one piece. That way no one is sitting there idly. You don't pay people to idle. You want to be Chairman? You gotta grind every last drop of sweat and blood out of your trainees.

- **Error-Proofing:** The idea that workers should draw immediate attention to defects, so that the bosses can come in and fix them.

Design-Measure Analyze Improve Control (Six Sigma)

Sigma = Standard Deviation. The idea is to target an error rate of 6 standard deviations from the average.

QI Tools *(Overview)*

The Big 5 *(expanded discussion with examples to follow)*

- **Brainstorming** – Generating a big list of ideas

- **Fishbone Diagram (Cause and Effect):** Categorize and organize contributing factors, in a cause and effect pathway.

- **Flow Charts:** A graphical map to show the steps / decision points involved in a process. There are two subtypes. "High Level" which describes a process from beginning to end. "Low Level" contains more details about the major steps.

- **Pareto Charts:** Lots of things are involved in the creation of a problem, but only some of them contribute in a manner that is actually responsible. In other words, changing one thing might fix a problem, even though 10 things contributed to it.

- **Shewhart Charts (Control Charts):** Is the process stable? Do we need to do a formal examination for quality? These are the questions a control chart (Shewhart) answers. The graph is generated by placing success on the numerator, and total opportunities on the denominator. The graph shows the changing process over time.

Other Tools *(still testable, but less high yield)*

- **Multi-voting** – People choose the highest priority problem. Based totally on popular opinion.

- **Nominal Group Technique (NGT)** - Used to deal with a big mouth in the room. Minimal conversation or interaction is tolerated. The technique has two stages: (1) Brainstorming by asking a question and having people write down their response. (2) Ideas are ranked by individuals, with the scores of the groups used to decide what is good.

- **Prioritization Matrix** – Things are ranked by specific criteria (how fixable, how serious, etc…). A matrix totaling all votes is then created.

- **Walkthrough** – Trying to spend a day in the shoes of your underling (or a patient). See if the problems are real, or bottlenecks in work flow can be identified.

Tool	"Catch Phrase" / "Buzzword"
Brainstorming	Identify all the Issues
Fishbone Diagram	Cause and Effect
Flow Charts	"Clarify the steps and decision points"
Pareto Charts	80% of problem, explained by 20% of causes
Shewhart Charts	Is the process "under control" or stable?
Multivoting	People's opinion of what is most important
Nominal Ground Technique (NGT)	No Big Mouths. Minimal talking, lots of idea writing.
Prioritization Matrix	Rank then and add them up

Fishbone Diagram (Cause and Effect):

This type of chart is used to organize the ideas that contribute to portions of a problem or process. The process of drawing one is essentially asking the question "cause and effect" over and over and over again.

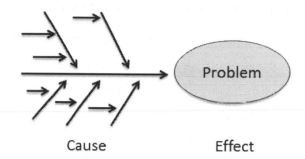

Cause   Effect

Example:

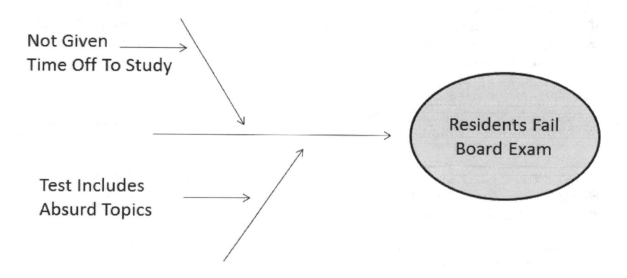

Not Given
Time Off To Study

Test Includes
Absurd Topics

Residents Fail
Board Exam

Flow Chart:

Flow charts use symbols chained together to illustrate a process. The standardized shapes for the major symbols are below.

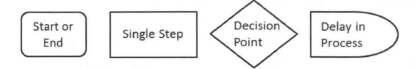

Processes can be high level ("get up go to work"), mid level ("get up, get in shower, eat, drive to work"), or low level ("get up, walk into bathroom, pee in toilet, flush toilet, start shower water").

Example:

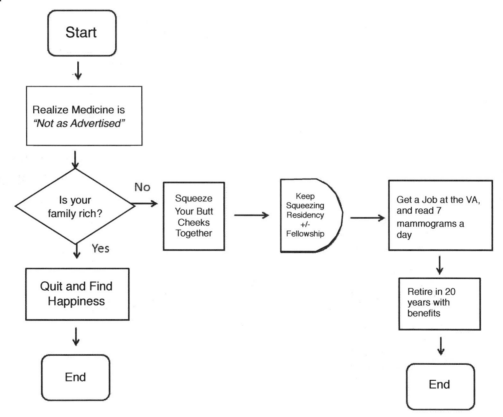

Testable Trivia:

- Flow charts are good for "cause and effect"
- Only use one arrow for yes, and one arrow for no.
- Draw the boxes first, then the lines
- It's OK to move the start and end boxes, after you start.

Pareto Charts

This is a chart named after Vifredo Pareto, who accomplished many great things in his life including popularizing the term "elite", marrying a women 30 years his junior (WIN!), and collecting a large number of cats – which he famously treated better than his house guests (he fed the cats first, and made his dinner guests wait). Oh, he also made a chart.

The chart contains both a line graph and a bar graph. The bars are ranked in descending order, creating a concave function. The entire **purpose of the chart is to highlight the most important factor among a set of factors.** The idea is that fixing the main cause, may fix the problem.

Example:

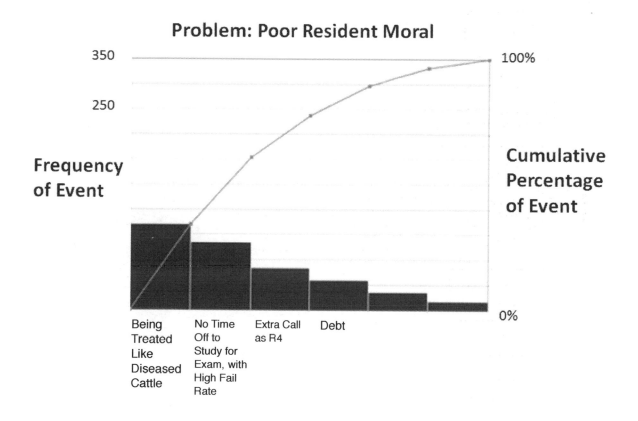

Shewhart Charts (Control Chart)

This is a "process-behavior" type of chart. The idea is to be able to look and see if a process is under control (with just stable variation), or not under control. Upper and lower "controls" are chosen based on the definition of success and failure for the system. Staying between the controls demonstrates a stable process.

Testable Trivia:

- What the chart looks like

- What is the numerator? Samples of Success

- What is the denominator? Total Opportunities

Example:

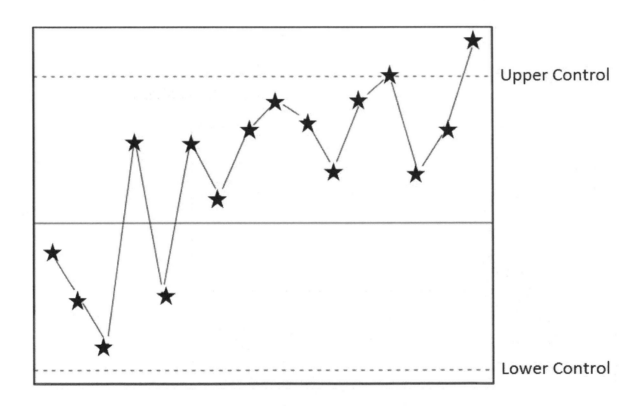

Section 2: MRI and CT Safety

MRI "Zones":

What are the 4 zones?

Zone I: No restriction. This is basically outside the building.

Zone II: No restriction. This is the waiting room and the dressing room. This is where you can screen patients and control access to Zone 3 and 4.

Zone III: Restricted Room. This is typically the control room, where the MRI tech does his/her thing. There should be some kind of a lock on the door between zone 2 and 3.

Zone IV: Restricted Room. This is the actual MRI scanner room (the same room as the magnet).

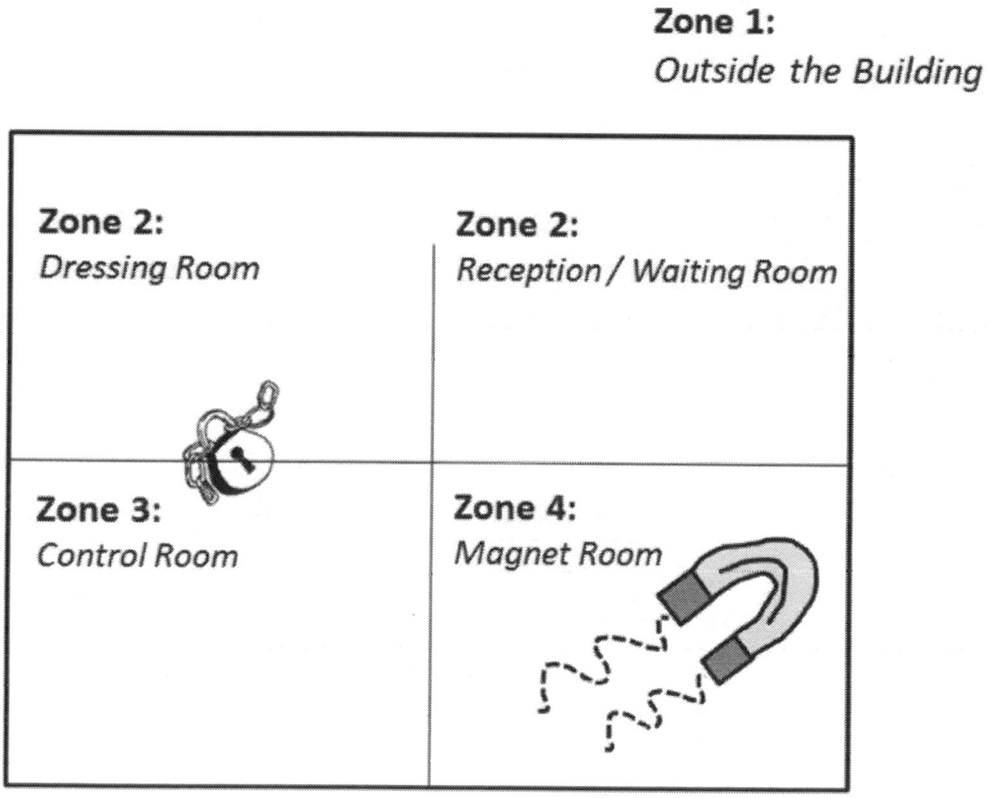

Zone 1:
Outside the Building

Zone 2: Dressing Room	**Zone 2:** Reception / Waiting Room
Zone 3: Control Room	**Zone 4:** Magnet Room

MRI Trivia:

Are there any exceptions for entry into restricted access zones? Access is restricted to zone 3 and 4 (without filling out the screening forms ect…). **There are NO exceptions to the guidelines restricting entry to zone 3 and 4**. Even if the patient codes in the scanner there are no exceptions (*per the Kanal article cited below*). The MRI techs should start CPR on the patient in the room (zone 4), stabilize the patient then get them out of zone 3 and 4 to a holding area where the code team can actually save them.

If there is a code in the scanner should you quench the magnet? Typically not. The magnetic field will still be around for a minute or two. Plus, that is really expensive and the bean counters who run the hospital will be pissed. Instead, do CPR then bring them out of Zone 3 and 4.

MRI Screening begins with? A focused history to identify patients who may have metal in them.

What if the Patient is insane, unconscious, or has terrible body odor and you can't initiate the screening process with him / her ? You will need to ask family members, consult the medical record, and possibly do screening x-rays (orbits etc…) as needed.

What is a magnet quench ? Quenching the magnet causes the liquid helium coolant to boil off. The helium is directed to the outdoors by means of a large pipe.

Is quenching dangerous ? It can be. (1) If the helium doesn't make it out the pipe correctly it can displace the oxygen in the room and cause asphyxiation. Because of this risk - everyone should evacuate the room. (2) It's very expensive, so you will likely be fired if you touch the button (make the tech do it - then later say you never told him to).

When is it ok to quench the magnet ? (1) If the patient or employee** is pinned down by a ferromagnetic object. Employee doesn't include residents/trainees. They must remain pinned down until they can free themselves (and then they must take call). (2) If there is a fire in the room.

Kanal, Emanuel, et al. "ACR guidance document for safe MR practices: 2007." American Journal of Roentgenology 188.6 (2007): 1447-1474.

CT Contrast – Reactions and Management:

Statistical Trivia – How Often Do Reactions Occur?

- Incidence of Any Contrast Reaction (mild or serious): 0.2-0.7 %

- Incidence of Serious Contrast Reactions: 0.01-0.02 %

Who gets contrast reactions?

- Greatest risk is prior reaction (5x increase for reaction).

- Atopy (2-3x increased risk of a serious reaction)

What is the idea behind premedicating?

- The goal is to block histamine. This is typically done with a steroid + an antihistamine.

Routine Premedication		
Method 1:	Prednisone: 50 mg by mouth at 13 hours, 7 hours, and 1 hour before contrast	Diphenhydramine (Benadryl): 50 mg IV (or PO) 1 hour before contrast
Method 2:	Methylprednisolone: 32 mg by mouth 12 hours and 2 hours before contrast	Diphenhydramine (Benadryl): 50 mg IV (or PO) 1 hour before contrast
Emergent Premedication		
Method 1:	Methylprednisolone 40 mg or hydrocortisone sodium succinate 200 mg IV Q4 until contrast study	Diphenhydramine (Benadryl) 50 mg IV 1 hour prior to contrast injection;
Method 2: * For Allergy to NSAIDS, or history of Asthma	Dexamethasone sodium 7.5 mg or betamethasone 6.0 mg IV Q4 until contrast study.	Diphenhydramine (Benadryl) 50 mg IV 1 hour prior to contrast injection
Method 3: * For People who can't / shouldn't get steroids – infected, or at risk for bowel perforation	Diphenhydramine 50 mg IV 1 hour prior to contrast injection.	

Contrast Reaction Management

Reaction	Treatment
Urticaria	Stop Injection
	Most cases don't need treatment
	H1 Blockers: Diphenhydramine (Benadryl) PO/IM/IV 25mg – 50mg
Severe Disseminated Urticaria	Epinephrine SC (1:1,000) 0.1 to 0.3 ml (=0.1 to 0.3 mg)
Facial or Laryngeal Edema	O2 6 to 10 liters/min (via mask).
	epinephrine SC or IM (1:1,000) 0.1 to 0.3 ml (=0.1 to 0.3 mg) or, especially if hypotension evident, epinephrine (1:10,000) slowly IV 1 to 3 ml (=0.1 to 0.3 mg). Can repeat epi up to maximum of 1mg.
Bronchospasm	O2 6 to 10 liters/min (via mask).
	Beta Agonist: Albuterol
	If unresponsive to Albuterol - epinephrine SC or IM (1:1,000) 0.1 to 0.3 ml (=0.1 to 0.3 mg) or, especially if hypotension evident, epinephrine (1:10,000) slowly IV 1 to 3 ml (=0.1 to 0.3 mg). Can repeat up to maximum of 1mg.
Hypotension with Tachycardia	Legs elevated 60 degrees or more (preferred) or Trendelenburg position.
	Give O2 6 to 10 liters/min (via mask).
	Rapid intravenous administration of large volumes of Ringer's lactate or normal saline.
	If unresponsive to fluids - epinephrine SC or IM (1:1,000) 0.1 to 0.3 ml (=0.1 to 0.3 mg) or, especially if hypotension evident, epinephrine (1:10,000) slowly IV 1 to 3 ml (=0.1 to 0.3 mg). Can repeat up to maximum of 1mg.
Hypotension with Bradycardia (vaso-vagal reaction)	Secure airway: give O2 6 to 10 liters/min (via mask).
	Legs elevated 60 degrees or more (preferred) or Trendelenburg position
	Rapid intravenous administration of large volumes of Ringer's lactate or normal saline.
	If unresponsive: Give atropine 0.6 to 1 mg IV slowly . Repeat atropine up to a total dose of 0.04 mg/kg (2 to 3 mg)
Seizure or Convulsion	Secure airway: give O2 6 to 10 liters/min (via mask).
	Diazepam (Valium) 5 mg IV (or more, as appropriate) or midazolam (Versed) 0.5 to 1 mg IV.
	If you need extended coverage – Phenytoin (Dilantin) infusion 15-18 mg/kg at 50mg/min.
	Monitor for respiratory depression when giving Benzos

Why is the concentration for IV Epi different than SubQ?

The way to think about this is that you need a large volume of fluid for IV - because you are going to push it around. Alternatively, you wouldn't want a large volume of fluid under the skin. The dose is actually the same (0.1 - 0.3mg) it's just the dilution volume that is different.

SC or IM: 1:1,000, 0.1 to 0.3 ml (0.1 to 0.3 mg)
IV: 1:10,000 , 1 to 3 ml (0.1 to 0.3 mg)

Contrast Induced Nephropathy (CIN):

Defining CIN?

The stone age ("historic") criteria is an absolute increase in the serum creatinine from by 0.5 mg/dL. There are more modern definitions that require an absolute increase of up to 2.0 mg/dL, or a percentage of change in the baseline serum creatinine of 25 to 50 percent – depending on the study. The reality is CIN is way way way over diagnosed, and there are at least 2 large studies showing that most things that are called "CIN" are just normal variation in Cr that occur in patients who are sick in the hospital.

How often does CIN occur? Real answer is almost never. If asked on the CORE, I would say something like less than 10% even with moderate kidney disease.

When does CIN occur? The typical course is a spike in Cr within 24 hours of getting contrast, peaking around day 4, then returning to baseline at day 10.

When should you check a Cr?

- Age >60;

- History of renal disease (dialysis, renal transplant, renal cancer)

- Solitary Kidney

- Bad Hypertension (that requires medication)

- Diabetes Mellitus

- Metformin

What is the deal with metformin? The trick is metformin is NOT a risk for developing CIN. However, if you do develop renal failure while on metformin you could get a lactic acidosis.

What do you do if you are on metformin? The typical recommendation is to stop the drug at the time of the study and hold in for 48 hours. If they didn't develop CIN – they can restart after 48hours.

How Does One Prevent the Plague of CIN? There are several techniques all of which are bogus. However, for the purpose of the CORE intravenous hydration, preferably with isotonic fluids such as 0.9% saline or Lactated Ringer's at 100 ml/hr for 6-12 hour before contrast administration and 4-12 hours after contrast administration is the best. The reason it "works" is that it artificially lowers the Cr on the labs.

Contrast Extravasation:

What is the typical outcome? Most of the time there is no significant sequelae.

Is the rate of injection a risk factor? No… but, it can make the severity worse.

What are the "severe" complications?

- Compartment Syndrome – This is the most common, and related to mechanical compression. The primary risk factor is the volume of contrast extravasation, into a small compartment (hand, foot, or ankle).

- Skin Ulceration / Necrosis –

What is the treatment? There is no consensus – so you shouldn't be asked. If you do get asked, I guess I'd say elevate the affected extremity above the heart.

Gadolinium Contrast agents:

Gd is easier than iodine contrast agents, with regard to necessary trivia. Just remember these things:

- Don't give Gd to patients with a GFR <30 or with acute kidney injury.

- Check a GFR (within 6 weeks is adequate) with patients with renal disease, transplant, over the age of 60, diabetes, or a history of hypertension.

Section 3: Radiation Safety – Buzzwords, Marketing, and Trivia

Buzzwords – All of which mean the same thing:

- *"Image Gently"* Pediatrics
- *"Image Wisely"* Adult equivalent
- *"Step Lightly"* Reduce radiation in pediatric IR. "Step lightly on the fluoro"
- *"ALARA"* As low as reasonably achievable. Basically try and minimize radiation dose.

Biologic Effects of Ionizing Radiation (BEIR) Committee – Also known as <u>BEIR 7 Report</u>

What were the sources of data used? Atomic Bomb Survivor data, medical radiation studies, occupational radiation studies, and environmental radiation studies. **The primary source was the bomb data.**

What was the primary task of this committee? To develop the best possible risk estimate for human exposure to low-dose (<100 mSv), low-LET ionizing radiation.

What did the BEIR 7 Report conclude? That there is a thing called a linear, no-threshold dose response between radiation and the development of cancer in humans.

More specifically, what does BEIR 7 accuse medical imaging of? Giving everyone cancer. BEIR 7 predicts that 1 in 100 will get a solid cancer or leukemia from a dose of 100mSv above background.

Is BEIR 7 legit? No… it's probably a load of monkey poop. If you look at how they get their data, they use a risk model that is "x" times excess relative risk + (1-"x") times the excess absolute risk. In this equation, "x" is determined by committee! In other words… they just made it up. Basically, all estimates are based on multiple models and assumption with confidence intervals that are subjective and partly based on opinion. Cancer estimates from BEIR 7 are not proven facts…. Having said all that, the test will probably want you to treat them as such. Who knows… **just say linear no-threshold based on bomb data.**

Section 4: "The Trainee Caused a Complication"

Any time I enter a patient care area, the first thing I do is look for the person I'm going to blame if something goes wrong- usually a tech or nurse. If I were working in academics, I would choose a "Trainee."

What is a "Trainee?" A Trainee is the new word for resident. It was developed by bureaucrats to help maintain the hierarchy of academic medicine, with the eventual goal of providing no salary or benefits (why would you pay the trainee?).

When can a "Trainee" be referred to as a Doctor? There are only two scenarios. (1) If there is a menial task that requires a physician signature (writing scripts, doing H&Ps, consenting patients, etc....) or (2) there has been a complication and someone needs to be blamed.

National Patient Safety Goals:

You need two identifiers when providing patient care / doing a procedure.

Labeling Medications: Current Medication Labeling Rules (*this isn't Nam there are rules*):

- Meds on and off the sterile field are labeled

- Meds are labeled even if they are the only ones on the field

- Drug Name and Strength (concentration) should be on the label

- You can NOT pre-label empty syringes

- Medications used throughout a procedure (pre-solution, normal saline for rinsing stuff, etc...) must be labeled – or the receiving container must be labeled.

- Exception to labeling rule is a scenario when you draw something up from the original container and immediately administer it.

Communicating Critical Results:

Per the National Patient Safety Goals (02.03.01) – Written procedures for dealing with critical results should be developed by the radiology group, which include to who from who, and the acceptable length of time between the read and the call.

What is this "Error" You Speak Of?

Types of Error: As stated above, most occur as a "system" and not individual. For the purpose of multiple choice, you can group these into two categories.

- Active Errors – Errors at the point of contact.

- Latent Errors – Errors which occur because of organizational failure (bad staffing, unsafe environment). An "accident waiting to happen."

Vocabulary of Error

Adverse Error: Any kind of iatrogenic injury. This doesn't necessarily mean an error occurred, it could be a side effect or therapy or known complication of the procedure. Examples include, drug allergy or post op infection.

Blunt End – The part of the health care system that is NOT in direct contact with patients.

Examples: Various bureaucrats, bean counters, chairmen. The people who set policy.

Sharp End – The part of the health care system that is in direct contact with stinky patients

Examples: Various Trainees, nurses etc…

Mistake: An error that occurs because of insufficient knowledge (you picked the wrong antibiotic, or chose the wrong test).

Slip: An error that occurs because of a lapse in concentration.

Near Miss *(Close Call)* – An event that could have caused an injury to the patient, and only didn't because of pure dumb luck.

Sentinel Event: An event that causes death , serious harm, or almost causes death/harm.

Classic Radiology Sentinel Event = whole body radiation dose of 15 Gy.

Why Errors Occur?

"To Err is Human" - This was a project started by the National Academy of Sciences' Institute of Medicine. The paper said most errors were system errors rather than individual errors. The result was the spending of 50 million dollars by congress to create a list of "never events" which require mandatory reporting.

Institute of Medicine ⟶ *patients die from system errors* ⟶ *list of never events.*

Behaviors that lead to error:

- **Human Error** – This is an unintentional and unpredictable behavior that causes an unwanted outcome. *You reached for the glass of milk, and spilled it.* These types of errors occur because of weakness in the system (the cup needed a lid, or the bottom of the cup should be been wider).

- **At Risk Behavior** – This is an unsafe habit, which the person thinks is a justified risk. *"This is just the way we do things here."* I always reach for my milk while I'm watching tv. It's ok, I won't spill it… I've been doing this for years.

- **Reckless Behavior** – This time the worker knows there is risk, and understands it is a real risk. They can't really defend why they did something. *I just thought it would be funny to balance the cup of milk on my nose.*

A Just Culture: This is a concept of accountability that distinguishes human errors, at risk behaviors, and reckless behaviors and addresses them accordingly.

Just Culture	
Human Error	Console the worker. Then try and fix the system.
At Risk	Don't Punish. Instead, fix the system based reason for behavior. Work to decrease the acceptance of such behavior from the staff.
Reckless	Punish!!! It's not revenge, it's punishment… according to department policy (placing the offender in the stockade).

What is this "Safety" You Speak Of?

Culture of Safety

The general concept is that the administration recognizes that what you do is high risk (needle sticks for HIV/ Hep C patients, constant threat of litigation, the ED being stupid, harassment from the trauma team). Because the administration agrees that things are high risk, it wants people to report misses or near misses so that they can be corrected. The culture of free reporting means that there is a blame-free culture. You won't get in trouble as long as you tell the truth. In the same vein as "all evaluations are anonymous." *Which of course, they are. Why would someone lie to you about that?*

Safety Champion: The Joint Commission describes this idea of a "safety champion." This is someone selected from each unit or department that receives special training to help advocate for safety and work environment awareness. They will help educate other members of the department and report them for "unsafe behaviors." ***Basically they run around and tattle.***

Environmental Safety Tours: The Joint Commission requires two environmental tours in the patient care area and one tour in non-patient care areas per year. The "safety champion" can be the one to do this.

Testable Trivia:

•   The title of safety champion should rotate among staff

•   The safety officer should train the safety champion

•   The safety officer can do the environmental tours (2 patient care, 1 non-patient care).

Stuff Nurses Do:

Medication Reconciliation - This is a task nurses who work on medical surgical floors will do to help reduce medication errors. Grandma will come in with a list of about 50 medications, many of which she isn't taking, many of which are duplicates with both generic and brand names listed separately (with different doses), etc....

The process of fixing this can be terrible, because if you ask Grandma what she takes she will probably tell you "I take a blue pill in the morning, and that orange one at night....".

Prior to discharge it's good to go through the list and make sure it makes sense, including the new medications she'll be on after discharge. Luckily, you are not a nurse or a medicine doctor, so you will never have to do this.

Buzzwords For Diagnosing and Preventing Errors

Human Factor Engineering – The idea that humans make mistakes, so you should build the system to minimize the risk of error.

Usability Testing – This is the idea of *testing systems in a real world condition.* The classic example is looking at the computerized provider order entry (CPOE) system, to see if it makes work harder (reducing bedside patient time) or actually creates more errors.

Workaround – This term describes workers not following the rules. They "work around" the rules, to get things done quicker.

Forcing Function – This term describes not allowing errors to occur to start with. For example, you don't stock lethal injection materials (concentrated potassium) in the code box.

Standardization – Making everything the same way, and **using lots and lots of check lists** is supposed to decrease the likelihood a trainee will make an error.

Resiliency Efforts –The general philosophy here is that trainees make errors and there is just no way to stop that. Instead, energy is focused on detecting errors early and stopping them before they progress to something worse.

Failure Mode and Effects Analysis (FEMA) - Prospectively identify error risk within a particular process

Root Cause Analysis - Retrospective; structured method used to analyze serious adverse events.

This vs That	
FEMA	Prospective
Root Cause Analysis	Retrospective

Section 5: "Getting Sued"

Since you made the terrible mistake of being a doctor, your punishment is to spend your career worrying about getting sued and eventually getting sued. This can only be prevented by (1) working at a VA, or (2) quitting medicine and going to law school (so you can do the suing).

What gets you sued?

- Errors in diagnosis are the most common cause of malpractice suits against Radiologists

- Imaging findings related to breast cancer is the most common organ related subject of malpractice suits against Radiologists

- Communication Errors (with referring M.D., or failure to recommend another test) is actually a much less frequent cause of litigation – when compared to interpretive error.

Whang, Jeremy S., et al. "The causes of medical malpractice suits against radiologists in the United States." Radiology 266.2 (2013): 548-554.

What must be proven?

All 5 Elements must be proven for a successful medical malpractice case:

1. A duty was owed: You owe that duty once you read that case, or do that procedure.

2. A duty was breached: You didn't follow the standard of care.

3. The breach caused an injury: Your failure to follow the standard of care is what hurt the patient.

4. Deviation from the accepted standard: You didn't follow the standard of care in your specialty (this is similar to #2).

5. Damage: The patient must have gotten hurt (physical or emotional). If they didn't get hurt, it doesn't matter if your were negligent or not.

Basically, it was your case, you missed the finding or didn't communicate a critical finding (or other violation of the standard of care), and the patient got hurt. If they didn't get hurt, then you are ok. If they got hurt but you followed the standard of care you are ok.

- If you drive an expensive car, you will also be more susceptible to character assassination, which will aid the prosecution.

Section 6: "Getting Paid"

The only reason to go to medical school and endure residency / fellowship is the chance to make enough money to buy a Porsche and/or Boat. This is still not guaranteed, as hospital administrators make more and more and doctors make less and less every year.

Step 1: Getting Credentialed

Testable Trivia revolves around two processes:

(1) **Focused Professional Practice Evaluation (FPPE)** – This is basically current medical staff checking your work (proctoring) you for the first few studies you read or a committee evaluating if you can do a new procedure or not.

(2) **Ongoing Professional Practice Evaluations (OPPE)** – The a continued review of your performance – typically q6 months, that is used for reappointment. Your department determines the scope of the review.

Step 2: Getting A Paycheck

Testable Trivia Regarding Payment:

Two Lists of Diseases/Procedures Made by Two Different Bodies for Billing:

1. Current Procedural Terminology Codes (CPT) – The **AMA editorial panel** is actually in charge of these. They create a "uniform" description of the procedure.

2. International Classification of Diseases (ICD) 9 – This is a list of diseases made by the **World Health Organization** (WHO). The "9th" version of this list is the most popular one.

Two Ways the Government Punishes you for Going to Medical School:

1. Physician Quality Reporting System (PQRS) – Medicare uses carrots (stick to come later) to force you to report "quality clinical data" on certain conditions.

2. Meaningful Use – Forcing you to have an electronic medical record, and then prove (by random button clicking) that you are using it.

Resource Based Relative Value System (RBRVS) – This is a system based on some Harvard study , that said doctors should get paid based on the time it took to do something and how difficult it was to do it. RBRVSs are adjusted based on geography with a "Geographic Practice Cost Indicator", so that you make more in LA than you do in rural South Dakota or New Mexico

Omnibus Budget Reconciliation Act of 1989 (OBRA 89) – This is the name of the Medicare payment reform law.

Participating vs Non-Participating Physicians

– Participating – If you agree to take what medicare gives you and not try and get the rest of the money owed to you by the patient.

– Non- Participating – You refuse to sign the agreement, and can attempt to collect the rest of the money from the patient. The government tries to discourage this by only paying you 95% of what is paid to the participating physicians.

Sustainable Growth Rate System (SGR) – This was put in place in 1997 to control the growth of Medicare. It's based on domestic product per capita. This is totally flawed, and would result in you making no money at all and being homeless eating out of the dumpster behind McDonalds. The only thing that keeps you from enjoying two day old Big Macs is a "patch fix" congress does yearly (at the stroke of midnight). The AMA wants a repeal of the SGR, but currently the AMA lacks enough funds to "convince" members of congress to act on its behalf.

Section 7: Radom Trivia

"Off Label"

- Using an approved drug / device for something other than its original intended use is called "off label" use.

- The FDA is in charge of monitoring the safety of medical devices and drugs

- The *"Practice of Medicine" doctrine* allows doctors to use things off label.

- For regular clinical work, off label use does NOT have to be disclosed while obtaining informed consent

- For research studies, off label use MUST be disclosed while obtaining consent

- If you are using a medication / device off label, you can't market the product as your own special product.

ACR Appropriateness Criteria

In an attempt to get promoted, various academic Radiologists got together in 1993 and formed committees to decide what tests are appropriate. The idea was to help ordering providers get the right test.

Testable trivia:

- Appropriateness Rating

    - Rating 1-3 = Usually NOT appropriate

    - Rating 4-6 = Might be appropriate

    - Rating 7-9 = Usually appropriate

- There is also a 1-6 Relative Radiation Score for each test.

CPR:

They have changed the CPR rules…. Again. Don't worry I'm sure the changes are evidence based.

Testable Trivia:

- *Current Sequence:* (1) Chest Compressions, (2) Airways, (3) Breathing. The American Heart Association believes it's critical to survival to begin circulating un- oxygenated blood first.

- Compression rate is 100/min, at 2 inches depth (to the beat of the disco song staying alive).

- Ratio is always 30:2 with one exception; the two person pediatric which is 15:2

Work Related Problems for Radiologists

Stress Over Proving You are a "Real Doctor"

- Improved by – getting control of your ego. Remember your alternative choice in medicine was to dedicate your life to poop, pus, and note writing.

Eye Strain "Asthenopia"

- According to an article from AJR 2005, written by a Canadian Academic Center – you can reduce eye strain by taking short breaks, reading less CTs, working less than 7 hours a day, and eliminating screen flicker. When I read this paper I had to laugh. Are you seriously that weak? Work hard! Make Money! Retire! In that order. Stop crying about your eyes hurting.

Carpal Tunnel Syndrome:

- Too much mousing

Back Pain

- Most common in IR – from the lead

Blank for scribbles / notes

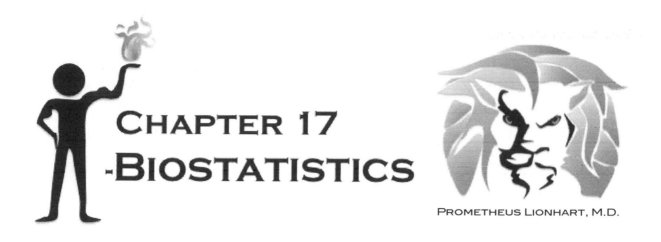

CHAPTER 17 -BIOSTATISTICS

PROMETHEUS LIONHART, M.D.

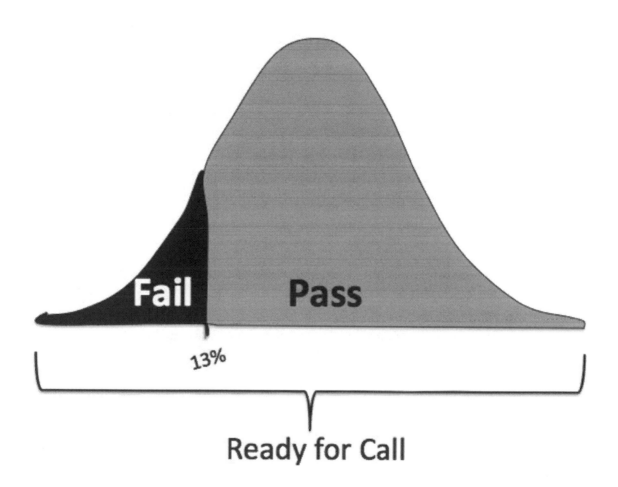

There is just no escape from this crap. It has been on every major certifying / board exam you've taken, and will be on every one to follow.

The Normal Distribution:

This will look familiar as it is how every "good test" will turn out. Naturally occurring phenomena will distribute as a bell-shaped "normal" or "Gaussian Distribution."

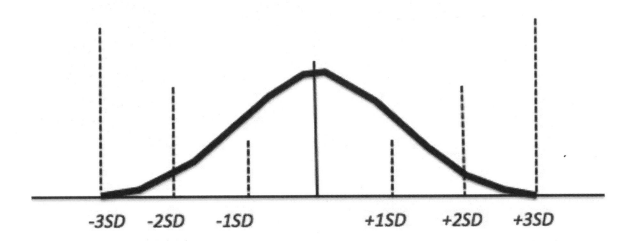

Data can be "skewed" to one side or the other.

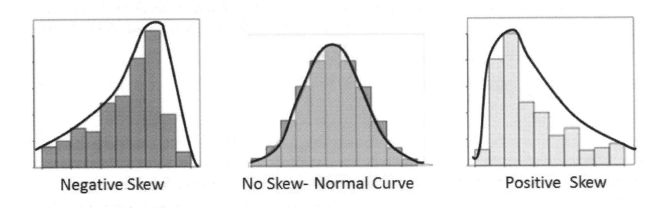

Negative Skew   No Skew- Normal Curve   Positive Skew

The "negative" or "positive" skewing is described by which side the tail is on. The relationship to the mean is the most likely testable trivia. A negative skew has the mean after the tail. A positive skew has the mean before the tail.

Precision and Accuracy:

Precision - This is the immunity to variation. "The dart hits the same spot every time." A wider confidence interval = a less precise study.

Accuracy (unbiased) - This is the immunity to systematic error or bias. "The dart hits the center."

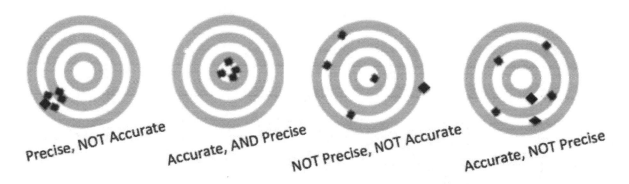

Precise, NOT Accurate   Accurate, AND Precise   NOT Precise, NOT Accurate   Accurate, NOT Precise

What is this "Statistical Significance" ?

You often hear people say "the study was significant, with a p value < 0.05." What the hell does that mean anyway? Basically, they are saying that the result is unlikely to have occurred by chance. You can flip a coin that lands on heads 50 times in a row, it's just not very likely to occur by chance. If you say the p value is < 0.05, then you are saying the likelihood it occurred by chance is less than 5%. In other words, the investigator is 95% sure the result did NOT occur by chance.

Correlation and Causality:

Just because two things seem to rise together (correlation), doesn't mean one is causing the other. The example I like to use is ice cream sales and death by drowning. You will find that the more ice cream is sold, the more people die in swimming pools and the ocean. Why is ice cream so deadly? Should we ban it? The people who believe the MMR vaccine causes autism probably think we should, but they don't understand the difference between correlation and causality.

When do people buy ice cream ? – The Summer When do people go swimming? - The Summer

Warm weather is actually the reason these things go up together, they are not actually causing each other.

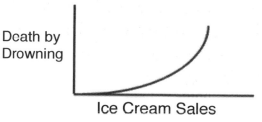

Statistical Epidemiology

Incidence: The number of NEW cases occurring in a particular time period.

$$\text{Incidence Rate} = \frac{\text{Number of NEW cases of disease}}{\text{Total Number of People at Risk}} \quad \text{Per unit time}$$

Prevalence: The number of cases of a certain disease in a particular moment in time.

$$\text{Prevalence Rate} = \frac{\text{Number of cases of disease}}{\text{Total Number of People at Risk}} \quad \text{At a particular time}$$

Sensitivity & Specificity

Both sensitivity and specificity measure validity (the ability to detect people with or without disease).

True Positive (TP) = Test shows cancer, Patient has cancer
False Positive (FP) = Test shows cancer, Patient does NOT have cancer.

* Same as a Type I error.

True Negative (TN) = Test shows NO cancer, Patient does NOT have cancer.

False Negative (FN) = Test shows NO cancer, Patient has cancer.

* Same as a Type II error.

Disease

	+	**−**
Test +	True Positive	False Positive *Type 1 Error*
−	False Negative *Type 2 Error*	True Negative

I want to discourage you from using the A, B, C, D method for doing statical problems. This can get you in hot water if the question writer flips the axis of the square (which they love to do). It's just better to understand what you are actually measuring.

Sensitivity = This is the *ability of the test to detect true disease.* In other words, the amount of true disease detected with the test / total people with the disease.

> True Positive / True Positive + False Negatives.

Specificity = The is the *ability of the test to detect people free of disease.* In other words, the amount of disease free people called negative by the test / total number of disease free people.

> True Negative / True Negative + False Positives

A very specific test rules in disease. (**SPIN** ; **SP**ecificity rules **IN**)

-- **Type 1 Error :** The fire alarm goes off, but there is no fire. - A false positive.

-- **Type 2 Error:** A fire burns, but the alarm does not go off. - A false negative. Obviously, this is the worst kind of error.

Accuracy = Think about this as how often the test was right:

True Positive + True Negative / TP + FP + TN + FN

Positive Predictive Value: This is the likelihood that a person with a positive test actually has the disease.

True Positive / True Positive + False Positives

Negative Predictive Value: This is the likelihood that a person with a negative test actually is disease free.

True Negative / True Negative + False Negative

Sensitivity and Specificity depend only on the characteristics of the test. Predictive value depends on the prevalence. This is a concept that multiple choice writers love!

The higher the prevalence of a disease the higher the PPV and the Lower the NPV. The lower the prevalence of a disease the lower the PPV and the higher the NPV.

For Example, Let's say there is a very rare disease called "The Fever." The symptoms of this include being paid very large amounts of money to screw over the next generation of your colleagues.

A very specific test might still have a low PPV because it's going to have alot of false positives. In other words if the prevalence is 1:300,000,000 and your false positive rate is 1:1,000,000 you are still going to have 1 true positive, and 299 false positives.

Validity – Is the test doing what it claims it does? An x-ray is a pretty valid test for looking for a fracture (it has the ability to show who has a fracture and who does not). Important qualities of a valid test are that it is – highly specific and highly sensitive.
Validity is similar to accuracy.

Power - Type II errors are bad (there is a fire, but the alarm doesn't go off). The ability to prevent this from happening is called "power." By convention a study needs a power of 0.8 (80% chance of the fire alarm going off for a fire). The most important thing to remember is that, the larger the sample size the greater the power. Larger protests have more power.

Risk:

Absolute Risk: The more common a disease is, the higher the risk of catching it. Most people will say that the incidence of a disease is the most important risk factor. That is why epidemiologists defined "absolute risk" as essentially the same thing as disease incidence.

The incidence of disease is 1:100, then the absolute risk is 1:100.

Relative Risk: Ever wondered how many times the guy with multi-drug resistant TB can cough on you on your plane ride to Chicago *(or Tucson)* to take the CORE exam before your PPD converts? This is the best way to think about relative risk – exposure to risk factors increases the risk of getting the disease.

   RR = Incidence of disease among persons exposed to risk factor / Incidence of   disease among people who did NOT get exposed to risk factor.

Absolute Risk Reduction: The general way to think about this is the difference between the people who did not get the drug (control group event rate) and the people who did get the drug (experimental group event rate). This is the inverse of number needed to treat.

Number Needed to Treat: How many drug addicts do you need to put in rehab before you actually get one clean? The math requires knowing the absolute risk reduction.

NNT = 100/Absolute Risk Reduction.

Attributable Risk: How much lung cancer is attributable to smoking?

   AR = (Incidence of disease in exposed) – (Incidence of disease in those NOT exposed.)

Odds Ratio: The absolute risk calculations require a prospective study. Odds ratio can be done using a **retrospective** study.

$$OR = \frac{\text{Odds that a case was exposed to the risk factor}}{\text{Odds that a control was exposed to the risk factor.}}$$

$$OR = \frac{(\text{Cases exposed to TB cougher on plane}) \times (\text{Cases of people not exposed})}{(\text{Controls exposed to the TB cougher on the plane}) \times (\text{Cases not exposed})}$$

ROC Curves:

People who write standardized tests have a strange obsession with ROC curves.

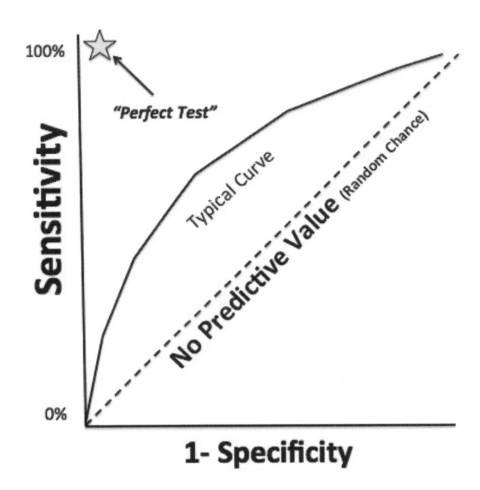

Questions You Can Ask About ROC Curves:

(1) What are the axes of the graph ? Sensitivity, and 1-Specificity
(2) What kind of a line would have no predictive value ? The straight one as above
(3) What kind of a line would occur from random chance? Same question, just different wording - still the straight one as above.
(4) Where is the "Ideal" or "Perfect" or "Gold Standard" test? Top left corner.
(5) When the accuracy improves how does the curve change? Shifts towards the upper left corner.

Blank for Notes / Scribbles

I'VE POURED ALL MY KNOWLEDGE INTO YOU.
WHEN YOU TAKE THE EXAM, MY SPIRIT WILL
TAKE THE EXAM WITH YOU.

THERE IS NO STOPPING US NOW
WE START, AND WE DON'T STOP

ALL YOUR STRENGTH
ALL YOUR POWER
ALL YOUR LOVE

EVERYTHING YOU GOT

-Tony "Duke" Evers

—-

What's Next For Prometheus Lionhart ? Check out <u>TitanRadiology.com</u> for updates

—Physics Review Course - Video Series - January 2016

—Expanded Stand Alone Physics Book - "The War Machine" - January 2016

—Flash Card App for I-Phone, I-Pad, and Android - January 2016

—"TOP 100" - CORE Rapid Review Book - February 2016

—"Titan Radiology Video Lecture Series" - <u>The Magnum Opus</u> - April 2016

44052675R00325

Made in the USA
Lexington, KY
21 August 2015